WATER FITNESS PROGRESSIONS

WATER FITNESS PROGRESSIONS

CHRISTINE ALEXANDER

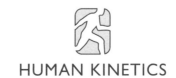

HUMAN KINETICS

Library of Congress Cataloging-in-Publication Data

Names: Alexander, Christine, 1950- author.
Title: Water fitness progressions / Christine Alexander.
Description: Champaign, IL : Human Kinetices, [2019] | Includes
  bibliographical references.
Identifiers: LCCN 2017044071 (print) | LCCN 2018003376 (ebook) | ISBN
  9781492562160 (ebook) | ISBN 9781492562153 (print)
Subjects: LCSH: Aquatic exercises.
Classification: LCC GV838.53.E94 (ebook) | LCC GV838.53.E94 A445 2019 (print)
  | DDC 613.7--dc23
LC record available at https://lccn.loc.gov/2017044071

ISBN: 978-1-4925-6215-3

The web addresses cited in this text were current as of November 2017, unless otherwise noted.

Acquisitions Editor: Michelle Maloney
Managing Editor: Caitlin Husted
Copyeditor: Bob Replinger
Permissions Manager: Martha Gullo
Graphic Designer: Dawn Sills
Cover Designer: Keri Evans
Cover Design Associate: Susan Allen
Photograph (cover): (top left) Getty Images/E+/kali9; (top right) Getty Images/E+/Fat Camera; (bottom left) Human Kinetics; (bottom right) Getty Images/Image Source
Photographs (interior): © Human Kinetics
Photo Asset Manager: Laura Fitch
Visual Production Assistant: Joyce Brumfield
Photo Production Manager: Jason Allen
Senior Art Manager: Kelly Hendren
Printer: Edwards Brothers Malloy

We thank the Jack Carter Pool in Plano, Texas, for assistance in providing the location for the photo shoot for this book.

Printed in the United States of America   10 9 8 7 6 5 4 3 2 1

The paper in this book is certified under a sustainable forestry program.

Human Kinetics
P.O. Box 5076
Champaign, IL 61825-5076
Website: www.HumanKinetics.com

In the United States, email info@hkusa.com or call 800-747-4457.
In Canada, email info@hkcanada.com.
In Europe, email hk@hkeurope.com.

For information about Human Kinetics' coverage in other areas of the world,
please visit our website: **www.HumanKinetics.com**   E7249

CONTENTS

CHAPTER 4 SHALLOW-WATER LESSON PLANS FOR CLASSES WITH TWO OBJECTIVES 137

PART II   DEEP-WATER EXERCISE   159

ACKNOWLEDGMENTS

I would like to give special thanks to the following people:

My husband, Jim, whose love and moral support were constant and whose computer skills kept this project from derailing on numerous occasions.

My water fitness class participants who graciously let me try out my lesson plan ideas on them.

Chris Alban, the pool manager at Jack Carter Pool, who allowed me to have the photo shoot at the facility.

Anne Hensarling, the coordinator at Oak Point Recreation Center where I teach, who not only is a pleasure to work for, but also facilitated the photo shoot at Jack Carter Pool.

Larry Fleming, the photographer who did a wonderful job with the photos.

My models, Amos Maxie and Sherry Silverman, who did a professional job of performing the exercises for the photos. Also the models for my first book, *Water Fitness Lesson Plans and Choreography*, whose photos were used again in this book—Johnnene Addison-Gay, Adam Alexander, Kathy Bolla, Rita Bryant, Anne Hensarling, and Amos Maxie.

Michelle Maloney and Caitlin Husted, my editors, and the staff at Human Kinetics, whose experience and encouragement in making this book a reality are very much appreciated.

HOW TO USE THIS BOOK

Step back and take a long view of your water fitness program. Are your classes on the same level year round? Or do you offer your participants an opportunity to improve their fitness? Overloading, or putting a greater-than-normal demand on the body's musculoskeletal and cardiorespiratory systems, improves fitness. Over time, however, the human body adapts to the workload it is given in an exercise program, and if no further progression is made, the class becomes a maintenance program. On the other hand, progressing too aggressively increases the risk of injury and chronic fatigue. An annual plan can be helpful in creating a program that gradually and systematically progresses your participants so that they have time to adapt safely to one fitness level before moving to the next.

One type of annual plan is periodization. Periodization is a training cycle used by athletes to achieve optimal development in all aspects of fitness. Periodization divides the year into a preseason, a transition season, a peak fitness season, and an active recovery season. Athletes arrange the cycle so that they achieve peak fitness during the season of their sport. Your participants may not be elite athletes, but it takes a certain amount of fitness to perform the activities of daily living. Why not train like athletes for the sport of daily life?

The purpose of this book is to explain how to use periodization within a water fitness class. Each season of the training cycle is explained in detail, including how to progress from lower-intensity interval training in the preseason to high-intensity interval training (HIIT) in the peak fitness season and how to progress from using the water's resistance for strength training in the preseason to using eccentric muscle actions with equipment in the peak fitness season. Participants learn how to use a scale of perceived exertion to judge whether they are working in the desired training zone (50 to 90 percent of their maximum heart rate).

The preseason lasts two to four months. The focus of this season is improving posture, learning to perform the exercises with good form, increasing range of motion, and using the properties of the water to create overload. Your classes will consist of cardiorespiratory training, low-intensity interval training, and strength training without equipment. You will have your participants stretch at the end of each class.

The transition season lasts two to four months. The focus of this season is improving the quality of participants' exercise by asking them to pay attention to how their arms and legs are moving the water. Participants will learn how to increase intensity beyond the levels used in the preseason to improve cardiorespiratory endurance and how to use equipment to increase resistance during strength training. Your classes will consist of cardiorespiratory training, moderate-intensity interval training, and strength training with equipment. High-intensity interval training will be introduced. Your participants will stretch at the end of each class.

The peak fitness season lasts two to four months. The focus of this season is to increase power and thus push the intensity into the anaerobic zone for short periods during the interval training and to use both concentric and eccentric contractions during strength training. Your classes will consist of cardiorespiratory training, high-intensity interval training, and strength training with equipment. Again, participants stretch at the end of each class.

The active recovery season lasts one to two months. The body needs rest to repair any microtrauma it suffered during the previous months of continuous training to avoid a cumulative injury. But rest does not mean that activity ends. Fitness continues as long as some training takes place, but fitness gains are lost if training stops altogether. Your classes at this time will consist of light cardiorespiratory training, core strength training, and fun activities such as games or relay races to provide a mental break. Stretching occurs at the end of each class.

The lesson plans in this book are designed to clearly demonstrate the progressions. Twelve lesson plans have the objective of improving cardiorespiratory fitness, and each of the plans has four versions. The first version is continuous cardio, the second version includes low-intensity intervals, the third version includes moderate-intensity intervals, and the fourth version includes high-intensity intervals. There are many ways to time the intervals: Nine different interval-timing techniques are demonstrated one or more times in these 12 lesson plans. Fifteen lesson plans have muscular strength and endurance as their objective. The techniques include using the water's resistance; using buoyant, drag, or rubberized equipment; using more than one piece of equipment in circuit classes; and performing core strength training. During active recovery, you can use the continuous cardio lesson plans and the core strength lesson plans. Also offered is a lesson plan of partner moves that is a lot of fun.

If you teach classes that meet only twice a week, you may find it difficult to work on progressions one objective at a time. To make the best use of your time, you need to combine objectives. A section of lesson plans for classes with two objectives meets this need. The 12 cardio lesson plans have been shortened to 30 minutes in this section. Next, aquatic endings includes 20 strength-training lesson plans of 20 minutes' duration and a variety of ideas for fun activities. The 30-minute cardio plans and the 20-minute aquatic endings can be mixed and matched any number of ways. Add a 5-minute warm-up and 5 minutes of stretching at the end to complete your one-hour class. If your classes meet three to five times a week, you will want to use this section for variety. The fun activities are good for active recovery season, but feel free to use them occasionally during the other seasons to give your class a mental break.

Table 1 provides an overview of the lesson plans for the preseason, the transition season, and the peak fitness season, and table 2 gives a list of options for the active recovery season. The following icons are used with the lesson plans in chapters 3, 4, 7, and 8 to indicate the season or seasons for each.

Preseason: **P**

Transition season: **T**

Peak fitness season: **PF**

Active recovery: **AR**

Periodization can be used for deep-water classes just as for shallow-water classes, but some of the exercises and techniques are different. All the topics covered in the periodization plan for shallow water are repeated and adapted for deep water in the second half of this book, including the lesson plans for classes with two objectives.

TABLE 1

Lesson Plans Overview

Preseason	Transition season	Peak fitness season
CONTINUOUS CARDIO		
Emphasize good form	Improve quality of movement	Increase power
INTERVALS		
Interval 30 30 seconds work 90 seconds recovery 1:3 ratio 6-8 sets	*Interval 30* 30 seconds work 60 seconds recovery 1:2 ratio 8-10 sets	*Interval 30* 30 seconds work 30 seconds recovery 1:1 ratio 10-12 sets
Interval 40 40 seconds work 80 seconds recovery 1:2 ratio 6-8 sets	*Interval 40* 40 seconds work 60 seconds recovery 1:1.5 ratio 8-10 sets	*Interval 40* 40 seconds work 40 seconds recovery 1:1 ratio 10-12 sets
Interval 60 60 seconds work 2 minutes recovery 1:2 ratio 6-8 sets	*Interval 60* 60 seconds work 90 seconds recovery 1:1.5 ratio 8-10 sets	*Interval 60* 60 seconds work 60 seconds recovery 1:1 ratio 10-12 sets
Reduced recovery time 60 seconds work 30 seconds recovery 2:1 ratio 4-6 sets	*Reduced recovery time* 2 minutes work 60 seconds recovery 2:1 ratio 3-4 sets	*Reduced recovery time* 3 minutes work 90 seconds recovery 2:1 ratio 2-3 sets
Rolling intervals 1 minute 50% 1 minute 60% 1 minute 70% 3-5 sets	*Rolling intervals* 1 minute 60% 1 minute 70% 1-minute 80% 3-5 sets	*Rolling intervals* 1 minute 70% 1 minute 80% 1 minute 90% 3-5 sets
Surges 45 seconds 60% 15 seconds 70% 1 minute recovery 1:1 ratio 4-8 sets	*Surges* 45 seconds 70% 15 seconds 80% 1 minute recovery 1:1 ratio 4-8 sets	*Surges* 45 seconds 80% 15 seconds 90% 1 minute recovery 1:1 ratio 4-8 sets
Random intervals For example: 30:30 seconds 45:45 seconds 15:15:15:15 rolling 1 minute recovery 45:45 seconds 30:30 seconds 1 cycle	*Random intervals* For example: 15:15:15:15 rolling 1 minute recovery 30:30 seconds 3× 15:15 seconds 4× 30:30:30:30 rolling 2 minutes recovery 1 cycle	*Random intervals* For example: 30:30:30:30 rolling 1 minute recovery 15:15:15:15 rolling 1 minute recovery 30:30 seconds 4× 20:10 seconds 8× Tabata 1 cycle

(continued)

TABLE 1 *(continued)*

Preseason	Transition season	Peak fitness season
Pyramid 15:45 seconds 20:45 seconds 25:45 seconds 30:45 seconds 1 or more cycles	*Pyramid* 15:30 seconds 20:30 seconds 25:30 seconds 30:30 seconds 1 or more cycles	*Pyramid* 15:15 seconds 20:15 seconds 25:15 seconds 30:15 seconds 1 or more cycles
Tabata Timing 20 seconds 70% 10 seconds recovery 8 sets 2:1 ratio 1 or more cycles	*Tabata Type* 20 seconds 80% 10 seconds recovery 8 sets 2:1 ratio 1 or more cycles	*Tabata Type* 20 seconds 90% 10 seconds recovery 8 sets 2:1 ratio 1 or more cycles
STRENGTH TRAINING		
Core strength Inertia Acceleration Action and reaction Concentric contractions	Buoyant equipment Drag equipment Rubberized equipment Concentric contractions	Buoyant equipment Drag equipment Rubberized equipment Concentric and eccentric contractions
STRETCH		
5 minutes	5 minutes	5 minutes

Adapted, by permission, from a handout distributed by Stephanie Thielen at a workshop called "Intelligent Intervals for the Deep" that was sponsored by the Metroplex Association of Aquatic Professionals on March 21, 2015.

TABLE 2

Active Recovery

Continuous cardio	Partner activities
Core strength	Dance moves
Balance	Modified synchronized swimming
Pilates	Games and relay races
Fun activities	Stretch

Beginning water fitness instructors may want to use this book to become familiar with various ways to do interval training and to learn how to use various types of equipment for strength training. Experienced instructors may wish to adopt periodization as a way to progress their participants to greater levels of fitness. Aquatic fitness personal trainers will also find some of these ideas helpful with their clients.

Periodization is typically considered an annual plan, but using it for shorter cycles of six months or four months is acceptable. After completing active recovery, the cycle begins again, only now your participants are starting from a level of greater fitness and have to work harder to achieve the desired percentage of their maximum heart rate. Congratulations! You have successfully progressed them toward their fitness goal.

PART I

SHALLOW-WATER EXERCISE

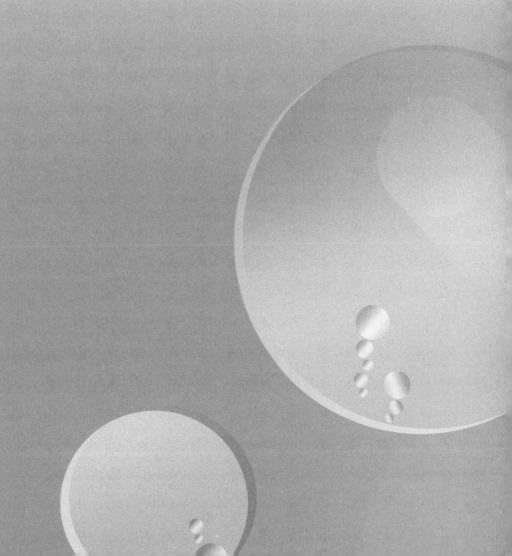

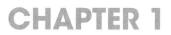

CHAPTER 1

Shallow-Water Periodization Stages

Everyone has a reason for exercising. Some people want to improve their overall health. Some want to lose weight. Some want to reduce stress. Some want to sleep better. Some want to boost their aerobic fitness. Some want to build strength. Some wish to age healthfully. Whatever their goal, performing the same workout over and over will not bring them the improvements they are looking for. Instructors who wish to help their participants meet their goals must offer progressions that enable them to improve their fitness. Periodization is a training tool that can be used to progress your participants to the next level gradually and systematically. Periodization is a cyclical plan that divides the year into preseason, transition season, peak fitness season, and active recovery season.

PRESEASON

The preseason establishes a baseline from which the following seasons progress. Your classes will include sessions of continuous cardiorespiratory fitness training, interval training to work on improving cardiorespiratory fitness, and strength training to work on improving muscular strength and endurance. You will want to emphasize good posture and performing the exercises correctly before you begin to increase resistance and add intensity in the following seasons. Exercises are performed correctly when the spine is in neutral—when the cervical, thoracic, and lumbar sections of the spine are aligned in their natural curves. Once the spine is in neutral, the next step is to brace the core, and only then are you ready to begin your workout. When the body is correctly aligned, you can maximize the use of the water's resistance. Failure to maintain neutral alignment while working the muscles of the arms and legs puts stress on the spine. Repeatedly performing an exercise incorrectly can cause microtrauma that eventually leads to an injury.

Teaching your class to perform exercises correctly requires you to be familiar with the muscles of the body and with movement terminology. This information is available in your water fitness instructor certification manual. Table 1.1 includes the major movements and the muscles most involved. Joint motion involves prime movers, which are responsible for initiating the motion. Assistors are also involved, though to a lesser degree, as are stabilizers, which maintain joint integrity during the motion. The table includes only the prime movers. All movements begin with the body in an athletic stance, that is, with the spine in neutral alignment, the arms down at the sides, the palms facing forward, and the feet hip-distance apart.

Joint Range of Motion

Knowing the normal joint range of motion will help you know what you can expect of healthy participants. But remember that when you train in water, the resistance is *in the*

TABLE 1.1

Major Movements and Muscles Involved

Joint	Joint motion	Muscles most involved
Scapula	Abduction	Serratus anterior
	Adduction	Trapezius, rhomboids
Shoulder	Flexion	Anterior deltoid, pectoralis major, biceps
	Extension or hyperextension	Latissimus dorsi, triceps
	Abduction	Middle deltoid
	Adduction	Latissimus dorsi, pectoralis major
	Horizontal abduction	Posterior deltoid
	Horizontal adduction	Pectoralis major, anterior deltoid
	Lateral rotation	Rotator cuff
	Medial rotation	Latissimus dorsi, rotator cuff
Elbow	Flexion	Biceps
	Extension	Triceps
Trunk	Flexion	Rectus abdominis
	Extension	Erector spinae
	Lateral flexion	Obliques
	Rotation	Obliques
	Core stabilization	Transversus abdominis
Hip	Flexion	Iliopsoas
	Extension or hyperextension	Gluteus maximus, hamstrings
	Abduction	Gluteus medius
	Horizontal abduction	Tensor fasciae latae
	Adduction	Adductors
Knee	Flexion	Hamstrings
	Extension	Quadriceps
Ankle	Plantar flexion	Gastrocnemius, soleus
	Dorsiflexion	Tibialis anterior

Adapted, by permission, from Aquatic Exercise Association, 2018, *Aquatic fitness professional manual,* 7th ed. (Champaign, IL: Human Kinetics), 70.

water, and even though a joint may have a range of a certain number of degrees, you will want to stop arm movement before the arm exits the water. Moving the arm into and out of the water with force puts a strain on the shoulder joint that could lead to an injury later. You will also want to limit the range of motion (ROM) of some movements for safety reasons. In shoulder abduction, impingement occurs between 80 and 120 degrees, and maintaining the shoulder within this area may provoke bursitis. The arms are out of the water in this degree of abduction anyway. Limiting shoulder abduction to 70 degrees is better (Ivens & Holder, 2011, p. 13). Shoulder adduction can continue beyond neutral 0 degrees if the hands are brought in front of the body. Participants, however, often round out their shoulders when they do this. Because you want to stress good posture, limit shoulder adduction to neutral 0 degrees or balance arm moves in front of the body with arm moves behind the body.

Bringing the arms to their full ROM in horizontal shoulder abduction during a chest stretch is acceptable. But forceful horizontal shoulder abduction exposes the head of the humerus to injury. Limit the ROM to 90 degrees by asking participants to keep their hands in their peripheral vision.

During hip flexion, as in a knee lift, the hip flexors tend to overpower the lower back if the ROM goes beyond 90 degrees. Cue to bring the upper leg parallel to the floor. Never touch a participant, especially to assist with his or her range of motion. A participant who has limitations in range of motion should be encouraged to see his or her doctor and get permission to participate in an exercise program. Table 1.2 lists joint range of motion with notations specific for use in the water.

Now that you have reviewed the prime movers for the basic joint movements and the normal range of motion specific to exercise in the water, we will look at how to perform the exercises used for cardiorespiratory fitness with good form.

Cardiorespiratory Fitness

Cardiorespiratory training is a constant through all four seasons. After all, the heart is the most important muscle in the body! During aerobic exercise, the muscles use oxygen to produce energy. The heart pumps blood to the lungs to collect the oxygen and then delivers it to the working muscles. Regular aerobic exercise both increases the ability of the lungs to hold air and strengthens the heart muscle so that it pumps a greater volume of blood with each stroke. As the cardiorespiratory system becomes more efficient, exercisers find that they are able to exercise longer. They experience many other health benefits as well, such as a reduced risk of coronary heart disease, adult onset diabetes, hypertension, and certain cancers (ACSM, 2017b). Therefore, one goal of the preseason is to be able to do continuous cardiorespiratory training at a moderate rate for 20 to 30 minutes without tiring. The American College of Sports Medicine (ACSM) recommends that adults get 150 minutes a week or more of moderate-intensity physical activity (ACSM, 2017b).

Basic Cardiorespiratory Exercises

The basic exercises used for cardiorespiratory training in a shallow-water class are walk, jog, kick, rocking horse, cross-country ski, and jumping jacks. All other moves are variations of these six exercises. Performing these exercises correctly means performing them with the spine in neutral. The following list describes the benefits as well as common mistakes to watch for.

WALK

Walk forward: *Benefit*: This movement is functional. Walk with the head up and the arms and legs moving naturally. *Common mistakes*: (1) leaning forward and (2) shortening the stride.

TABLE 1.2

Joint Movement Range of Motion

Joint	Joint motion	ROM
Shoulder	Flexion	150-180 degrees (In chest-deep water, shoulder flexion should stop at 80 degrees.)
	Extension	To neutral 0 degrees
	Hyperextension	50-60 degrees
	Abduction	180 degrees (In chest-deep water, stop at 70 degrees. Shoulder impingement occurs between 80 and 120 degrees.)
	Adduction	50 degrees (Participants often round out their shoulders when bringing palms together in front; stop at neutral 0 degrees.)
	Horizontal abduction	130 degrees (Stop at 90 degrees to avoid risk of shoulder injury when working against the water's resistance.)
Elbow	Flexion	140-150 degrees
	Extension	To neutral 0 degrees
Hip	Flexion	100-120 degrees (Stop at 90 degrees to avoid stress on the lower back.)
	Extension	To neutral 0 degrees
	Hyperextension	30 degrees
	Abduction	40-50 degrees
	Adduction	0-30 degrees
Knee	Flexion	130-150 degrees
	Extension	0-10 degrees
Ankle	Plantar flexion	40-50 degrees
	Dorsiflexion	20 degrees

Walk backward: *Benefit*: This exercise strengthens the muscles of the back. Maintain a normal stride. *Common mistake*: sitting down and pushing the body backward with the feet instead of walking tall.

JOG

Knee-high jog: *Benefit*: This exercise works multiple leg muscles, including the powerful iliopsoas, more commonly called the hip flexors. This exercise is good for burning calories. Beginners can do the move successfully. *Common mistakes*: (1) wobbling the shoulders from side to side, which takes the spine out of neutral, (2) flexing the elbows instead of pumping the arms from the shoulders, (3) bringing the knees too high, which may aggravate the sciatic nerve, and (4) jogging on the toes, which keeps the calf muscles tight.

Crossover knees: *Benefit*: This exercise works the obliques. *Common mistake*: bringing opposite elbow to knee because twisting while flexing forward is hard on the back.

Straddle jog: *Benefit*: Jogging with the hips open works the gluteus medius. *Common mistake*: jogging with the feet too far apart, which makes this exercise the same as running tires.

Run tires: *Benefit*: The hips are open wider than with straddle jog, increasing the range of motion. *Common mistake*: leaning the trunk from side to side, which puts stress on the lower back. Instead, the core muscles should be stabilized to put the focus on working the legs.

Ankle touch or inner-thigh lift: *Benefit*: This move improves hip flexibility by working on a diagonal. Hip flexibility is important for reducing the risk of falling. *Common mistakes*: (1) performing the exercise from a narrow instead of a wide stance, which makes it the same as a knee-high jog, and (2) leaning forward to touch the foot instead of bringing the foot up to the hand, which puts stress on the lower back. Calling the exercise an inner-thigh lift reduces this tendency.

Hopscotch: *Benefit*: This exercise works the hamstrings. *Common mistake*: leaning to the side to reach down to the foot instead of bringing the foot up toward the hand, which puts stress on the lower back.

Heel jog: *Benefit*: This exercise is another one for the hamstrings. *Common mistake*: bringing the knee up in front instead of lifting the heel up in back, which makes the exercise similar to a knee-high jog.

Bicycle: *Benefit*: A suspended jog can be awkward to perform, and therefore a suspended bicycle is used instead. This exercise works multiple leg muscles. *Common mistake*: Some participants have difficulty with suspended moves.

KICK

Kick forward: *Benefit*: The kick forward uses the quadriceps and hip flexors. *Common mistakes*: (1) sitting down when traveling backward, which reduces the range of motion, and (2) power popping the knees, that is, adding force at the end of the kick, which is hard on the knee joint.

High kick: *Benefit*: The high kick increases the range of motion, therefore increasing intensity. *Common mistakes*: (1) leaning backward to get the toes out of the water, which takes the spine out of neutral alignment, and (2) emphasizing the upward motion at the expense of the downward motion, which works the powerful hip flexors more than the weaker gluteus maximus.

Kick side to side: *Benefit*: This kick works the adductors and gluteus medius. *Common mistake*: performing the exercise with the feet apart and simply shifting the weight from foot to foot, eliminating the work for the targeted muscles.

Skate kick: *Benefit*: The kick backward works the gluteus maximus. *Common mistakes*: (1) bending the knee, which takes the work out of the gluteus maximus and puts it in the hamstrings, and (2) arching the back, which puts stress on the lower back. To avoid arching the back, lean forward slightly from the hips.

ROCKING HORSE

Rocking horse: *Benefit*: This exercise works the hip flexors, gluteus maximus, hamstrings, and quadriceps. It also challenges balance by taking the body off axis. *Common* *mistakes*: (1) arching the back, which takes the spine out of neutral, and (2) performing the rocking horse with straight legs to increase intensity, which causes the hip flexors to overpower the lower back.

CROSS-COUNTRY SKI

Cross-country ski: *Benefit*: This exercise works hip flexors and gluteus maximus, as well as the shoulders. It is a long-lever, high-intensity move, which burns calories. *Common mistakes*: (1) You want full hip flexion and hyperextension, but some people keep the back foot under them or perform an alternating lunge, limiting the range of motion. (2) The arm movement contributes to the intensity, but some people reduce it by pushing the hands forward instead of swinging the arms through their full range of motion.

Cross-country ski suspended: *Benefit*: The suspended ski also works hip flexors and gluteus maximus. Suspended exercises increase the intensity for many. *Common mistakes*: (1) doing a suspended kick forward, which is much easier than moving the legs from the hips through their full range of motion, and (2) being unable to perform suspended moves.

JUMPING JACKS

Jumping jacks: *Benefit*: Jacks work the adductors and gluteus medius. *Common mistakes*: (1) trying to make the legs go too far apart, which is hard on the hip joints, and (2) taking the arms in and out of the water, which is hard on the shoulders.

You can create many variations of these exercises. Here are some examples:

- Try different arm movements, such as standing row, arm swing, lat pull-down, clap hands, arm curl, and forearm press. Use only one arm, both arms in unison, alternating arms, or no arms.
- Vary the tempo. Water tempo is the normal speed used in water. Land tempo is faster, but you want to be sure not to lose your range of motion. Half water tempo adds a bounce on every other beat. You can also add variations in tempo such as pauses, doubles, and syncopate. An example of a pause is 3× and hold. Single, single, double means one right, one left, two right, and so on. Syncopate means slow, slow, quick, quick, quick.
- Change the working position, also called the impact option. Exercises can be performed upright with some rebounding, in the neutral position with the hips and knees flexed to submerge the body to shoulder depth, suspended with the feet not touching the floor, and grounded or keeping one foot on the floor at all times.
- Add turns. You can do quarter turns, half turns, or full turns. Diagonal turns are quarter turns toward the right corner and then toward the left corner.
- Combine exercises. Putting two or more exercises together creates a new exercise.

Not every variation will work with every exercise, but using even a few variations will increase the number of exercises in your repertoire.

Exercisers are able to judge how hard they are working by using perceived exertion. One scale of perceived exertion (see table 1.3) uses numbers from 1 to 10. Each number corresponds to a percentage of maximum exertion.

The target heart rate for aerobic exercise is 50 to 80 percent of the maximum heart rate. Participants who are working somewhat easy (50 percent), with moderate effort (60 percent), somewhat hard (70 percent), and hard (80 percent) are working within their target heart rate. During the preseason, you will ask your participants to work at a minimum of

TABLE 1.3

Scale of Perceived Exertion

Level 1	No effort
Level 2	Little effort
Level 3	Very easy
Level 4	Easy
Level 5	Somewhat easy
Level 6	Moderate
Level 7	Somewhat hard
Level 8	Hard
Level 9	Very hard
Level 10	Maximum effort

Adapted, by permission, from Aquatic Exercise Association, 2018, *Aquatic fitness professional manual,* 7th ed. (Champaign, IL: Human Kinetics), 12.

50 percent of their maximum exertion during the continuous cardiorespiratory training sessions.

Interval Training

Interval training is an effective way to improve cardiorespiratory fitness. During interval training, the exerciser works in alternating periods of higher and lower intensity. The higher intensity is called work, and the lower intensity is called recovery. One period of work plus one period of recovery is called a set. A group of sets is called a cycle. The length of the work compared with the length of the recovery is referred to as the work–recovery ratio. The recovery needs to be long enough that the class participant is able to recover sufficiently so that he or she can again increase intensity for the next work period. The recovery exercises can be a low-intensity version of the exercise used during the work, a functional movement such as walking, or full range of motion movements to promote flexibility. Exercising at a level of exertion that the participant is able to sustain for only a short time improves the heart's muscular strength.

Interval training is appropriate for beginners and fit participants alike. Beginners will be able to increase their exertion for short periods because the exertion is followed by a period of active recovery. One way to cue for interval training in the preseason is to ask participants to increase their exertion from 50 percent (somewhat easy) to 60 percent of maximum levels (moderate). Remember that one person's moderate effort may not be the same as another's. For safety's sake, encourage your participants to modify the intensity to a level that is challenging for them rather than try to keep up with other participants.

When you ask participants to increase their intensity, most likely they will go faster, but speed is not the only way to increase intensity. So rather than just encouraging them to work harder, you can use cues that tell participants how to change an exercise to make it more intense. Begin with exercises that use large-muscle groups in the legs. Save small movements, complex moves, and core challenges for the warm-up, the cool-down, or the recovery period. You want to use exercises that will put a demand on the heart muscle and make it beat faster. Then add one or more intensity variables. Five intensity variables can be used for shallow-water exercise:

1. **Range of motion**. Increasing the range of motion by changing an exercise from a short-lever move, with elbows and knees bent, to a long-lever move, with arms and legs fully extended (but not locked), is one way to increase intensity. Exercises can be performed with larger arm or leg movements, or with the feet farther apart, or

you can cross the midline of the body. Perform the long-lever moves at the same speed as the short-lever moves for the highest intensity.

2. **Speed**. Any exercise becomes more intense when you change from water tempo to land tempo. The temptation, however, is to reduce the range of motion when increasing speed. Tiny moves are not an effective way to increase intensity. An exercise should not be performed so fast that the range of motion is lost or that good form is compromised.

3. **Suspended moves**. This is a working position. The suspended working position is difficult for many people, so it is often used as a way to increase intensity. But suspended moves are easy for people who are natural floaters. For this group you can still go suspended, but you should add one of the other intensity variables to the exercise.

4. **Acceleration**. (a) Acceleration can mean pushing off the floor in a rebounding or jumping move. (b) But it can also mean pushing hard against the water's resistance in a power move. If you are increasing intensity by rebounding, offer a similar power move for those who are unwilling or unable to jump.

5. **Travel**. Newton's law of inertia states that an object will remain at rest or in motion with constant velocity unless acted on by a net external force. Starting the body moving, stopping it once it is moving, or changing a movement requires more effort than continuing with the same movement. You can travel forward, backward, sideways, or on a diagonal. You can travel in patterns, such as a circle, square, bowtie pattern, zigzag, scatter pattern, or with quick change of direction.

Let's look again at the basic exercises to see how these intensity variables can be used with each of them during interval training. Walking is not included in this list because it is used mainly for warming up and cooling down. The numbers following the name of the exercise represent the intensity variable being used. Not all variables can be used with every exercise.

JOG

Knee-high jog: (1) Run (use a long stride). Steep climb (like climbing a ladder out of the pool. (2) Knee-high jog, faster. Sprint. Steep climb, faster. (4b) Power run (pull the water forcefully with cupped hands). Steep climb with power. (5) Knee-high jog, travel. Run. Sprint. Power run.

Straddle jog: (3) Frog, suspended. (4a) Frog jump. Frog jump with hands up. (4b) Frog jump with double-arm press-down. (5) Straddle jog travel. Frog jump, travel.

Run tires: (4a) Squat and jump. (4b) Squat and power leg (squat and lift one knee as you return to standing; extend that knee and power press it down, transitioning into the next squat). (5) Run tires travel.

Inner-thigh lift: (1) Inner-thigh lift with full range of motion (ROM). (2) Inner-thigh lift, faster. (4b) Inner-thigh lift with power. Inner-thigh lift with double arms (extend both arms to one side and then touch the opposite inner thigh with both hands). (5) Inner-thigh lift, travel.

Hopscotch: (1) Hopscotch with full range of motion (ROM). (2) Hopscotch, faster. (4b) Hopscotch with power. (5) Hopscotch, travel.

Heel jog: (4a) Skateboard jump. (5) Heel jog, travel.

Bicycle: (1) Bicycle with full range of motion (ROM) (large circles), suspended. (2) Bicycle, faster, suspended. (4b) Bicycle with power, suspended. (5) Bicycle, suspended, travel.

KICK

Kick forward: (1) High kick. (2) Kick forward, faster. Front kick (karate), faster. (3) Flutter kick, suspended. (4b) Knee lift, straighten, and power press-down. High kick, power down. High kick with power. Kick and lunge. Kick and lunge with double-arm press-down. Front kick (karate). (5) Kick forward, travel. High kick, travel.

Kick side to side: (1) Kick side to side, arms and legs opposite. (2) Kick side to side, faster. Side kick (karate), faster. (4b) Kick side to side, arms sweep side to side. Kick side to side with power, grounded (add power to the adduction phase of the kick). Side kick (karate). (5) Kick side to side, travel. Side kick (karate), travel sideways.

Skate kick: (1) Skate kick with full range of motion (ROM). (2) Skate kick, faster. (4b) Skate kick with power. Knee lift and lunge. (5) Skate kick, travel.

ROCKING HORSE

Rocking horse: (1) Rocking horse with a front kick. (5) Rocking horse, travel.

CROSS-COUNTRY SKI

Cross-country ski: (1) Cross-country ski with full range of motion (ROM). Cross-country ski with full range of motion (ROM), neutral position. Cross-country ski with rotation. (2) Mini ski, faster. Cross-country ski, faster. Cross-country ski, faster, suspended. (3) Cross-country ski, suspended. (4b) Cross-country ski with power. Cross-country ski with power, neutral position. Cross-country ski, arms sweep side to side. Cross-country ski with rotation, hands together. (5) Cross-country ski, travel.

JUMPING JACKS

Jumping jacks: (1) Jacks cross. (2) Mini jacks, faster. Jumping jacks, faster. Jumping jacks, faster, suspended. (3) Jumping jacks, suspended. (4a) Jumping jacks, landing feet out only. (4b) Jumping jacks with power, neutral position (arms sweep out and in, add power to both abduction and adduction.) Jacks cross with power, grounded (lift leg side, cross front, lift side and down; repeat other side. (5) Jumping jacks, travel.

Timing the Intervals You can time intervals in many ways. During the preseason, you may wish to intersperse cycles of interval training among periods of continuous cardiorespiratory training. In effect, the cardio serves as a long period of recovery between the cycles of interval sets. The goal is to pull the interval sets together gradually and place them in the middle or at the end of your continuous cardio.

In general, your participants will aim for 60 percent of maximum effort (moderate) during the preseason. But occasionally introduce them to higher levels of intensity—70 percent (somewhat hard) in a rolling interval, a surge, or Tabata. Toward the end of the preseason, let them try working at 80 percent (hard) in a random interval set. An intensity of 80 percent of maximum effort is considered high-intensity interval training (HIIT).

The following are options for timing intervals in the preseason (Thielen, 2015):

INTERVAL 30

30 seconds of work to 90 seconds of recovery (1:3 ratio), 6 to 8 sets

INTERVAL 40

40 seconds of work to 80 seconds of recovery (1:2 ratio), 6 to 8 sets

TABATA

Tabata is an interval format first developed by Dr. Izumi Tabata in Japan in 1996. He asked speed skaters to work at greater than maximal intensity for 20 seconds and then rest for 10 seconds eight times in a 4-minute exercise cycle. The result was a remarkable improvement in cardiorespiratory fitness. Tabata as Dr. Tabata designed it is called True Tabata. Obviously, you would not ask participants in a water fitness class to perform any exercise at greater than 100 percent of maximum intensity. But Tabata modified for nonathletes has become quite popular. One modification is called Tabata Type, in which the intensity level is reduced to 80 to 90 percent. Although you can use a single high-intensity exercise for the work, you can also use two or more high-intensity exercises in your eight-set cycle. Rest consists of standing in place and catching your breath. Because the intensity level is submaximal, you can choose to perform more than one Tabata cycle in a class. You will want to wait until the transition season to introduce your class to Tabata Type intervals.

Another modification of Tabata is called Tabata Timing. Tabata Timing uses the format of 20 seconds of work to 10 seconds of recovery eight times per cycle, but the work consists of aerobic intervals or other objectives such as strength training. The recovery period can be a lower-intensity exercise rather than standing in place and catching your breath because the work period may not be intense enough to warrant complete rest. You can perform as many cycles of Tabata Timing as you choose, including using it for an entire class.

INTERVAL 60

60 seconds of work to 2 minutes of recovery (1:2 ratio), 6 to 8 sets

REDUCED RECOVERY TIME

60 seconds of work to 30 seconds of recovery (2:1 ratio), 4 to 6 sets

ROLLING INTERVALS

1 minute at 50 percent, 1 minute at 60 percent, and 1 minute at 70 percent of maximum effort, 3 to 5 sets

SURGES

45 seconds at 60 percent, 15 seconds at 70 percent of maximum effort, and 1 minute of recovery (1:1 ratio), 4 to 8 sets

RANDOM INTERVALS

30 seconds of work to 30 seconds of recovery

45 seconds of work to 45 seconds of recovery

15 seconds at 50 percent of maximum effort, 15 seconds at 60 percent, 15 seconds at 70 percent, and 15 seconds at 80 percent to 1 minute of recovery (rolling interval)

45 seconds of work to 45 seconds of recovery

30 seconds of work to 30 seconds of recovery

1 cycle

PYRAMID

15 seconds of work to 45 seconds of recovery

20 seconds of work to 45 seconds of recovery

25 seconds of work to 45 seconds of recovery

30 seconds of work to 45 seconds of recovery

1 or more cycles

TABATA TIMING

20 seconds of work at 70 percent of maximum effort to 10 seconds of recovery

8 sets (2:1 ratio), 1 or more cycles

Muscular Strength and Endurance

Strength training is an important component of the periodization program. Some participants may wonder why they should strength train. Children's muscles grow larger and stronger as their bodies grow, and this muscle growth continues into adulthood until around age 30. After reaching a peak, muscle mass begins to decline with age. The prescription for preventing or reversing this loss of muscle mass is strength training. Maintaining or increasing muscular fitness can help prevent osteoporosis, decrease the risk of heart disease, reduce the risk of falling, and enhance the quality of life. The American College of Sports Medicine recommends that every adult perform activities that maintain or increase muscular strength and endurance for a minimum of two days a week. Adults over 65 should strength train two to three times a week (ACSM, 2017c). Strength training involves training both the muscles of the core and the muscles of the limbs to improve muscular strength and endurance.

Neutral alignment is possible when the muscles that affect the spine, including the shoulder girdle, the trunk muscles, and the pelvic girdle, are balanced in strength. In modern life, we spend a lot of time seated in front of the computer, television, or steering wheel of our cars, in a position referred to as passive forward flexion. As we age, gravity affects us as well. If nothing is done to keep the core muscles strong, we become bent over, unable to stand up straight, and prone to poor balance and falls. Participants who may be able to achieve neutral alignment, but who have difficulty maintaining it, should therefore begin their fitness program by focusing on core strength training. Any participant who is unable to achieve neutral posture may need to be referred to a doctor.

The core refers to the postural muscles of the trunk: transversus abdominis, rectus abdominis, internal and external obliques, erector spinae, latissimus dorsi, trapezius, rhomboids, serratus anterior, gluteus maximus, and hip abductors and adductors. The trapezius is involved in scapular stabilization. Strong hip abductors are important for maintaining balance. These muscles work together to maintain good posture and to support and move the shoulders, the back, and the hips. Obviously, working the core is not limited to working the rectus abdominis!

In functional movement, the stabilizers activate before the prime movers do. Specifically, the core muscles engage before the arms and legs move. The water is the perfect place to work on core stabilization because immersion activates the core stabilizers. Some of the best exercises for training the core are functional exercises that mimic activities of daily living, such as walking forward and backward, walking in multiple directions, running forward and backward, and running in multiple directions. Cross-country ski is another good core exercise that uses long levers with alternating arm and leg movement to create balance. You can challenge core muscles in a variety of ways, such as the following: (1) dropping into the neutral position, (2) keeping the feet grounded and moving the arms in sweeping motions, (3) performing off-axis moves such as the rocking horse, (4) pausing, holding a position, and balancing, and (5) keeping one foot grounded while the other leg moves.

Avoid exercises that take the spine out of neutral alignment. Do not run or perform a cross-country ski while leaning forward. Avoid leaning forward to touch the toes during a front kick. Forward flexion with rotation, such as a knee lift with opposite elbow to knee, puts a strain on the lower back. Prone flutter kicks at the pool wall result in hyperextension of the back. Pay careful attention to neutral alignment in your participants and demonstrate good posture at all times. In the pool the water movement constantly challenges core stabilization, so more postural cues are necessary. Use multiple cues to reinforce good posture. The classic cue is "Ears over shoulders, over hips, over ankles." You can also ask class participants to walk as if they have a book on their heads, to keep their chests up and their shoulders down, to relax their shoulders and brace the core, and to stand tall. Have frequent posture checks and repeat your cues over and over.

Although knowing movement terminology is important, you will not use those terms with class participants. Exercises have a variety of names because terms are not standardized in the aquatics industry. For the purpose of this book, the terms in table 1.4 will be used for strength-training exercises.

Muscle Pairs

If you refer to table 1.1 earlier in the chapter, you will notice that the body's muscles are organized in pairs of opposing muscle groups. Often one muscle in a pair is stronger than the opposing muscle. Although you will want to work both sets of opposing muscles (see table 1.5), you should cue your participants to place more force in the direction of the weaker muscle. You also want to be sure to stretch the stronger muscle.

Muscular Contractions

There are three types of muscle actions: isotonic, isometric, and isokinetic. In isotonic contractions, the muscle shortens and lengthens and movement occurs at the joint. In isometric contractions, muscle tension occurs but no movement occurs at the joint and muscle length does not change. Isokinetic muscle actions occur at a consistent rate of speed regardless of the muscular force being used. Isokinetic muscle actions require specialized equipment and are not possible in water exercise. The type of muscle action that occurs during strength training in water is an isotonic contraction. During an isotonic contraction, the muscle contracts, or shortens, and then lengthens, causing movement at a joint. The shortening phase is called a concentric contraction, and the lengthening phase is called an eccentric action. Eccentric actions are not called contractions because the muscle is lengthening rather than contracting. In water, the muscles are working against resistance in every direction. Both muscles in a muscle pair work concentrically. Eccentric actions will not occur unless certain types of equipment are used. Gains in strength are possible with concentric contractions alone. Eccentric actions are associated with delayed onset muscle soreness, which almost never happens in water exercise. This consideration may be important for participants who are new to strength training or who have a history of poor compliance to a fitness routine because they don't like the muscle soreness afterward.

Properties of Water

To produce gains in strength, greater-than-normal stress must be placed on the working muscles. Participants can move gently through the water in ways that do not put any stress on the limbs. Therefore, a person who is serious about improving his or her muscular strength must be intentional about overloading the muscles. Remember that the spine must be in neutral alignment before overloading the muscles in any strength-training exercise. In the preseason, muscles are overloaded by taking advantage of the properties of water.

TABLE 1.4

Strength Training Exercise Names

Exercise science terminology	Common terms
Scapula adduction	Standing row, crawl stroke, bowstring pull, shoulder blade squeeze
Shoulder flexion	Double-arm lift, arm swing forward
Shoulder extension or hyperextension	Double-arm press-down, arm swing back
Shoulder abduction	Arm lift to sides
Shoulder adduction	Lat pull-down
Shoulder horizontal abduction	Clap hands out, shoulder sweep out, breaststroke
Shoulder horizontal adduction	Clap hands in, shoulder sweep in, reverse breaststroke, chest fly, chest press, crossovers
Shoulder lateral rotation	Forearm press out
Shoulder medial rotation	Forearm press in
Elbow flexion	Arm curl
Elbow extension	Triceps extension, push forward, triceps kick back
Elbow flexion with shoulder abducted 70 degrees	Close doors, side arm curl, elbow sweep in
Elbow extension with shoulder abducted 70 degrees	Open doors, elbow sweep out
Trunk flexion	Crunch
Trunk extension	Spine extension
Trunk lateral flexion	Lateral flexion, hip hike
Trunk rotation	Upper-body twist, lower-body twist
Hip flexion	Kick forward, knee swing forward
Hip extension or hyperextension	Kick back, hip extension, knee lift straighten and power press-down, knee swing back, standing leg press, seated leg press
Hip abduction	Kick side, dog hike
Hip adduction	Return kick side to center, standing leg press to the side
Hip horizontal abduction	Clamshells open, jumping jacks open neutral position
Hip horizontal adduction	Clamshells close, jumping jacks close neutral position
Knee flexion	Hamstring curl
Knee extension	Quad kick
Hip flexion and knee flexion, heels on floor	Squat
Hip flexion and knee flexion with hip extension and knee flexion	Lunge
Plantar flexion	Up on toes, point feet
Dorsiflexion	Flex feet

TABLE 1.5

Opposing Muscles

Muscle	Opposing muscle	Stronger muscle
Middle deltoid	Latissimus dorsi	Latissimus dorsi
Posterior deltoid	Pectoralis major	Pectoralis major
Biceps	Triceps	Biceps
Rectus abdominis	Erector spinae	Erector spinae
Gluteus medius	Adductors	Adductors
Hamstrings	Quadriceps	Quadriceps
Gastrocnemius	Tibialis anterior	Gastrocnemius

Buoyancy   The Archimedes principle states that a body will float if it displaces water weighing more than its own weight. Buoyancy is the upward force exerted on lighter-than-water objects submerged in water, including many participants and their limbs. Buoyancy helps objects float toward the surface of the water. Buoyancy also resists movement of buoyant objects toward the bottom of the pool. But buoyancy does not act on all participants equally. People with a greater percentage of body fat tend to float, but muscular people may have a greater tendency to sink, because muscle is denser than fat and may be heavier than the amount of water displaced. These people will be affected more by gravity than by buoyancy.

What this means in practice is that movements toward the surface of the water (shoulder flexion, shoulder abduction, elbow flexion, hip flexion, hip abduction, knee flexion, and plantar flexion) are buoyancy assisted for most people. Movements toward the pool floor (shoulder extension, shoulder adduction, elbow extension, hip extension, hip adduction, knee extension, and dorsiflexion) are buoyancy resisted. The opposite may be true for very muscular participants. The downward phase of squats and lunges are more difficult for buoyant people, whereas the upward phase of squats and lunges are more difficult for muscular people. Movement that is parallel to the water's surface (scapula abduction and adduction, shoulder horizontal abduction and adduction, shoulder rotation, and hip horizontal abduction and adduction) is buoyancy neutral. The effects of buoyancy can be counteracted in some cases by a change of position. Elbow flexion and extension can be done with the shoulders abducted at 70 degrees, making the movement buoyancy neutral. Knee flexion can be done in a seated position, making it buoyancy resisted. Trunk flexion in a standing position is not considered buoyancy resisted, and in fact the weight of the trunk may put stress on the lower back during standing trunk flexion.

Newton's Law of Inertia   Newton's law of inertia states that an object will remain at rest or in motion with constant velocity unless acted on by a net external force. Starting the body moving, stopping it once it is moving, or changing a movement requires more effort than continuing with the same movement. This effect is more pronounced in the water than on land because the water's resistance tends to slow movement quickly. This resistance is called drag resistance. The law of inertia can be used to create overload by changing movements or changing direction frequently. But the body is not the only thing affected by inertia. The water also has inertia. When a group travels for some distance through the water, the water moves with the group. Take advantage of the water's inertia by reversing direction. This action will feel as if you are moving upstream. The combined effect of the body's inertia and the water's inertia increases intensity.

Frontal Resistance   Frontal resistance creates overload by increasing drag resistance. The larger the frontal surface area presented to the resistance of the water, the greater the energy required to move through the water. A larger surface area can be created by traveling forward with the arms stretched to the side or by traveling forward with the legs farther apart. Traveling sideways presents less frontal resistance, except for very obese participants. You can increase frontal resistance while traveling sideways by performing exercises in the sagittal plane, such as a cross-country ski.

Hand Positions   Hand positions can assist in creating overload. A hand sliced sideways through the water or a closed fist encounters minimal resistance. A flat palm encounters more resistance. But a cupped hand position with the fingers relaxed and slightly apart will pull water more effectively and encounter the most resistance.

Lever Length   Lever length is another factor in creating overload for strength training. The longer the lever, the greater the drag resistance and the more force the muscle must use to move the limb. Although shoulder movement can be performed with the elbow bent, greater resistance is encountered when the elbow is extended (but not locked) and the wrist is in the neutral position. Although hip movement can be performed with the knee bent, greater resistance is encountered when the knee is extended (but not locked) and the ankle is plantar flexed.

Newton's Law of Acceleration   Newton's law of acceleration states that the rate at which a body changes speed is directly related to the force applied. The law of acceleration can be used to create overload by pushing harder, or applying more force, against the water's resistance with the arms or legs. The harder you push the water, the harder the water pushes back. Double speed produces quadruple the force. But you are not simply trying to move faster; the goal is to move the limb through a greater range of motion at the same tempo or faster. The law of acceleration can be used to overcome the effects of buoyancy because force can be applied in any direction, including upward. The law of acceleration is the primary means for overloading the muscles during strength training in water. It should be used consistently and intentionally, even when other means of increasing intensity are added. You want to accelerate through most of your range of motion, but you must also decelerate near the end of the movement to prevent the joint from going beyond its normal range of motion. A brief pause before moving the limb in the opposite direction will allow the acceleration to be more powerful and the overload more effective.

Newton's Law of Action and Reaction   Newton's law of action and reaction states that every action causes an equal and opposite reaction. Newton discovered that forces occur in pairs, which he named action and reaction. These forces are obvious in water. For example, when you perform the action of sweeping the arms to the right, the reaction is that the body moves to the left. Swimmers use this law with their swim strokes. They use impeding arm and leg movements to use the law of action and reaction to create overload. An arm movement that propels the body forward while traveling backward increases the intensity. An arm movement that propels the body backward while traveling forward increases the intensity. A leg movement that propels the body forwards while traveling backward increases the intensity. A leg movement that propels the body backward while traveling forward increases the intensity. Arm and leg movements that propel the body forward while traveling backward add even more intensity, as do arm and leg movements that propel the body backward while traveling forward.

In the preseason, inertia, frontal resistance, hand positions, lever length, acceleration, and action and reaction are used to overload the muscles. Participants should be competent using the properties of water before resistance equipment is added in the transition season. Perform 8 to 10 exercises for the major muscle groups in a strength-training session. Aim for at least one set of 8 to 15 repetitions of each exercise. If you use music, choose something

ASSISTED AND RESISTED MOVEMENT

Forward Assisted or Backward Resisted Arm Movement:
Standing row
Unison arm swing back
Double-arm press-down
Breaststroke
Shoulder sweep out
Forearm press out
Triceps kick back

Forward Resisted or Backward Assisted Arm Movement:
Push forward
Unison arm swing forward
Double-arm lift
Reverse breaststroke
Shoulder sweep in
Forearm press in
Arm curl

Forward Assisted or Backward Resisted Leg Movement:
Heel jog
Skate kick
Knee lift, straighten, and power press-down

Forward Resisted or Backward Assisted Leg Movement:
Quad kick
Kick forward

that is 134 beats per minute or slower. Exercisers will lose their range of motion if they try to strength train to the beat of music faster than 134 beats per minute (Yazigi, 2011).

Flexibility

Stretch at the end of each class to increase range of motion. Choose either dynamic stretches, in which a joint slowly moves through its full range of motion, or static stretches, in which participants hold the stretch for 10 to 20 seconds. Spend at least 5 minutes on stretching.

DYNAMIC STRETCHES

Middle trapezius (upper back) and pectoralis major (pectorals): Round out the back and stretch the chest; sweep one arm across the chest and bowstring pull back.

Pectoralis major (pectorals): Stretch one arm to the side and walk in a circle away from the arm.

Deltoids (shoulders): One arm swings forward and back; arms sweep side to side.

Latissimus dorsi and obliques: Climb a rope.

Iliopsoas (hip flexors) and gluteus maximus: One leg swings forward and back.

Gluteus medius (outer thigh): Crossover step.

Hip adductors (inner thigh) and gluteus medius (outer thigh): One leg lifts side, crosses front, lifts side, and crosses back.

Ankle: Circle the ankle.

STATIC STRETCHES

Upper trapezius (neck): Bring your ear toward your shoulder; look over your shoulder.

Middle trapezius (upper back): Hug yourself; round out your back as if hugging a barrel.

Pectoralis major (pectorals): Clasp hands behind your back.

Latissimus dorsi: Raise one or both arms straight up.

Erector spinae (lower back): Perform a posterior pelvic tilt and round out the lower back.

Triceps: Raise one arm up and bend the elbow; support the arm with the other hand above the elbow.

Iliopsoas (hip flexors): From a stride position perform a posterior pelvic tilt.

Gluteus maximus: Lift one knee and support it with the hand under the thigh.

Hamstrings: Place one heel on the floor in front of you with the toes pointing up and the knee straight and then lean forward until you feel the stretch; lift one knee and straighten the leg, support the leg with one hand under the thigh, or rest the foot on the pool wall.

Gluteus medius (outer thigh): Put one ankle on the opposite knee and sit down.

Hip adductors (inner thigh): Yoga tree pose (lateral hip stretch); lunge to the side.

Quadriceps: Lift one foot up behind the body with the knee pointed down and add a posterior pelvic tilt; the foot may be supported by hand if the range of motion allows, or it may be supported on the pool wall (the back is to the wall).

Gastrocnemius: In a stride position lower the back heel to the floor.

Preseason Lesson Plans

In the periodization program you devote some time to each of the requirements for cardiorespiratory fitness, strength, and flexibility, but unless your class meets five days a week, you will not be able to meet all the requirements in class. Encourage your participants to get additional exercise on the days that the class does not meet. A schedule might look like the following:

TWO ONE-HOUR CLASSES A WEEK

1. 5 minutes warm-up, 30 minutes cardiorespiratory training, 20 minutes strength training or core strength training *or* 50 minutes strength training, 5 minutes stretching
2. 5 minutes warm-up, 50 minutes cardiorespiratory training with intervals, 5 minutes stretching

THREE ONE-HOUR CLASSES A WEEK

1. 5 minutes warm-up, 50 minutes cardiorespiratory training, 5 minutes stretching
2. 5 minutes warm-up, 50 minutes strength training or core strength training, 5 minutes stretching
3. 5 minutes warm-up, 50 minutes cardiorespiratory training with intervals, 5 minutes stretching

FIVE ONE-HOUR CLASSES A WEEK

1. 5 minutes warm-up, 50 minutes cardiorespiratory training, 5 minutes stretching
2. 5 minutes warm-up, 50 minutes strength training, 5 minutes stretching
3. 5 minutes warm-up, 50 minutes cardiorespiratory training with intervals, 5 minutes stretching
4. 5 minutes warm-up, 50 minutes strength training or core strength training, 5 minutes stretching
5. 5 minutes warm-up, 50 minutes cardiorespiratory training *or* cardiorespiratory training with intervals, 5 minutes stretching

TRANSITION SEASON

The transition season progresses from the baseline established in the preseason. Continue to emphasize good posture and correct performance of the exercises, although by now you should see improvements in your participants' form. Neutral spine and bracing the core has become second nature to them.

The focus of this season is improving the quality of their exercise by paying attention to how the arms and legs move the water. You want them to become more aware of how they use their hand positions to push and pull the water and how the water moves in reaction to their leg exercises. As their awareness grows, they will have more control of their body movements. Being able to manipulate the water intentionally improves stability, helps control travel, and allows participants to use acceleration at will to increase intensity for intervals and strength training. During the transition season, cardiorespiratory training continues, interval training continues at a higher intensity including occasional HIIT sessions, and equipment is introduced in the sessions that focus on muscular strength.

Cardiorespiratory Fitness

Your participants should now be able to do continuous cardiorespiratory training at 50 percent of maximum effort for 30 minutes without tiring. Compliment them for their improvement in endurance. Begin to draw their attention to the quality of their movement. Relaxed fluid moves should now become more intentional. Remind them that the resistance of water is much greater than the resistance of air and encourage them to push it, pull it, and move it around with their arms and legs. Have them drag the water with them when they travel. You will be asking them to increase their exertion from 50 percent to 60 percent of maximum. They should work with moderate effort during their sessions of continuous cardiorespiratory training. They need to establish a base fitness level, which means that they need to be able to work at 60 percent of maximum effort for 30 minutes without tiring to be able to add regular sessions of high-intensity interval training (HIIT) to their workout schedule.

To increase the intensity, you can use interval training. Interval-training intensities increase from 60 percent of maximum effort to 70 percent (somewhat hard). You may still occasionally intersperse cycles of interval training between periods of cardiorespiratory training, but more often you will put all your intervals together in the middle or at the end of the cardio. You will also begin to include HIIT once every two weeks or even once a week toward the end of the transition season.

HIIT involves working at 80 percent of maximum effort or greater. After you reach 90 percent of maximum effort, you cross the anaerobic threshold. Working at 90 percent of maximum effort improves both aerobic and anaerobic fitness. During aerobic exercise, the muscles use oxygen to produce energy. In anaerobic exercise your body's demand for oxygen exceeds the oxygen supply available. Anaerobic exercise, therefore, is not dependent on oxygen from breathing but instead relies on energy sources that are stored in the muscles. The recovery period in anaerobic exercise is important. If the recovery period is shorter than the high-intensity period, then the body is unable to achieve full anaerobic recovery. Therefore, in most cases the recovery needs to be longer than the work. Besides improving fitness, HIIT has been shown to improve blood pressure, cardiovascular health, insulin sensitivity, cholesterol profiles, and abdominal fat and body weight. HIIT burns more calories than continuous cardiorespiratory training, especially after the workout. This occurs because the heart and lungs work hard to supply oxygen to the working muscles and after the exercise ends, the body has excess oxygen to consume. About two hours are needed to use up the excess oxygen. This postexercise period adds around 15 percent more calories to the overall workout energy expenditure (ACSM, 2017a).

HIIT in the transition season includes rolling intervals and surges during which participants get up to 80 percent of maximum effort (hard). In random intervals you might ask your participants to work at 80 percent to 90 percent (very hard) for 15 to 30 seconds. Introduce your participants to a Tabata Type class performed at 80 percent of maximum effort. This format has a recovery period shorter than the work period. Do not cue an active recovery but instead let the participants stand in place to catch their breath. Include a transition period of 1 to 2 minutes of moderate activity between Tabata cycles.

If your participants have been following the progression of gradually increasing intensity levels up to this point, then they should be ready for HIIT. Nevertheless, you want to encourage everyone to modify the intensity of the work intervals to their preferred challenging level. Safety is always a priority. Ask everyone to focus on their own optimal training intensities rather than try to keep up with other participants.

The following are options for interval training during the transition season (Thielen, 2015):

INTERVAL 30

30 seconds of work to 60 seconds of recovery (1:2 ratio), 8 to 10 sets

INTERVAL 40

40 seconds of work to 60 seconds of recovery (1:1.5 ratio), 8 to 10 sets

INTERVAL 60

60 seconds of work to 90 seconds of recovery (1:1.5 ratio), 8 to 10 sets

REDUCED RECOVERY TIME

2 minutes of work to 1 minute of recovery (2:1 ratio), 3 to 4 sets

ROLLING INTERVALS

1 minute at 60 percent, 1 minute at 70 percent, and 1 minute at 80 percent of maximum effort, 3 to 5 sets

SURGES

45 seconds at 70 percent, 15 seconds at 80 percent of maximum effort, and 1 minute of recovery (1:1 ratio), 4 to 8 sets

RANDOM INTERVALS

15 seconds at 60 percent of maximum effort, 15 seconds at 70 percent, 15 seconds at 80 percent, and 15 seconds at 90 percent to 1 minute of recovery (rolling interval)

30 seconds of work to 30 seconds of recovery, 3 sets

15 seconds of work to 15 seconds of recovery, 4 sets

30 seconds at 60 percent of maximum effort, 30 seconds at 70 percent, 30 seconds at 80 percent, and 30 seconds at 90 percent to 1 minute of recovery (rolling interval)

1 cycle

PYRAMID

15 seconds of work to 30 seconds of recovery

20 seconds of work to 30 seconds of recovery

25 seconds of work to 30 seconds of recovery

30 seconds of work to 30 seconds of recovery

1 or more cycles

TABATA TYPE

20 seconds of work at 80 percent of maximum effort to 10 seconds of recovery

8 sets (2:1 ratio), 1 or more cycles

Muscular Strength and Endurance

In the transition season equipment is added to the program. Strength training in the water can be accomplished using only the properties of water. The muscular contractions are always concentric. As mentioned previously, gains in strength are possible with concentric contractions alone as long as greater-than-normal stress is placed on the muscle being trained. It is a misconception that eccentric muscle actions are better than concentric contractions at building muscle strength (AEA, 2018, p. 54). Eccentric muscle actions, however, can be added by using certain types of equipment. Equipment also increases the resistance beyond what is possible using only the properties of water.

Equipment Types

Three types of equipment are commonly available for use in shallow water: buoyant, drag, and rubberized equipment. In addition, some instructors may have access to aquatic steps. Before adding any equipment, remind your participants that they need to maintain neutral posture at all times to avoid injury.

Buoyant Equipment   Buoyant equipment uses the buoyancy of the water for resistance. The most popular forms of buoyant equipment are foam dumbbells and noodles. Buoyant equipment floats, so the resistance occurs when the equipment is plunged toward the pool floor. The muscular contraction is concentric. When the buoyant equipment is raised, the same muscle lengthens against the resistance in an eccentric action. For example, in elbow extension the triceps shortens in a concentric contraction to press the equipment toward the pool floor. Then, to prevent the equipment from popping out of the water, the triceps maintains its tension as it lengthens in a controlled manner. The opposing muscle, the biceps, is not involved. This action is the opposite of using weighted equipment on land. In the same example, during elbow flexion the biceps shortens in a concentric contraction to lift the weight against gravity. Then, to avoid dropping the weight, the biceps maintains its tension as it lengthens in a controlled manner. The opposing muscle, the triceps, is not involved.

What this means is that only one muscle in a muscle pair is worked with buoyant equipment. When using weighted equipment on land, changing positions to work the other muscle of the pair is possible, but in water many of those positions are not possible because they involve going underwater, or at least getting into an awkward position in which it is difficult to maintain neutral alignment. When buoyant equipment is moved parallel to the floor, such as when targeting the pectoralis major, then the drag forces of the water come into play. But the main muscular contraction is an isometric contraction of the latissimus dorsi and lower trapezius to hold the buoyant equipment under water (AEA, 2018 p. 86). In the case of targeting the pectoralis major, movements parallel to the floor can be avoided by standing in a lunge position and leaning forward 45 degrees with the spine in neutral alignment. The shoulders can now be horizontally adducted in a chest fly. The equipment can also be plunged diagonally downward to work the pectoralis major and triceps in a chest press. You must carefully observe your participants to make sure that they are able to maintain a neutral spine in this position. If they cannot, avoid these exercises.

Squats and lunges are a special case. These complex multijoint exercises involve almost all of the leg muscles. In the downward phase of a squat or lunge, the hips flex, lengthening the hamstrings and gluteus maximus in an eccentric muscle action. The knees flex, lengthening the quadriceps in an eccentric muscle action. The ankles dorsiflex, lengthening the gastrocnemius in an eccentric muscle action. When you stand back up, the hips extend, shortening the hamstrings and gluteus maximus in a concentric contraction. The knees extend, shortening the quadriceps in a concentric contraction. And the ankles plantar flex, shortening the gastrocnemius in a concentric contraction. Holding buoyant dumbbells in the hands with the arms fully extended at the sides adds resistance during the eccentric phase of the movement, which is the opposite of holding weighted dumbbells on land. Many participants who are unable to perform squats and lunges on land will be able to

EXERCISE SAFETY WITH FOAM DUMBBELLS

Foam dumbbells are a handheld piece of buoyant equipment. Submerging them requires the shoulder stabilizers to contract. Holding the dumbbells underwater for extended periods or performing too many repetitions puts undue stress on the shoulder stabilizers. Therefore, limit each set of upper-body exercises to 8 to 15 repetitions or fewer if the participant cannot maintain good shoulder alignment.

Good postural alignment must also be maintained. A participant who has to throw his or her body weight into the exercise has selected foam dumbbells that are too large. Watch for participants who are elevating the shoulders. This action is a second indication that the equipment is too large.

A third indication is a loss of range of motion when the participant tries to increase the speed of the exercise. Replace the foam dumbbells with smaller ones or perform the exercise without equipment. The movement should be performed smoothly, at the participant's full range of motion.

Participants may also unconsciously grip the handles tightly, putting stress on the wrists and fingers. Give cues to keep the wrist in neutral and relax the grip. After every set, allow 30 to 60 seconds to rest and encourage them to relax their shoulders and stretch their fingers.

Never use foam dumbbells as a flotation device. When the body is suspended between dumbbells held in the hands with the arms fully abducted, the shoulders are unacceptably loaded and the tendons are pinched (Ivens & Holder, 2011, p. 12). When the body is suspended from dumbbells placed under the arms, nerve damage may occur (Ivens & Holder, 2011, p. 15). Use foam dumbbells as a piece of resistance equipment only.

perform them in water because buoyancy reduces the stress on the hip and knee joints. The depth of the water dictates how far down the participant can go in a squat or lunge.

Table 1.6 shows which muscles are worked with buoyant equipment.

Drag Equipment Drag equipment increases the drag forces of the water by increasing surface area and creating turbulence. The most popular piece of drag equipment is webbed gloves. Drag equipment includes paddles and handheld equipment with multiple planes to increase turbulence. Paddles have fan blades that can be opened or closed to adjust the resistance. Kickboards can also be used as a piece of drag equipment.

The movement of the arms and legs with drag equipment feels natural, and for that reason, some participants prefer drag equipment to buoyant equipment. The muscular contraction with drag equipment is concentric in all directions, working both muscles in a muscle pair. But eccentric action of the opposing muscle also occurs at the end of the range of motion, slowing down the movement as the limb prepares to change direction (AEA, 2010, p. 121). For example, in elbow flexion the biceps shortens in a concentric contraction, but near the end of the range of motion, the triceps fires eccentrically to slow the motion so that the arm can stop and change direction. Then, the triceps contracts concentrically to extend the elbow.

Movement parallel to the floor using drag equipment does not involve any isometric contractions of the latissimus dorsi or lower trapezius, as when using buoyant equipment. Therefore, no special body positions are required to target any muscle group, making drag equipment ideal for those who are unable to maintain neutral alignment in a lunge position while leaning forward 45 degrees. Squats and lunges are similar to the same exercises on land, involving concentric and eccentric muscle actions. Hold the drag equipment in the hands with the arms fully extended at the sides. If possible, use an area of the pool that is waist deep.

Table 1.7 shows the muscle contractions with drag equipment.

Rubberized Equipment Rubberized equipment works the same in water as on land. The resistance comes from the equipment itself rather than from buoyancy or the drag forces of the water. Rubberized equipment is available as straight bands, loops, and tubes. Pool chemicals and sunlight tend to break down rubberized equipment fairly quickly, so it must be inspected frequently. Chlorine-resistant rubberized equipment is now available.

EXERCISE SAFETY WITH HANDHELD DRAG EQUIPMENT

With handheld drag equipment, participants need to keep the wrist neutral rather than flex and extend it. Cue straight wrists and a loose grip. Good postural alignment must be maintained. A participant who has to throw his or her body weight into the exercise has selected equipment that is too large.

Watch for participants who are elevating the shoulders. This action is a second indication that the equipment is too large. A third indication is a loss of range of motion when the participant tries to increase the speed of the exercise. The participant should open the fan blades on the paddles or replace the multiplane drag equipment with a smaller size or perform the exercise without equipment.

The movement should be performed smoothly, with equal force in both directions, at the participant's full range of motion. After every set allow 30 to 60 seconds to rest and encourage participants to relax their shoulders and stretch their fingers.

TABLE 1.6

Muscle Actions With Buoyant Equipment in Shallow Water

Motion	Muscle action	Note
Chest press (push)	Concentric pectoralis major, serratus anterior, anterior deltoid, and triceps	Lunge position, lean forward 45 degrees
Chest press (pull)	Eccentric pectoralis major, serratus anterior, anterior deltoid, and triceps	Lunge position, lean forward 45 degrees
Standing row	Isometric latissimus dorsi and lower trapezius, concentric middle trapezius, and rhomboids	Drag forces used
Shoulder flexion	Eccentric latissimus dorsi and triceps	
Shoulder extension or hyperextension	Concentric latissimus dorsi and triceps	
Shoulder abduction	Eccentric latissimus dorsi and pectoralis major	
Shoulder adduction	Concentric latissimus dorsi and pectoralis major	
Shoulder horizontal abduction	Eccentric pectoralis major and anterior deltoid	Lunge position, lean forward 45 degrees
Shoulder horizontal adduction	Concentric pectoralis major and anterior deltoid	Lunge position, lean forward 45 degrees
Shoulder lateral rotation	Isometric latissimus dorsi and lower trapezius, concentric rotator cuff	Drag forces used
Shoulder medial rotation	Isometric latissimus dorsi and lower trapezius, concentric rotator cuff	Drag forces used
Elbow flexion	Eccentric triceps	
Elbow extension	Concentric triceps	
Hip flexion	Eccentric gluteus maximus and hamstrings	Foot on a noodle
Hip extension	Concentric gluteus maximus and hamstrings	Foot on a noodle
Standing leg press (down)	Concentric gluteus maximus, hamstrings, and quadriceps	Foot on a noodle
Standing leg press (return)	Eccentric gluteus maximus, hamstrings, and quadriceps	Foot on a noodle
Hip abduction or standing leg press to side	Eccentric adductors	Foot on a noodle
Hip adduction or standing leg press to side	Concentric adductors	Foot on a noodle
Squat (down)	Eccentric hamstrings, gluteus maximus, quadriceps, and gastrocnemius	Buoyant equipment in hands
Squat (return)	Concentric hamstrings, gluteus maximus, quadriceps, and gastrocnemius	Buoyant equipment in hands

(continued)

TABLE 1.6 *(continued)*

Motion	Muscle action	Note
Lunge (down)	Eccentric hamstrings, gluteus maximus, quadriceps, and gastrocnemius	Buoyant equipment in hands
Lunge (return)	Concentric hamstrings, gluteus maximus, quadriceps, and gastrocnemius	Buoyant equipment in hands
Plantar flexion, calf raise	Eccentric tibialis anterior	Buoyant equipment in hands
Dorsiflexion	Concentric tibialis anterior	

Adapted from Aquatic Exercise Association, 2018, *Aquatic fitness professional manual,* 7th ed. (Champaign, IL: Human Kinetics), 86-87.

Both regular rubberized equipment and chlorine-resistant rubberized equipment will last longer if it is rinsed in fresh water after each use.

The band needs to be anchored to something, such as the nonworking arm, the leg or foot, a partner, or something attached to the pool such as a ladder. Stepping on a band or attaching a loop around the legs in the pool may be difficult for some participants. Attaching multiple bands to a single ladder is impractical in a class setting. Instructors must take into consideration their participants' abilities when designing a class using rubberized equipment.

The muscle being worked depends on the location of the anchor. The muscular contraction is concentric away from the anchor point and eccentric toward the anchor point. Position the body so that it is stabilized with the spine in neutral before beginning the exercise. Table 1.8 shows the muscle contractions with rubberized equipment.

Aquatic Steps   When you stand on an aquatic step, a larger percentage of your body is out of the water, so the effects of buoyancy are reduced and the effects of gravity are greater. The load on the legs increases because they must support a higher percentage of body weight. Squats and lunges can go deeper than they do for the same exercises performed on the pool floor. Hopping onto the step and back down to the floor, as when performing jumping jacks with the feet together in the center of the step and apart on the floor on either side of the step, overloads the leg muscles effectively. Be sure to use aquatic steps rather than regular steps. Aquatic steps have rubber on the bottom to reduce sliding around on the pool floor.

Strength Reps and Sets

Perform 8 to 10 exercises for the major muscle groups in a strength-training session. Aim for two or three sets of 8 to 15 repetitions of each exercise. Cue to relax the shoulders and the grip after each set with equipment. As when using the properties of water for strength training, if you use music while using equipment, choose something that is 134 beats per minute or slower (Yazigi, 2011). Exercisers will not be able to move the equipment through their full range of motion and keep up with music that is too fast.

Flexibility

Be sure to end all of your transition season classes with at least five minutes of stretching, focusing on the major muscles used during the class.

Transition Season Lesson Plans

Three sessions per week of 20 to 60 minutes of vigorous-intensity exercise meets the American College of Sports Medicine guidelines for cardiorespiratory exercise (ACSM, 2017b). By increasing the intensity of the interval sessions in the periodization program,

TABLE 1.7

Muscle Actions With Drag Equipment in Shallow Water

Motion	Muscle action
Chest press	Concentric pectoralis major, serratus anterior, anterior deltoids, and triceps
Standing row	Concentric trapezius and rhomboids
Shoulder flexion	Concentric anterior deltoid, pectoralis major, and biceps
Shoulder extension or hyperextension	Concentric latissimus dorsi and triceps
Shoulder abduction	Concentric middle deltoid
Shoulder adduction	Concentric latissimus dorsi and pectoralis major
Shoulder horizontal abduction	Concentric posterior deltoid
Shoulder horizontal adduction	Concentric pectoralis major and anterior deltoid
Shoulder lateral rotation	Concentric rotator cuff
Shoulder medial rotation	Concentric latissimus dorsi and rotator cuff
Elbow flexion	Concentric biceps
Elbow extension	Concentric triceps
Trunk rotation	Concentric obliques
Squat (down)	Eccentric hamstrings, gluteus maximus, quadriceps, and gastrocnemius
Squat (return)	Concentric hamstrings, gluteus maximus, quadriceps, and gastrocnemius
Lunge (down)	Eccentric hamstrings, gluteus maximus, quadriceps, and gastrocnemius
Lunge (return)	Concentric hamstrings, gluteus maximus, quadriceps, and gastrocnemius
Plantar flexion	Concentric gastrocnemius and soleus
Dorsiflexion	Concentric tibialis

Adapted from Aquatic Exercise Association, 2018, *Aquatic fitness professional manual*, 7th ed. (Champaign, IL: Human Kinetics), 86-87.

your class comes closer to meeting these guidelines, but unless your class meets five days a week, you will not be able to meet all the requirements for cardiorespiratory fitness, strength, and flexibility in class.

Encourage your participants to get additional exercise on the days that the class does not meet. A schedule might look like the following:

TWO ONE-HOUR CLASSES A WEEK

1. 5 minutes warm-up, 30 minutes cardiorespiratory training, 20 minutes strength training *or* 50 minutes of strength training, 5 minutes stretching

2. 5 minutes warm-up, 50 minutes cardiorespiratory training with intervals (HIIT every other week), 5 minutes stretching

TABLE 1.8

Muscle Actions With Rubberized Equipment in Shallow Water

Motion	Muscle action	Note
Chest press (push)	Concentric pectoralis major, serratus anterior, anterior deltoids, and triceps	Band wrapped around back
Chest press (return)	Eccentric pectoralis major, serratus anterior, anterior deltoids, and triceps	
Standing row (pull)	Concentric trapezius and rhomboids	Anchor in front
Standing row (return)	Eccentric trapezius and rhomboids	
Shoulder flexion	Concentric anterior deltoid, pectoralis major, and biceps	Anchor in back
Shoulder extension	Eccentric anterior deltoid, pectoralis major, and biceps	
Shoulder flexion	Eccentric latissimus dorsi and triceps	Anchor in front
Shoulder extension	Concentric latissimus dorsi and triceps	
Shoulder abduction	Eccentric latissimus dorsi and pectoralis major	High anchor
Shoulder adduction	Concentric latissimus dorsi and pectoralis major	
Shoulder abduction	Concentric middle deltoid	Low anchor
Shoulder adduction	Eccentric middle deltoid	
Shoulder horizontal abduction	Eccentric pectoralis major and anterior deltoid	Anchor in back
Shoulder horizontal adduction	Concentric pectoralis major and anterior deltoid	
Shoulder horizontal abduction	Concentric posterior deltoid	Anchor in front
Shoulder horizontal adduction	Eccentric posterior deltoid	
Shoulder lateral rotation	Concentric rotator cuff	Pull band apart, elbows anchored at waist
Shoulder medial rotation	Eccentric rotator cuff	
Elbow flexion	Eccentric triceps	High anchor
Elbow extension	Concentric triceps	
Elbow flexion	Concentric biceps	Low anchor
Elbow extension	Eccentric biceps	
Trunk lateral flexion	Concentric or eccentric obliques	Low anchor
Hip flexion	Concentric iliopsoas	Anchor in back
Hip extension	Eccentric iliopsoas	
Hip flexion	Eccentric gluteus maximus and hamstrings	Anchor in front
Hip extension	Concentric gluteus maximus and hamstrings	
Hip abduction	Concentric gluteus medius	Medial anchor
Hip adduction	Eccentric gluteus medius	

Motion	Muscle action	Note
Hip abduction	Eccentric adductors	Lateral anchor
Hip adduction	Concentric adductors	
Horizontal hip abduction	Concentric tensor fasciae latae	Loop around thighs
Horizontal hip adduction	Eccentric tensor fasciae latae	
Knee flexion	Eccentric quadriceps	Anchor in back
Knee extension	Concentric quadriceps	
Knee flexion	Concentric hamstrings	Anchor in front
Knee extension	Eccentric hamstrings	
Plantar flexion	Concentric gastrocnemius and soleus	Foot on band
Dorsiflexion	Eccentric gastrocnemius and soleus	

Adapted from Aquatic Exercise Association, 2018, *Aquatic fitness professional manual,* 7th ed. (Champaign, IL: Human Kinetics), 87.

THREE ONE-HOUR CLASSES A WEEK

1. 5 minutes warm-up, 50 minutes cardiorespiratory training, 5 minutes stretching
2. 5 minutes warm-up, 50 minutes strength training, 5 minutes stretching
3. 5 minutes warm-up, 50 minutes cardiorespiratory training with intervals (HIIT every other week), 5 minutes stretching

FIVE ONE-HOUR CLASSES A WEEK

1. 5 minutes warm-up, 50 minutes cardiorespiratory training with intervals, 5 minutes stretching
2. 5 minutes warm-up, 50 minutes strength training, 5 minutes stretching
3. 5 minutes warm-up, 50 minutes cardiorespiratory training, 5 minutes stretching
4. 5 minutes warm-up, 50 minutes strength training, 5 minutes stretching
5. 5 minutes warm-up, 50 minutes cardiorespiratory training with intervals (HIIT every other week), 5 minutes stretching

PEAK FITNESS SEASON

At last, you have arrived at the season for peak fitness. The preseason and the transition season have prepared your participants for the highest level of fitness that they will achieve this year. Peak fitness can be maintained for a few months, but it cannot be sustained indefinitely before the body will need to rest. Peak fitness will be different for everyone. But your participants should notice that the exercises seem easier even though they are performing more repetitions. Compliment them on their good posture and ability to perform the exercises correctly. Draw their attention to the improvement in the quality of their moves, because they are now better able to push and pull and drag the water with them while maintaining a braced core. The focus of this season is to increase their power to go beyond the intensity levels they achieved in the previous season, including short periods in their anaerobic zone. Your classes will consist of cardiorespiratory training, HIIT, and strength training with equipment using concentric and eccentric muscle actions but focusing on the eccentric actions.

Cardiorespiratory Fitness

Your participants should now be able to do continuous cardiorespiratory training at 60 percent of maximum effort for 30 minutes without tiring. They may have noticed that as long as they maintain neutral posture, they can safely increase the intensity of their arm and leg movements. They may have to work a little harder to achieve a moderate level of effort. Now is the time for them to lengthen their stride and add more power to their movements. Ask them to increase their exertion from 60 percent to 70 percent of maximum. They should be working somewhat hard during their sessions of continuous cardiorespiratory training.

Now that a base fitness level has been established, interval-training intensities can increase from 70 percent of maximum effort to 80 percent (hard). Your participants may also be ready to cross the anaerobic threshold regularly, so you will include more frequent cycles in which they work at 90 percent of maximum effort (very hard). To work at this level, you will need to employ additional strategies for increasing intensity. Instead of using one intensity variable, use two, such as full range of motion with power, speed with power, or power with travel.

Another strategy is to work in two planes at the same time. You can do this by alternating one move in the frontal plane, such as a frog jump, with another move in the sagittal plane, such as tuck ski. A second way to work in two planes is to combine a leg move in one plane with an arm move in a different plane. Examples include kick side to side (frontal plane) with arms sweeping side to side (transverse plane), cross-country ski (sagittal plane) with rotation, hands together (transverse plane), and high kick (sagittal plane) clap over (transverse plane) and under (frontal plane). You will no longer intersperse cycles of interval training between periods of cardiorespiratory training. You will instead perform all your interval cycles together.

All of your intervals during peak fitness are HIIT, but not all HIIT intervals are anaerobic. Rolling intervals, surges, random intervals, and Tabata Type intervals include sets in which you ask your participants to work at 90 percent of maximum effort for periods of 15 seconds up to 1 minute. Remember that 90 percent of maximum effort is different for everyone and that some may not be able to achieve that level of effort for 1 minute or even 15 seconds. Encourage all participants to modify the intensity of the work intervals to their preferred challenging level and focus on their own optimal training.

The following are options for interval training during peak fitness (Thielen, 2015):

INTERVAL 30

30 seconds of work to 30 seconds of recovery (1:1 ratio), 10 to 12 sets

INTERVAL 40

40 seconds of work to 40 seconds of recovery (1:1 ratio), 10 to 12 sets

INTERVAL 60

60 seconds of work to 60 seconds of recovery (1:1 ratio), 10 to 12 sets

REDUCED RECOVERY TIME

3 minutes of work to 90 seconds of recovery (2:1 ratio), 2 to 3 sets

ROLLING INTERVALS

1 minute at 70 percent, 1 minute at 80 percent, and 1 minute at 90 percent of maximum effort, 3 to 5 sets

SURGES

45 seconds at 80 percent, 15 seconds at 90 percent of maximum effort, and 1 minute of recovery (1:1 ratio), 4 to 8 sets

RANDOM INTERVALS

30 seconds at 60 percent of maximum effort, 30 seconds at 70 percent, 30 seconds at 80 percent, and 30 seconds at 90 percent to 1 minute of recovery (rolling interval)

15 seconds at 60 percent of maximum effort, 15 seconds at 70 percent, 15 seconds at 80 percent, and 15 seconds at 90 percent to 1 minute of recovery (rolling interval)

30 seconds of work to 30 seconds of recovery, 4 sets

20 seconds of work to 10 seconds of recovery, 8 sets (Tabata)

1 cycle

PYRAMID

15 seconds of work to 15 seconds of recovery

20 seconds of work to 15 seconds of recovery

25 seconds of work to 15 seconds of recovery

30 seconds of work to 15 seconds of recovery

1 or more cycles

TABATA TYPE

20 seconds of work at 90 percent of maximum effort to 10 seconds of recovery (2:1 ratio)

8 sets, 1 or more cycles

Muscular Strength and Endurance

In the transition season, equipment was added to the program. Strength training without equipment involves only concentric contractions. Drag equipment involves a minor amount of eccentric action. Buoyant and rubberized equipment involve both concentric and eccentric muscle actions. Gains in strength are possible with concentric contractions alone. Eccentric actions can also be used to improve strength, and they add variety to a strength-training program. Eccentric actions may also improve muscle coordination and balance (ACSM, 2017c).

During peak fitness, you will continue to use equipment when your participants are strength training. Now, however, you will emphasize the eccentric action. For this you will choose either buoyant or rubberized equipment. When they are using buoyant equipment, ask them to dynamically press the equipment down under the water and then pause for two seconds. Participants should control the upward movement so that it takes about four seconds to return to the starting position. Watch for elevated shoulders when using buoyant equipment. This action is an indication that the participants selected equipment that is too large for them.

When they are using rubberized equipment, ask participants to pull the equipment away from the anchor point as fully as range of motion allows and then pause for two seconds. They should control the release so that it takes about four seconds to return to the anchor point. Remember to cue to relax the shoulders and the grip after each set with equipment. Be aware that delayed onset muscle soreness is common 24 to 48 hours after eccentric exercise, so begin slowly. Start with eight repetitions of each exercise and gradually increase the number of repetitions over time.

During the transition season, you aimed for two or three sets of 8 to 15 repetitions of each exercise. During peak fitness you will aim for three sets. You have several options for performing the three sets and incorporating eccentric actions.

1. Perform the first set without equipment. Perform the second set with buoyant or rubberized equipment without emphasizing the eccentric actions. Perform the third set with the pause and slow return.
2. Perform one set without equipment. Perform the second set with drag equipment. Perform the third set with buoyant or rubberized equipment using the pause and slow return.
3. Perform two sets with buoyant or rubberized equipment without emphasizing the eccentric action. Perform the third set with the pause and slow return.
4. Perform one set without equipment. Then perform two sets with buoyant or rubberized equipment using the pause and slow return.
5. Perform one set with buoyant or rubberized equipment without emphasizing the eccentric action. Then perform two sets using the pause and slow return.

If you use music with your strength-training sessions, choose something that is 134 beats per minute or slower (Yazigi, 2011). Exercisers will not be able to move the equipment through their full range of motion and keep up with music that is faster than 134 beats per minute.

Flexibility

Be sure to end all of your peak fitness classes with at least five minutes of stretching, focusing on the major muscles used during the class.

Peak Fitness Season Lesson Plans

Three sessions per week of 20 to 60 minutes of vigorous-intensity exercise meets the American College of Sports Medicine guidelines for cardiorespiratory exercise (ACSM, 2017b). By including HIIT, your class comes closer to meeting these guidelines, but unless your class meets five days a week, you will not be able to meet all the requirements for cardiorespiratory fitness, strength, and flexibility in class. Encourage your participants to get additional exercise on the days that the class does not meet. A schedule might look like the following:

TWO ONE-HOUR CLASSES A WEEK

1. 5 minutes warm-up, 30 minutes cardiorespiratory training, 20 minutes strength training *or* 50 minutes strength training, 5 minutes stretching
2. 5 minutes warm-up, 50 minutes cardiorespiratory training with HIIT, 5 minutes stretching

THREE ONE-HOUR CLASSES A WEEK

1. 5 minutes warm-up, 50 minutes cardiorespiratory training with HIIT, 5 minutes stretching
2. 5 minutes warm-up, 50 minutes strength training, 5 minutes stretching
3. 5 minutes warm-up, 50 minutes cardiorespiratory training with HIIT, 5 minutes stretching

FIVE ONE-HOUR CLASSES A WEEK

1. 5 minutes warm-up, 50 minutes cardiorespiratory training with HIIT, 5 minutes stretching
2. 5 minutes warm-up, 50 minutes strength training, 5 minutes stretching
3. 5 minutes warm-up, 50 minutes cardiorespiratory training with HIIT, 5 minutes stretching
4. 5 minutes warm-up, 50 minutes strength training, 5 minutes stretching
5. 5 minutes warm-up, 50 minutes cardiorespiratory training with HIIT, 5 minutes stretching

ACTIVE RECOVERY SEASON

Your participants have worked hard for most of the year. Now it is time to rest. Their muscles may have suffered from microtrauma caused by the months of continuous training. Their bodies need time to repair so that the microtrauma does not lead to a cumulative injury. They also need to rest to restore their energy reserves. But you do not have to cancel class. Fitness will continue as long as some training continues, so this period is called the active recovery season. Classes consist of low-intensity continuous cardiorespiratory training, core strength training including balance exercises and Pilates, and fun activities such as partner classes, dance moves, modified synchronized swimming, games, and relay races. Be sure to stretch at the end of every class.

Active Recovery Season Lesson Plans

A schedule might look like the following:

TWO ONE-HOUR CLASSES A WEEK

1. 5 minutes warm-up, 30 minutes light cardiorespiratory training, 20 minutes core strength training, 5 minutes stretching
2. 5 minutes warm-up, 30 minutes light cardiorespiratory training, 20 minutes fun activities, 5 minutes stretching

THREE ONE-HOUR CLASSES A WEEK

1. 5 minutes warm-up, 30 minutes light cardiorespiratory training, 20 minutes core strength training, 5 minutes stretching
2. 5 minutes warm-up, 50 minutes core strength training, 5 minutes stretching
3. 5 minutes warm-up, 30 minutes light cardiorespiratory training, 20 minutes fun activities, 5 minutes stretching

FIVE ONE-HOUR CLASSES A WEEK

1. 5 minutes warm-up, 30 minutes light cardiorespiratory training, 20 minutes fun activities, 5 minutes stretching
2. 5 minutes warm-up, 50 minutes core strength training, 5 minutes stretching
3. 5 minutes warm-up, 50 minutes light cardiorespiratory training, 5 minutes stretching
4. 5 minutes warm-up, 30 minutes light cardiorespiratory training, 20 minutes fun activities, 5 minutes stretching
5. 5 minutes warm-up, 50 minutes core strength training, 5 minutes stretching

References

ACSM. (2017a). *High intensity interval training.* Retrieved from www.acsm.org/docs/brochures/high-intensity-interval-training.pdf

ACSM. (2017b). Quantity and quality of exercise for developing and maintaining cardiorespiratory, musculoskeletal, and neuromotor fitness in apparently healthy adults: Guidance for prescribing exercise. *Medicine & Science in Sports & Exercise 43*(7). Retrieved from http://journals.lww.com/acsm-msse/Fulltext/2011/07000/Quantity_and_Quality_of_Exercise_for_Developing.26.aspx

ACSM. (2017c). *Resistance training for health and fitness.* Retrieved from www.acsm.org/docs/brochures/resistance-training.pdf

AEA. (2010). *Aquatic fitness professional manual, sixth edition.* Champaign, IL; Human Kinetics.

AEA. (2018). *Aquatic fitness professional manual, seventh edition.* Champaign, IL; Human Kinetics.

Ivens, P., & Holder, C. (2011). *Do no harm.* Retrieved from www.aquaaerobics.com

Thielen, Se. (2015, March 21). *Intelligent intervals for the deep.* Presented at Metroplex Association of Aquatic Professionals Continuing Education Training, Plano, TX.

Yazigi, F. (2011, May 11). *Aquatic research review.* International Aquatic Fitness Conference, Orlando, FL.

CHAPTER 2

Shallow-Water Exercises and Cues

This chapter is a list of exercises used in the shallow-water lesson plans in chapter 3. The list includes the basic cardiorespiratory exercises of walk, squats and lunges, jog, kick, rocking horse, cross-country ski, and jumping jacks with multiple variations of each basic exercise. Wall exercises round out the cardio exercises. Following these are strength exercises for the upper body, abdominals, obliques, and lower body. Finally is a list of balance exercises. Cues or descriptions of the exercise are included for those exercises that may need additional explanation. These exercises can be used to create new classes for cardiorespiratory fitness or strength training. Choose variations that use a full range of motion, speed, the suspended working position, or acceleration and power when higher intensity is desired. Travel will also increase the intensity. Add equipment with the strength exercises to increase the resistance.

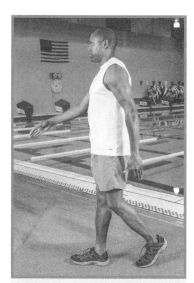

FIGURE 2.1 Walk forward.

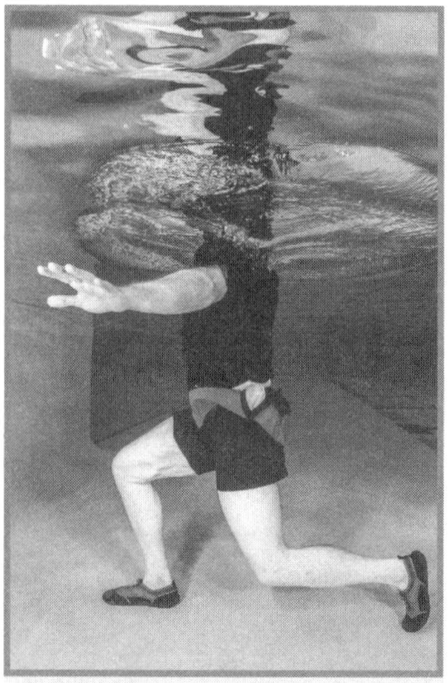

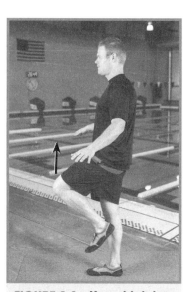

FIGURE 2.2 Lunge.

CARDIORESPIRATORY EXERCISES

1. WALK

Walk forward—walk upright with good posture (see figure 2.1)

Walk forward, big steps

Step forward with R foot first

Step forward with L foot first

Walk backward

Walk backward, big steps

Walk on toes

Walk on heels

Walk on a tightrope

Crossover step—step across the midline

Crossover step 3× and half turn

Step sideways

Crab walk sideways—lunge to the side like a crab walking sideways

2. SQUATS AND LUNGES

Squat—keep heels on the floor

Squat on one foot

Squat and jump

Squat and power leg—squat and lift one knee as you return to standing; extend that knee and power press it down, transitioning into the next squat

Lunge (see figure 2.2)

Knee lift and lunge

Kick and lunge

Lunge walk

3. JOG

Knee-high jog—bring the knee up to hip level and land toe-ball-heel (see figure 2.3)

Knee-high jog, faster

Run—use a long stride

Sprint—run at top speed

Power run—pull the water forcefully with cupped hands

Run 3× and hurdle

Steep climb—like climbing a ladder out of the pool

Steep climb, faster

Steep climb with power

Leap—lift one leg and leap forward

Jump backward—feet push off the floor traveling backward, tuck, and land

Log jump forward and back—feet are together; hop forward and back

FIGURE 2.3 Knee-high jog.

Log jump side to side—feet are together; hop side to side

Knee-high jog with toes in

Knee-high jog with toes out

Knee lift, doubles—lift each knee 2×

Knee-high jog 3× and hold

Knee-high jog, syncopate—slow, slow, quick, quick, quick

Knee-high jog, neutral position

Hip curl, suspended—pull both knees toward chest and push out

Crossover knees—knees cross the midline

Straddle jog—hips are open, but feet are close together (see figure 2.4)

Frog jump

Frog jump with hands up

Frog jump, neutral position

Frog, suspended—frog jump without landing on the floor

Run tires—hips are open and feet are wide apart, like running through tires at football practice

Run tires, faster

In, in, out, out—alternate feet in and out

Inner-thigh lift or ankle touch—bring the inner thigh toward the opposite hand

Inner-thigh lift, full ROM

Inner-thigh lift, faster

Inner-thigh lift with power

Inner-thigh lift with double arms—extend both arms to one side and then touch the opposite inner thigh with both hands

Inner-thigh lift and squat

Inner-thigh lift, one side

Inner-thigh lift, doubles—inner-thigh lift toward opposite hand 2× on each side

Hopscotch—touch the heel in back with the opposite hand; if you can't reach the heel, just aim for it

Hopscotch, full ROM

Hopscotch, faster

Hopscotch with power

Hopscotch, one side

Hopscotch, doubles—touch heel 2× on each side

Heel jog—keep knees under hips and curl the hamstrings (see figure 2.5)

Skip rope—heel up and kick forward, as if skipping a rope

Skateboard—stand with one foot as if on a skateboard and pedal with the other foot

Skateboard jump—lunge, jump up, lunge

Heel jog 3× and hold

Hitchhike—lean side to side, lifting heels and signaling hitchhike with thumbs

Bicycle, suspended

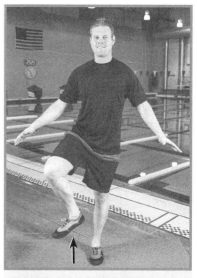

FIGURE 2.4 **Straddle jog.**

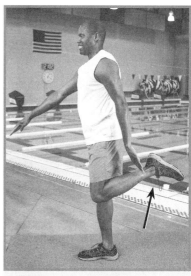

FIGURE 2.5 **Heel jog.**

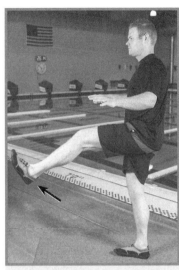

FIGURE 2.6 **Kick forward.**

Bicycle, full ROM, suspended—large circles

Bicycle, faster, suspended

Bicycle with power, suspended

4. KICK

Kick forward—keep knees soft (see figure 2.6)

Kick forward, faster

Front kick (karate)—lift the knee and kick forward through the heel

Front kick (karate), faster

Knee lift, straighten, and power press-down

High kick

High kick and return—bring the foot to center before beginning the next kick

High kick, power down

High kick with power

High kick, clap over and under—clap the hands over the leg and then under the leg

Kick forward, doubles—kick 2× with each leg

Kick forward, doubles, one low and one high

Chorus line kick—knee, down, kick, down

Kick and squat

Kick forward, neutral position

Kick forward, faster, neutral position

One leg kicks forward, neutral position

Kick forward, suspended

Hold one leg up; other leg kicks forward, suspended

Hold one leg up; other leg kicks forward 3× suspended and down

Mermaid, suspended—like pumping a swing, suspended

Flutter kick, suspended—flutter kick from the hips, not the knees

Crossover kick—kick across the midline

Crossover kick, doubles—kick across the midline 2× with each leg

Crossover kick, doubles, one low and one high

Crossover kick and sweep out—kick across the midline and then sweep the foot out to the side

Skate kick, crossover kick, sweep out, and center—kick back, kick across the midline, and then sweep the foot out to the side

Crossover kick and sweep out, doubles—kick across the midline and then sweep the foot out to the side 2× with each leg

Crossover kick, neutral position

Crossover kick and sweep out, neutral position

One leg sweeps out and in, neutral position

Kick forward 3×, crossover kick 1×, neutral position

Kick forward 3× and hold; one leg sweeps out and in 1×, neutral position

Hold one leg up; other leg kicks forward and sweeps out, suspended

Kick to the corners

Kick side to side—feet return to center after each kick to the side (see figure 2.7)

Kick side to side, arms and legs opposite

Kick side to side, faster

Kick side to side; arms sweep side to side

Kick side to side with power, grounded—add power to the adduction phase of the kick

Kick side to side, doubles—kick 2× with each leg

Side kick (karate)—lift the knee and kick to the side through the heel

Side kick (karate) one side—leg stays up

Side kick (karate), faster

Skate kick—kick backward with the leg straight; lean forward slightly to avoid arching the back (see figure 2.8)

Skate kick, full ROM

Skate kick, faster

Skate kick and return—bring the foot to center before beginning the next kick

Skate kick with power

In-line skate—keep the feet wide and step behind the opposite foot with alternating legs

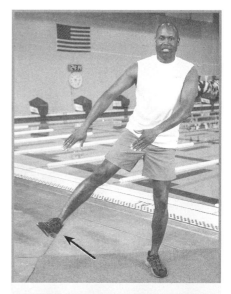

FIGURE 2.7 **Kick side to side.**

5. ROCKING HORSE

Rocking horse—rock from the front foot to the back foot; avoid arching the back (see figure 2.9)

Rocking horse to the side—hips are open; rock from side to side, knee up on one side and heel up on the other

Rocking horse 3× and hold

Rocking horse with a front kick—add a quad kick when you lift the knee in front

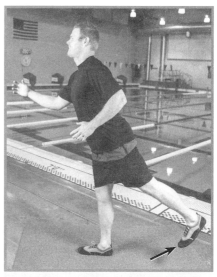

FIGURE 2.8 **Skate kick.**

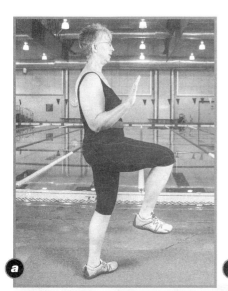 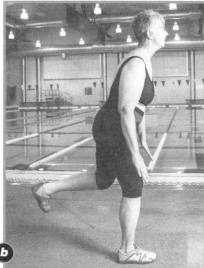

FIGURE 2.9 **Rocking horse: (*a*) start and (*b*) finish.**

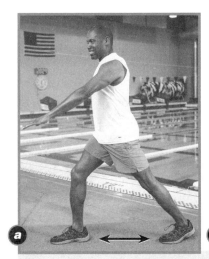 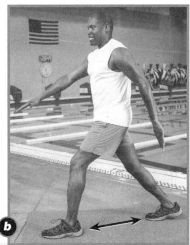

FIGURE 2.10 Cross-country ski: (*a*) start and (*b*) finish.

6. CROSS-COUNTRY SKI

Cross-country ski—start in a lunge position and then switch legs (see figure 2.10)

Cross-country ski, full ROM

Cross-country ski with rotation—the arm reaches across the midline

Cross-country ski with rotation, hands together

Mini ski—short range of motion

Mini ski, faster

Cross-country ski, faster

Cross-country ski with power

Cross-country ski; arms sweep side to side

Cross-country ski, slow

Cross-country ski with feet wide

Cross-country ski 3× and hold

Cross-country ski 3× and bounce center

Cross-country ski single, single, double

Cross-country ski, doubles—bounce on each side 2×

Cross-country ski 3-1/2× and half turn—ski R, L, R, L, R, L, R, and half turn

Tuck ski

Tuck ski, neutral position

Tuck ski with rotation—the arm reaches across the midline

Cross-country ski, tuck, diagonal turn and center—cross-country ski, tuck, hold the tuck, and turn 45 degrees toward a corner, return to center

Cross-country ski, neutral position

Cross-country ski, full ROM, neutral position

Cross-country ski with power, neutral position

Cross-country ski, pause in center on toes, neutral position

Cross-country ski, suspended—make sure the legs go backward as well as forward

Cross-country ski, faster, suspended

Cross-country ski 3×, suspended and touch center

7. JUMPING JACKS

Jumping jacks—keep the arms underwater (see figure 2.11)

Mini jacks—short range of motion

Mini jacks, faster

Jumping jacks, faster

Jumping jacks, land feet out only

Jumping jacks with arms out of the water

Mini cross—using short range of motion, cross the ankles

Jacks cross—begin with the feet apart and then cross the thighs

Jacks cross, faster

Jacks cross with power, grounded—lift leg side, cross front, lift side and down, and repeat other side

Jacks cross, R leg in front

Jacks cross, L leg in front

Jacks cross 3-1/2× and half turn—cross, out, cross, out, cross, out, cross, and half turn

Jumping jacks with diagonal turn—turn 45 degrees toward a corner when the feet come apart, feet come together in the center, turn 45 degrees to the opposite corner when the feet come apart again

Jumping jacks with toes in

Jumping jacks with toes out

Jumping jacks, syncopate—slow, slow, quick, quick, quick

Jumping jacks, doubles—bounce out 2× and in 2×

Jumping jacks squat—squat as the feet come apart

Jacks tuck

Jacks tuck, neutral position

Jumping jacks, neutral position

Jumping jacks with power, neutral position—arms sweep out and in; add power to both abduction and adduction

Jumping jacks, heels out and toes in center, neutral position

Jumping jacks, suspended

Jumping jacks, faster, suspended

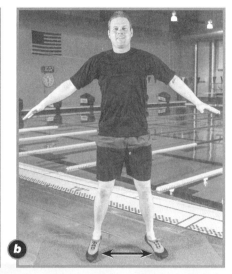

FIGURE 2.11　**Jumping jacks: (*a*) start and (*b*) finish.**

8. WALL EXERCISES

Wall push-ups

Climb the wall, one foot on the wall and one on the floor—right foot on the wall and left foot on the floor, then switch to left foot on the wall and right foot on the floor

Climb the wall, both feet on the wall and down to the floor—right and left feet on the wall, hop down to the floor with both feet

Push off the wall with both feet (see figure 2.12) and run back

Push off the wall with one foot (see figure 2.13), tuck, and breaststroke back

Jump back, jump forward, jump on the wall, and jump down

Jump and jump tuck, hands on the wall

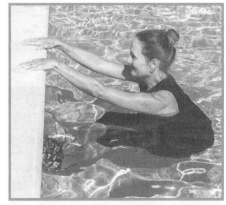

FIGURE 2.12　**Push off the wall with both feet.**

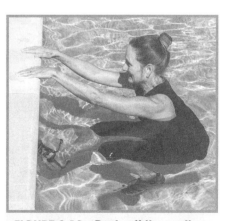

FIGURE 2.13　**Push off the wall with one foot.**

STRENGTH EXERCISES

9. UPPER BODY

Scapula adduction

Standing row

Seated row—on a noodle

Kayak row—paddle with both hands, alternate right and left sides

Crawl stroke (see figure 2.14)

Bowstring pull—hold the bow in front with one hand and pull the bowstring with the other hand

Bowstring pull to the side—hold the bow to the side with one hand and pull the bowstring with the other hand

Shoulder blade squeeze

Shoulder flexion and extension

Double-arm lift

Arm swing

Unison arm swing

Double-arm press-down (see figure 2.15)

Pumping arms

Shoulder abduction and adduction

Arm lift to sides

Arm lift to sides with elbows bent

Lat pull-down (see figure 2.16)

Lat pull-down with elbows bent

Arms cross in front and in back

Palms touch in front and in back

Palms touch in back

Windshield wiper arms—swing the arms side to side in front of the thighs

Shoulder horizontal abduction and adduction

Clap hands

Shoulder sweep, out or in (see figure 2.17)

Arms sweep side to side

Breaststroke—do the breaststroke with thumbs up to protect the shoulders

Reverse breaststroke

Chest fly—with equipment

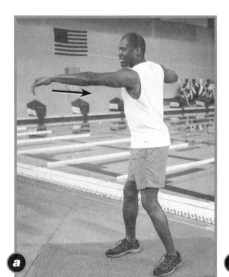
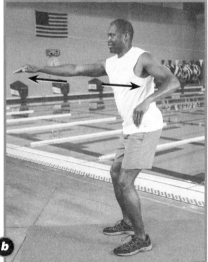

FIGURE 2.14   **Crawl stroke: (*a*) start and (*b*) finish.**

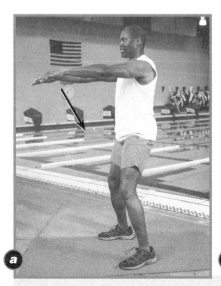
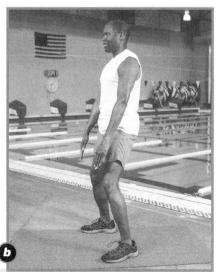

FIGURE 2.15   **Double-arm press-down: (*a*) start and (*b*) finish.**

Chest press—push forward with the hands shoulder-distance apart

Crossovers—hands cross at chest level

Shoulder lateral rotation

Forearm press (see figure 2.18)

Forearm press side to side

Resistor arms

Elbow flexion and extension

Arm curl

Triceps extension

Triceps kick back—with elbows back, press back

Push forward—push forward with the hands in front of the chest

Unison push forward

Push across—push across the midline

Reach side to side—reach arms to side and then curl alternating arms toward the armpit

Open and close doors—arm curl with shoulders abducted (see figure 2.19)

Side arm curl—one-arm curls with shoulder abducted

Elbow sweep—one-arm triceps extension with shoulder abducted

Jog press—press alternating hands down at the sides

Unison jog press

Punch forward and side

Punch down

Punch across

Other arm and hand movements

Jab—punch forward

Cross—punch across the midline

Hook—curving punch toward the midline

Upper cut—upward punch

Tennis backhand

Tennis forehand

Baseball swing

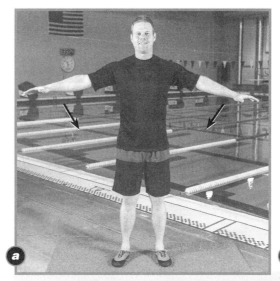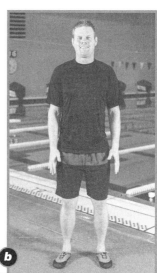

FIGURE 2.16 Lat pull-down: (*a*) start and (*b*) finish.

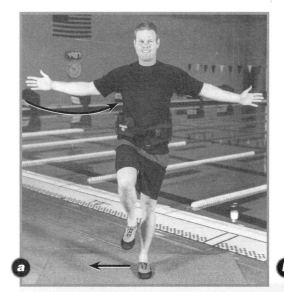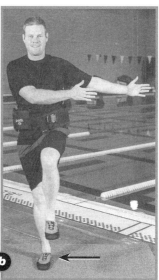

FIGURE 2.17 Shoulder sweep in: (*a*) start and (*b*) finish.

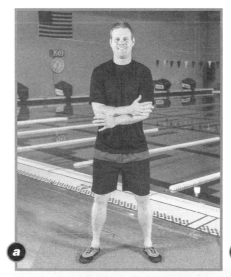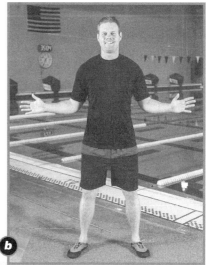

FIGURE 2.18 Forearm press: (*a*) start and (*b*) finish.

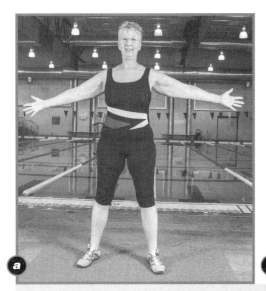 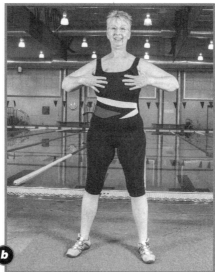

FIGURE 2.19 Open and close doors: (a) start and (b) finish.

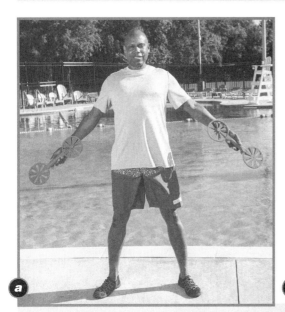 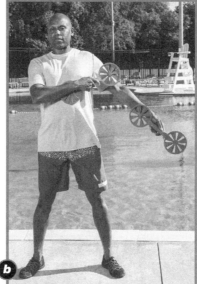

FIGURE 2.20 Bring arm across to opposite shoulder: (a) start and (b) finish.

Golf swing

Bring one arm across to opposite shoulder—start with arms down at sides (see figure 2.20)

Bring one arm down to opposite hip—start with arms to sides 70 degrees

Stir the soup

Paddlewheel

Hand waves—hands are just above the surface of the water

Pronate and supinate—palms up, palms down

Finger flicks—bend and straighten the fingers

Circle thumbs

Scull—sweep in with the thumbs slightly up and sweep out with the thumbs slightly down

Propeller scull—make figure eights with the hands in front of the body to travel backward or the hands down at the sides to travel forward

10. ABDOMINALS

Brace core, arms down, turbulent hand movements

Pelvic tilt

Tuck, mermaid, tuck, down and tuck, unison kick to the corners, tuck, down

Pike—extend legs in an L position; keep the knees together, suspended or noodle in posterior sling

Crunch, V position—bring chest toward the knees, noodle in posterior sling

Pull one knee toward chest, lift and lower other leg—noodle in posterior sling

Flex one foot and lower, point it, and lift—noodle in posterior sling

Fall forward, tuck, and stand—fall forward with the arms near the surface of the water, go into a suspended tuck position, land with the feet under the body (see figure 2.21)

Fall forward and hold position, then pull back—dumbbells on surface of water

Plank—hold noodle or dumbbells under the shoulders; the body is in a 45-degree angle with the spine in alignment

Plank scissors—one leg is hyperextended

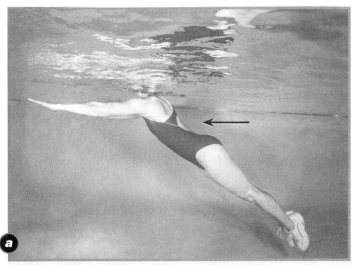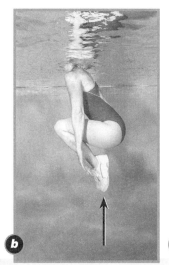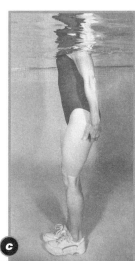

FIGURE 2.21 **Fall forward, tuck, and stand:** (*a*) **start,** (*b*) **finish,** (*c*) **stand.**

11. OBLIQUES

Lateral flexion

Hip hike—lift one hip and then the other hip

Climb a rope

Side extension—tuck and extend legs to one side, tuck and down; keep the knees together

Upper-body twist—rotate the upper body side to side

Lower body twist—rotate the lower body side to side

Pelvic circles

Hula hoop

Pull one knee toward chest, hip roll—noodle in posterior sling

Side fall, tuck, and stand—fall to the side with the arms near the surface of the water, go into a suspended tuck position, and land with the feet under the body

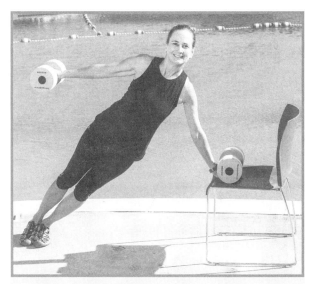

FIGURE 2.22 **Side plank.**

Side plank—hold noodle or dumbbell under one shoulder; the body is leaning in a 45-degree angle to the side with the spine in alignment (see figure 2.22)

Side plank pliers—top leg is abducted

12. LOWER BODY

Quad kick—lift the knee and kick from the knee

Side quad kick—lift the knee to the side and kick from the knee

One knee swings forward and back

Knee swing forward, back, forward, and down

Knee lift and kick back—lift the knee in front and swing it back, extending the leg

Tap heel in front and toe in back

One leg kicks forward

One leg kicks forward and back

One leg kicks side

One leg kicks side and crosses midline

One leg kicks side, crosses front, kicks side, crosses back

One leg kicks back

Hip extension

Knee lift, straighten, and power press-down

Hamstring curl—keep knees under hips and curl the hamstrings

Dog hike—hip abduction with knee flexed

Clamshells—horizontal hip abduction and adduction with knee flexed

Up on toes and down

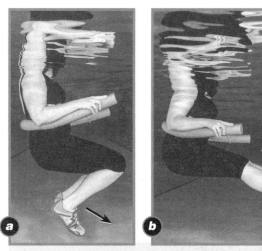

FIGURE 2.23 **Mermaid: (*a*) start and (*b*) finish.**

Jump and land toe-ball-heel

Ankle circles

Bicycle—on a noodle

Bicycle one leg only—on a noodle

Seated leg press—press the heels forward as if sitting in a leg press machine, on a noodle

Seated kick—on a noodle

Mermaid—on a noodle (see figure 2.23)

Seated flutter kick—on a noodle

Seated jacks—on a noodle

Point and flex feet—on a noodle

Hip extension—foot on a noodle

Standing leg press—foot on a noodle

Standing leg press to the side—foot on a noodle

13. BALANCE

Stand on one foot

Stand on one foot and turn head R and L

Stand on one foot, raise one arm, raise the other arm, and balance

Stand on one foot with eyes closed

Stand on one foot, raise one arm, raise the other arm, and close eyes

Yoga tree pose—stand on one foot and lift the other knee to the side with that foot on the other leg anywhere between the knee and the ankle

Hop forward and back on one foot

Lift knee, extend knee, flex knee, and lower

Warrior II—lunge to the side with arms extended side to side (see figure 2.24)

Warrior III—balance on one leg with other leg extended back, arms forward

Walk with hands on hips

Knee lift, straighten, and step

Walk three steps, pause, stand on one foot

Knee-high jog 3×, pause, stand on one foot

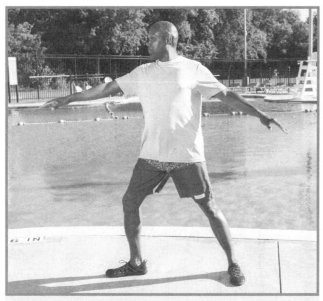

FIGURE 2.24 **Warrior II.**

CHAPTER 3

Shallow-Water Lesson Plans for Classes With a Single Objective

The following lesson plans are divided into three sections:

Section 1. The objective for the 12 lesson plans in the first section is cardiorespiratory fitness. Each lesson plan has four versions:

1. Continuous cardio
2. Preseason intervals
3. Transition season intervals
4. Peak fitness intervals

Section 2. The objective for the 15 lesson plans in the second section is strength training. Four lesson plans use the properties of water for strength training, three lessons use buoyant equipment, two lessons use drag equipment, one lesson uses rubberized equipment, two circuit classes use a variety of equipment, and three lesson plans focus on core strength. The lesson plans that use the properties of water for strength training will mainly be used in the preseason. The lesson plans that focus on eccentric muscle actions will mainly be used in the peak fitness season. The remaining lesson plans can be used during the transition season or the peak fitness season. The core strength lesson plans are especially helpful during the preseason if you have participants who need to work on their posture. Core strength is also a focus during the recovery season.

Section 3. This single lesson plan of fun partner activities is designed for the recovery season. Additional fun activities can be found in chapter 4.

SECTION 1: CARDIORESPIRATORY FITNESS

▶ Shallow-Water Cardio Lesson Plan 1

 MOVEMENT IN TWO PLANES

EQUIPMENT
None

TEACHING TIP
This lesson plan alternates sets of exercises in the sagittal plane with sets of exercises in the frontal plane. The exercises in the frontal plane begin with ankle touch or inner-thigh lift (see figure 3.1). Perform the exercise with the spine in neutral, bringing the ankle up toward the hand. If your participants tend to lean forward to reach the ankle, call the exercise an inner-thigh lift instead.

WARM-UP
Knee-high jog
Run tires
Rocking horse to R side
Kick side to side
Rocking horse to L side
Jumping jacks
Inner-thigh lift
Hopscotch
Straddle jog

A SET
R quad kick, travel sideways R
Knee-high jog with paddlewheel

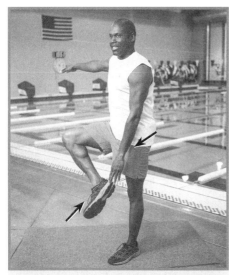

FIGURE 3.1 Ankle touch or inner-thigh lift.

L quad kick, travel sideways L
Knee-high jog with paddlewheel
Knee-high jog, travel backward
Kick forward, travel forward
Knee-high jog, travel backward
Kick forward, neutral position, travel forward
Jump backward
Knee-high jog, travel forward
Knee lift, straighten and power press-down, travel forward
Knee-high jog with breaststroke and knee-high jog, push forward, alternate
Knee-high jog, faster and knee-high jog, alternate

B SET
Inner-thigh lift
Jumping jacks
Frog jump, neutral position
Jacks tuck
Hopscotch

C SET
Cross-country ski, travel sideways R
Knee-high jog with hand waves
Cross-country ski, travel sideways L
Knee-high jog with hand waves
Knee-high jog travel backward
Cross-country ski, neutral position, travel forward
Knee-high jog, travel backward
Cross-country ski, suspended, travel forward
Cross-country ski, travel backward
Knee-high jog, travel forward
Lunge walk
Knee-high jog with standing row and knee-high jog with unison jog press, alternate
Knee-high jog, faster and knee-high jog, alternate

D SET
Inner-thigh lift
Jumping jacks
Frog jump, neutral position
Jacks tuck
Hopscotch

E SET
Rocking horse to R side, travel sideways R
Knee-high jog with finger flicks
Rocking horse to L side, travel sideways L

Knee-high jog with finger flicks

Knee-high jog, travel backward

Skip rope, travel forward

Knee-high jog, travel backward

Bicycle, suspended, travel forward

Jump backward

Knee-high jog, travel forward

Skateboard R

Skateboard L

Knee-high jog with double-arm press-down and knee-high jog with arm curl, alternate

Knee-high jog, faster and knee-high jog, alternate

F SET

Inner-thigh lift

Jumping jacks

Frog jump, neutral position

Jacks tuck

Hopscotch

COOL-DOWN

Walk forward with hands on hips

Step forward with R foot first

Step forward with L foot first

Walk on a tightrope

R leg kicks forward and back, no bounce

L leg kicks forward and back, no bounce

Fall forward, tuck, and stand

Side fall, tuck, and stand

Stretch: hip flexors, quadriceps, gastrocnemius, hamstrings, inner thigh, outer thigh

▶ Shallow-Water Interval Lesson Plan 1

INTERVAL 30

EQUIPMENT

None

TEACHING TIP

Shallow-water cardio lesson plan 1 is modified to include interval training. Interval 30 in the preseason is 30 seconds of work to 90 seconds of recovery (1:3 ratio). The intensity level is 60 percent.

Level 6 (60 percent HR max)—Moderate

WARM-UP

Knee-high jog

Run tires

Rocking horse to R side

Kick side to side

Rocking horse to L side

Jumping jacks

Inner-thigh lift

Hopscotch

Straddle jog

A SET

R quad kick, travel sideways R

Knee-high jog with paddlewheel

L quad kick, travel sideways L

Knee-high jog with paddlewheel

Work: Kick and lunge R (30 seconds)

Recovery: Knee-high jog, travel backward (30 seconds)

Kick forward (30 seconds)

Knee-high jog, travel forward (30 seconds)

Work: Kick and lunge L (30 seconds)

Recovery: Jump backward (30 seconds)

Kick forward (30 seconds)

Knee-high jog, travel forward (30 seconds)

Knee-high jog with breaststroke and knee-high jog, push forward, alternate

Knee-high jog, faster and knee-high jog, alternate

B SET

Inner-thigh lift

Jumping jacks

Frog jump, neutral position

Jacks tuck

Hopscotch

C SET

Cross-country ski, travel sideways R

Knee-high jog with hand waves

Cross-country ski, travel sideways L

Knee-high jog with hand waves

Work: Cross-country ski, full ROM (30 seconds)

Recovery: Knee-high jog, travel backward (30 seconds)

Rocking horse R (30 seconds)

Knee-high jog, travel forward (30 seconds)

Work: Cross-country ski, full ROM, neutral position (30 seconds)

Recovery: Jump backward (30 seconds)

Rocking horse L (30 seconds)

Knee-high jog, travel forward (30 seconds)

Knee-high jog with standing row and knee-high jog with unison jog press, alternate

Knee-high jog, faster and knee-high jog, alternate

D SET

Inner-thigh lift

Jumping jacks

Frog jump, neutral position

Jacks tuck

Hopscotch

E SET

Rocking horse to R side, travel sideways R

Knee-high jog with finger flicks

Rocking horse to L side, travel sideways L

Knee-high jog with finger flicks

Work: Bicycle, full ROM, suspended (30 seconds)

Recovery: Knee-high jog, travel backward (30 seconds)

Skateboard R (30 seconds)

Knee-high jog, travel forward (30 seconds)

Work: Bicycle, full ROM, suspended (30 seconds)

Recovery: Jump backward (30 seconds)

Skateboard L (30 seconds)

Knee-high jog, travel forward (30 seconds)

Knee-high jog with double-arm press-down and knee-high jog with arm curl, alternate

Knee-high jog, faster and knee-high jog, alternate

F SET

Inner-thigh lift

Jumping jacks

Frog jump, neutral position

Jacks tuck

Hopscotch

COOL-DOWN

Walk forward with hands on hips

Step forward with R foot first

Step forward with L foot first

Walk on a tightrope

R leg kicks forward and back, no bounce

L leg kicks forward and back, no bounce

Fall forward, tuck, and stand

Side fall, tuck, and stand

Stretch: hip flexors, quadriceps, gastrocnemius, hamstrings, inner thigh, outer thigh

► Shallow-Water Interval Lesson Plan 1

INTERVAL 30

EQUIPMENT

None

TEACHING TIP

Interval 30 in the transition season is 30 seconds of work to 60 seconds of recovery (1:2 ratio). The intensity level is 70 percent.

Level 7 (70 percent HR max)—Somewhat hard

WARM-UP

Knee-high jog

Run tires

Rocking horse to R side

Kick side to side

Rocking horse to L side

Jumping jacks

Inner-thigh lift

Hopscotch

Straddle jog

A SET

R quad kick, travel sideways R

Knee-high jog with paddlewheel

L quad kick, travel sideways L

Knee-high jog with paddlewheel

Work: Kick forward, faster (30 seconds)

Recovery: Knee-high jog, push forward (30 seconds)

Kick forward (30 seconds)

Work: High kick (30 seconds)

Recovery: Jump backward (30 seconds)

Kick forward, travel forward (30 seconds)

Work: Flutter kick, suspended (30 seconds)

Recovery: Jump backward (30 seconds)

Kick forward, neutral position, travel forward (30 seconds)

Knee-high jog with breaststroke and knee-high jog, push forward, alternate

Knee-high jog, faster and knee-high jog, alternate

B SET

Inner-thigh lift

Jumping jacks

Frog jump, neutral position

Jacks tuck

Hopscotch

C SET

Cross-country ski, travel sideways R

Knee-high jog with hand waves

Cross-country ski, travel sideways L

Knee-high jog with hand waves

Work: Cross-country ski, faster (30 seconds)

Recovery: Knee-high jog with unison jog press (30 seconds)

　　Cross-country ski (30 seconds)

Work: Cross-country ski, suspended (30 seconds)

Recovery: Jump backward (30 seconds)

　　Cross-country ski, travel forward (30 seconds)

Work: Cross-country ski, faster, suspended (30 seconds)

Recovery: Jump backward (30 seconds)

　　Cross-country ski, neutral position, travel forward (30 seconds)

Knee-high jog with standing row and knee-high jog with unison jog press, alternate

Knee-high jog, faster and knee-high jog, alternate

D SET

Inner-thigh lift

Jumping jacks

Frog jump, neutral position

Jacks tuck

Hopscotch

E SET

Rocking horse to R side, travel sideways R

Knee-high jog with finger flicks

Rocking horse to L side, travel sideways L

Knee-high jog with finger flicks

Work: Bicycle, faster, suspended (30 seconds)

Recovery: Knee-high jog with arm curl (30 seconds)

　　Skip rope (30 seconds)

Work: Jumping jacks, suspended (30 seconds)

Recovery: Jump backward (30 seconds)

　　Rocking horse R, travel forward (30 seconds)

Work: Bicycle, faster, suspended (30 seconds)

Recovery: Jump backward (30 seconds)

　　Rocking horse L, travel forward (30 seconds)

Knee-high jog with double-arm press-down and knee-high jog with arm curl, alternate

Knee-high jog, faster and knee-high jog, alternate

F SET

Inner-thigh lift

Jumping jacks

Frog jump, neutral position

Jacks tuck

Hopscotch

COOL-DOWN

Walk forward with hands on hips

Step forward with R foot first

Step forward with L foot first

Walk on a tightrope

R leg kicks forward and back, no bounce

L leg kicks forward and back, no bounce

Fall forward, tuck, and stand

Side fall, tuck, and stand

Stretch: hip flexors, quadriceps, gastrocnemius, hamstrings, inner thigh, outer thigh

▶ Shallow-Water Interval Lesson Plan 1

INTERVAL 30

PF

EQUIPMENT

None

TEACHING TIP

Interval 30 in the peak fitness season is 30 seconds of work to 30 seconds of recovery (1:1 ratio). The intensity level is 80 percent. Level 8 is high-intensity interval training (HIIT). For safety's sake, encourage your participants to modify the intensity to a level that is challenging for them rather than try to keep up with other participants.

　　Level 8 (80 percent HR max)—Hard

WARM-UP

Knee-high jog

Run tires

Rocking horse to R side

Kick side to side

Rocking horse to L side

Jumping jacks

Inner-thigh lift

Hopscotch

Straddle jog

A SET

R quad kick, travel sideways R

Knee-high jog with paddlewheel

L quad kick, travel sideways L

Knee-high jog with paddlewheel

Kick forward

Kick forward, doubles

Kick forward, doubles, one low and one high

Knee-high jog with breaststroke and knee-high jog, push forward, alternate

Knee-high jog, faster and knee-high jog, alternate

B SET

Inner-thigh lift

Jumping jacks

Frog jump, neutral position

Jacks tuck

Hopscotch

C SET

Cross-country ski, travel sideways R

Knee-high jog with hand waves

Cross-country ski, travel sideways L

Knee-high jog with hand waves

Cross-country ski

Cross-country ski, doubles

Cross-country ski, single, single, double

Knee-high jog with standing row and knee-high jog with unison jog press, alternate

Knee-high jog, faster and knee-high jog, alternate

D SET

Inner-thigh lift

Jumping jacks

Frog jump, neutral position

Jacks tuck

Hopscotch

E SET

Rocking horse to R side, travel sideways R

Knee-high jog with finger flicks

Rocking horse to L side, travel sideways L

Knee-high jog with finger flicks

Skateboard R

Skateboard L

Skip rope

Knee-high jog with double-arm press-down and knee-high jog with arm curl, alternate

Knee-high jog, faster and knee-high jog, alternate

G SET INTERVALS

Work: Kick and lunge R with double-arm press-down (30 seconds)

Recovery: Knee-high jog (30 seconds)

Work: Kick and lunge L with double-arm press-down (30 seconds)

Recovery: Kick forward (30 seconds)

Work: High kick with power (30 seconds)

Recovery: Kick forward, neutral position (30 seconds)

Work: Cross-country ski with power, neutral position (30 seconds)

Recovery: Knee-high jog (30 seconds)

Work: Cross-country ski with power (30 seconds)

Recovery: Cross-country ski (30 seconds)

Work: Cross-country ski with rotation (30 seconds)

Recovery: Cross-country ski, neutral position (30 seconds)

Work: Bicycle with power, suspended (30 seconds)

Recovery: Skateboard R (30 seconds)

Work: Bicycle with power, suspended (30 seconds)

Recovery: Skateboard L (30 seconds)

Work: Skateboard jump R (30 seconds)

Recovery: Knee-high jog (30 seconds)

Work: Skateboard jump L (30 seconds)

Recovery: Knee-high jog (30 seconds)

F SET

Inner-thigh lift

Jumping jacks

Frog jump, neutral position

Jacks tuck

Hopscotch

COOL-DOWN

Walk forward with hands on hips

Step forward with R foot first

Step forward with L foot first

Walk on a tightrope

R leg kicks forward and back, no bounce

L leg kicks forward and back, no bounce

Fall forward, tuck, and stand

Side fall, tuck, and stand

Stretch hip flexors, quadriceps, gastrocnemius, hamstrings, inner thigh, outer thigh

▶ Shallow-Water Cardio Lesson Plan 2

TURNS AND CIRCLES

EQUIPMENT

None

TEACHING TIP

Add interest and fun to your lesson plan with turns and circles. Practicing the turns in slow motion during the warm-up may be helpful. For the jacks cross 3-1/2× and half turn (see figure 3.2), cue, "Cross, out, cross, out, cross, out, cross and turn." For the cross-country ski 3-1/2× and half turn (see figure 3.3), cue, "Ski R, L, R, L, R, L, R, and turn." The cool-down uses travel in a bowtie pattern, which includes traveling diagonally to a corner. Turning to the corner and jogging forward is not the same as traveling diagonally. Instead, continue to face forward while moving diagonally toward the corner.

WARM-UP

Instructor's choice

A SET

Knee-high jog, R shoulder sweep out 2× and L shoulder sweep out 2×

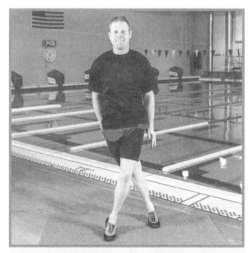

FIGURE 3.2   **Jacks cross.**

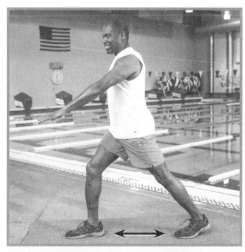

FIGURE 3.3   **Cross-country ski.**

Knee-high jog with unison arm swing

Jumping jacks, doubles 1×, jacks cross 2×

Knee-high jog with reverse breaststroke, travel backward

Rocking horse R, travel forward

Knee-high jog with reverse breaststroke, travel backward

Rocking horse L, travel forward

Knee-high jog with standing row, travel backward

Skip rope, travel forward

Knee-high jog with standing row, travel backward

Skip rope, travel forward

Crossover kick

Crossover kick, doubles

Jacks cross 3-1/2× and half turn

Jacks cross, R leg in front, circle clockwise

Jacks cross, L leg in front, circle counterclockwise

Knee-high jog

B SET

Knee-high jog with double-arm press-down 2× and lat pull-down 2×

Jumping jacks with unison arm swing

Cross-country ski and mini ski, alternate

Jump backward

Jacks tuck with breaststroke, travel forward

Jump backward

Jacks tuck with breaststroke, travel forward

Knee-high jog with standing row, travel backward

Inner-thigh lift, travel forward

Knee-high jog with standing row, travel backward

Inner-thigh lift, travel forward

Crossover kick, doubles

Crossover kick, doubles, one low and one high

Cross-country ski 3-1/2× and half turn

Cross-country ski, suspended, circle clockwise and counterclockwise

Knee-high jog

C SET

Knee-high jog, punch down R, L, and punch across R, L

Cross-country ski with unison arm swing

Jumping jacks and mini cross, alternate

Knee-high jog with reverse breaststroke, travel backward

Cross-country ski, travel forward

Knee-high jog with reverse breaststroke, travel backward

Cross-country ski, travel forward

Knee-high jog with standing row, travel backward

Leap forward

Knee-high jog with standing row, travel backward

Leap forward

Crossover kick, doubles, one low and one high

Crossover kick and sweep out

Jacks cross 3-1/2× and half turn

Jacks cross, R leg in front, circle clockwise

Jacks cross, L leg in front, circle counterclockwise

Knee-high jog

D SET

Knee-high jog, open and close doors: open R, open L, close R, close L, and open close 2×

Run tires with unison arm swing

Cross-country ski, doubles 1×, tuck ski 1×

Jump backward

Frog jump, neutral position, travel forward

Jump backward

Frog jump, neutral position, travel forward

Knee-high jog with standing row, travel backward

Hopscotch, travel forward

Knee-high jog with standing row, travel backward

Hopscotch, travel forward

Crossover kick and sweep out

Skate kick, crossover kick, sweep out and center

Cross-country ski 3-1/2× and half turn

Cross-country ski, suspended circle clockwise and counterclockwise

Knee-high jog

COOL-DOWN

(Travel in a bowtie pattern)

Knee-high jog, travel backward

Knee-high jog, travel diagonally to front L corner

Knee-high jog, travel backward

Knee-high jog, travel diagonally to front R corner

Knee-high jog, travel diagonally backward to back L corner

Knee-high jog, travel forward

Knee-high jog, travel diagonally backward to back R corner

Knee-high jog, travel forward

Walk backward

Walk diagonally to front L corner

Walk backward

Walk diagonally to front R corner

Walk diagonally backward to back L corner

Walk forward

Walk diagonally backward to back R corner

Walk forward

Walk diagonally backward to back L corner, look R

Walk diagonally forward to front R corner, look L

Stand on one foot with eyes closed

Stretch: shoulders, pectorals, hip flexors, gastrocnemius, hamstrings, outer thigh

▶ Shallow-Water Interval Lesson Plan 2

INTERVAL 40   ⓟ

EQUIPMENT

None

TEACHING TIP

Shallow-water cardio lesson plan 2 is modified to include interval training. Interval 40 in the preseason is 40 seconds of work to 80 seconds of recovery (1:2 ratio). The intensity level is 60 percent.

Level 6 (60 percent HR max)—Moderate

WARM-UP

Instructor's choice

A SET

Knee-high jog, R shoulder sweep out 2× and L shoulder sweep out 2×

Knee-high jog with unison arm swing

Jumping jacks, doubles 1×, jacks cross 2×

Knee-high jog with reverse breaststroke, travel backward

Rocking horse R, travel forward

Knee-high jog with reverse breaststroke, travel backward

Rocking horse L, travel forward

Work: Knee lift and lunge R (40 seconds)

Recovery: Crossover knees (20 seconds)

Knee-high jog (20 seconds)

Crossover knees (20 seconds)

Knee-high jog (20 seconds)

Work: Knee lift and lunge L (40 seconds)

Recovery: Heel jog (20 seconds)

Knee-high jog (20 seconds)

Heel jog (20 seconds)

Knee-high jog (20 seconds)

Jacks cross 3-1/2× and half turn

Jacks cross, R leg in front, circle clockwise

Jacks cross, L leg in front, circle counterclockwise

B SET

Knee-high jog with double-arm press-down 2× and lat pull-down 2×

Jumping jacks with unison arm swing

Cross-country ski and mini ski, alternate

Jump backward

Jacks tuck with breaststroke, travel forward

Jump backward

Jacks tuck with breaststroke, travel forward

Work: Jacks cross (40 seconds)

Recovery: Straddle jog (20 seconds)

Knee-high jog (20 seconds)

Straddle jog (20 seconds)

Knee-high jog (20 seconds)

Work: Jacks cross (40 seconds)

Recovery: Squat (20 seconds)

Knee-high jog (20 seconds)

Squat (20 seconds)

Knee-high jog (20 seconds)

Cross-country ski 3-1/2× and half turn

Tuck ski, circle clockwise and counterclockwise

C SET

Knee-high jog, punch down R, L, and punch across R, L

Cross-country ski with unison arm swing

Jumping jacks and mini cross, alternate

Knee-high jog with reverse breaststroke, travel backward

Cross-country ski, travel forward

Knee-high jog with reverse breaststroke, travel backward

Cross-country ski, travel forward

Work: Cross-country ski, full ROM (40 seconds)

Recovery: Heel jog (20 seconds)

Knee-high jog (20 seconds)

Heel jog (20 seconds)

Knee-high jog (20 seconds)

Work: Cross-country ski, full ROM, neutral position (40 seconds)

Recovery: Rocking horse R (20 seconds)

Knee-high jog (20 seconds)

Rocking horse L (20 seconds)

Knee-high jog (20 seconds)

Jacks cross 3-1/2× and half turn

Jacks cross, R leg in front, circle clockwise

Jacks cross, L leg in front, circle counterclockwise

D SET

Knee-high jog, open and close doors: open R, open L, close R, close L, and open close 2×

Run tires with unison arm swing

Cross-country ski, doubles 1×, tuck ski 1×

Jump backward

Frog jump, neutral position, travel forward

Jump backward

Frog jump, neutral position, travel forward

Work: Skate kick, full ROM (40 seconds)

Recovery: Skateboard R (20 seconds)

Knee-high jog (20 seconds)

Skateboard L (20 seconds)

Knee-high jog (20 seconds)

Work: Skate kick, full ROM (40 seconds)

Recovery: Lunge R (20 seconds)

Knee-high jog (20 seconds)

Lunge L (20 seconds)

Knee-high jog (20 seconds)

Cross-country ski 3-1/2× and half turn

Tuck ski, circle clockwise and counterclockwise

COOL-DOWN

(Travel in a bowtie pattern)

Knee-high jog, travel backward

Knee-high jog, travel diagonally to front L corner

Knee-high jog, travel backward

Knee-high jog, travel diagonally to front R corner

Knee-high jog, travel diagonally backward to back L corner

Knee-high jog, travel forward

Knee-high jog, travel diagonally backward to back R corner

Knee-high jog, travel forward

Walk backward

Walk diagonally to front L corner

Walk backward

Walk diagonally to front R corner

Walk diagonally backward to back L corner

Walk forward

Walk diagonally backward to back R corner

Walk forward

Walk diagonally backward to back L corner, look R

Walk diagonally forward to front R corner, look L

Stand on one foot with eyes closed

Stretch: shoulders, pectorals, hip flexors, gastrocnemius, hamstrings, outer thigh

▶ Shallow-Water Interval Lesson Plan 2

INTERVAL 40

EQUIPMENT

None

TEACHING TIP

Interval 40 in the transition season is 40 seconds of work to 60 seconds of recovery (1:1.5 ratio). The intensity level is 70 percent.

Level 7 (70 percent HR max)—Somewhat hard

WARM-UP

Instructor's choice

A SET

Knee-high jog, R shoulder sweep out 2× and L shoulder sweep out 2×

Knee-high jog with unison arm swing

Jumping jacks, doubles 1×, jacks cross 2×

Knee-high jog with reverse breaststroke, travel backward

Rocking horse R, travel forward

Knee-high jog with reverse breaststroke, travel backward

Rocking horse L, travel forward

Knee-high jog with double-arm press-down 2× and lat pull-down 2×

Jumping jacks with unison arm swing

Cross-country ski and mini ski, alternate

Jump backward

Jacks tuck with breaststroke, travel forward

Jump backward

Jacks tuck with breaststroke, travel forward

Jacks cross 3-1/2× and half turn

Jacks cross, R leg in front, circle clockwise

Jacks cross, L leg in front circle, counterclockwise

Knee-high jog

B SET

Knee-high jog, punch down R, L, and punch across R, L

Cross-country ski with unison arm swing

Jumping jacks and mini cross, alternate

Knee-high jog with reverse breaststroke, travel backward

Cross-country ski, travel forward

Knee-high jog with reverse breaststroke, travel backward

Cross-country ski, travel forward

Knee-high jog, open and close doors: open R, open L, close R, close L, and open close 2×

Run tires with unison arm swing

Cross-country ski, doubles 1×, tuck ski 1×

Jump backward

Frog jump, neutral position, travel forward

Jump backward

Frog jump, neutral position, travel forward

Cross-country ski 3-1/2× and half turn

Cross-country ski, suspended, circle clockwise and counterclockwise

Knee-high jog

C SET INTERVALS

Work: Steep climb, faster (40 seconds)

Recovery: Crossover knees (30 seconds)

Knee-high jog (30 seconds)

Work: Knee-high jog, faster (40 seconds)

Recovery: Knee-high jog, neutral position (30 seconds)

Knee-high jog (30 seconds)

Work: Mini jacks, faster (40 seconds)

Recovery: Straddle jog (30 seconds)

Knee-high jog (30 seconds)

Work: Jumping jacks, faster (40 seconds)

Recovery: Jumping jacks, neutral position (30 seconds)

Knee-high jog (30 seconds)

Work: Mini ski, faster (40 seconds)

Recovery: Heel jog (30 seconds)

Knee-high jog (30 seconds)

Work: Cross-country ski, faster (40 seconds)

Recovery: Tuck ski (30 seconds)

Knee-high jog (30 seconds)

Work: Frog, suspended (40 seconds)

Recovery: Squat (30 seconds)

Knee-high jog (30 seconds)

Work: Bicycle, faster, suspended (40 seconds)

Recovery: Lunge R (30 seconds)

Knee-high jog (30 seconds)

Work: Bicycle, faster, suspended (40 seconds)

Recovery: Lunge L (30 seconds)

Knee-high jog (30 seconds)

COOL-DOWN

(Travel in a bowtie pattern)

Walk backward

Walk diagonally to front L corner

Walk backward

Walk diagonally to front R corner

Walk diagonally backward to back L corner

Walk forward

Walk diagonally backward to back R corner

Walk forward

Walk diagonally backward to back L corner, look R

Walk diagonally forward to front R corner, look L

Stretch: shoulders, pectorals, hip flexors, gastrocnemius, hamstrings, outer thigh

▶ Shallow-Water Interval Lesson Plan 2

PF

INTERVAL 40

EQUIPMENT

None

TEACHING TIP

Interval 40 in the peak fitness season is 40 seconds of work to 40 seconds of recovery (1:1 ratio). The intensity level is 80 percent. Level 8 is high-intensity interval training (HIIT). For safety's sake, encourage your participants to modify the intensity to a level that is challenging for them rather than try to keep up with other participants.

Level 8 (80 percent HR max)—Hard

Jacks cross with power, grounded (see figure 3.4) may be a new move for some. Cue to lift the leg to the side, cross it in front, lift again to the side, and bring it down to center; then repeat on the other side.

WARM-UP

Instructor's choice

A SET

Knee-high jog, R shoulder sweep out 2×, and L shoulder sweep out 2×

Knee-high jog with unison arm swing

Jumping jacks, doubles 1×, jacks cross 2×

Knee-high jog with reverse breaststroke, travel backward

Rocking horse R, travel forward

Knee-high jog with reverse breaststroke, travel backward

Rocking horse L, travel forward

Knee-high jog with double-arm press-down 2× and lat pull-down 2×

Jumping jacks with unison arm swing

Cross-country ski and mini ski, alternate

Jump backward

Jacks tuck with breaststroke, travel forward

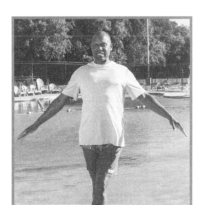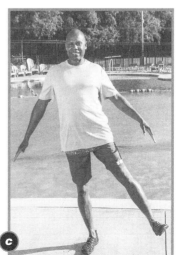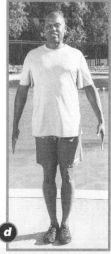

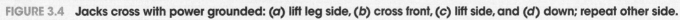

FIGURE 3.4 Jacks cross with power grounded: (*a*) lift leg side, (*b*) cross front, (*c*) lift side, and (*d*) down; repeat other side.

Jump backward

Jacks tuck with breaststroke, travel forward

Jacks cross 3-1/2× and half turn

Knee-high jog

B SET

Knee-high jog, punch down R, L, and punch across R, L

Cross-country ski with unison arm swing

Jumping jacks and mini cross, alternate

Knee-high jog with reverse breaststroke, travel backward

Cross-country ski, travel forward

Knee-high jog with reverse breaststroke, travel backward

Cross-country ski, travel forward

Knee-high jog, open and close doors: open R, open L, close R, close L, and open close 2×

Run tires with unison arm swing

Cross-country ski, doubles 1×, tuck ski 1×

Jump backward

Frog jump, neutral position, travel forward

Jump backward

Frog jump, neutral position, travel forward

Cross-country ski 3-1/2× and half turn

Knee-high jog

C SET INTERVALS

Work: Steep climb with power (40 seconds)

Recovery: Crossover knees (20 seconds)

Knee-high jog (20 seconds)

Work: Power run (40 seconds)

Recovery: Knee-high jog, neutral position (20 seconds)

Knee-high jog (20 seconds)

Work: Power run (40 seconds)

Recovery: Knee-high jog, neutral position (20 seconds)

Knee-high jog (20 seconds)

Work: Jacks cross with power, grounded (40 seconds)

Recovery: Straddle jog (20 seconds)

Knee-high jog (20 seconds)

Work: Frog jump (40 seconds)

Recovery: Jumping jacks, neutral position (20 seconds)

Knee-high jog (20 seconds)

Work: Squat and jump (40 seconds)

Recovery: Jumping jacks, neutral position (20 seconds)

Knee-high jog (20 seconds)

Work: Cross-country ski with rotation (40 seconds)

Recovery: Heel jog (20 seconds)

Knee-high jog (20 seconds)

Work: Cross-country ski with power (40 seconds)

Recovery: Tuck ski (20 seconds)

Knee-high jog (20 seconds)

Work: Cross-country ski with power, neutral position (40 seconds)

Recovery: Tuck ski (20 seconds)

Knee-high jog (20 seconds)

Work: Bicycle with power, suspended (40 seconds)

Recovery: Lunge R and L, alternate (20 seconds)

Knee-high jog (20 seconds)

Work: Bicycle with power, suspended, travel forward (40 seconds)

Recovery: Skateboard R (20 seconds)

Knee-high jog (20 seconds)

Work: Bicycle with power, suspended, travel forward (40 seconds)

Recovery: Skateboard L (20 seconds)

Knee-high jog (20 seconds)

COOL-DOWN

(Travel in a bowtie pattern)

Walk backward

Walk diagonally to front L corner

Walk backward

Walk diagonally to front R corner

Walk diagonally backward to back L corner

Walk forward

Walk diagonally backward to back R corner

Walk forward

Walk diagonally backward to back L corner, look R

Walk diagonally forward to front R corner, look L

Stand on one foot with eyes closed

Stretch: shoulders, pectorals, hip flexors, gastrocnemius, hamstrings, outer thigh

▶ Shallow-Water Cardio Lesson Plan 3

INCREASING COMPLEXITY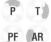

EQUIPMENT

None

TEACHING TIP

Another way to organize a lesson plan is to start with a set of basic exercises. Repeat those same exercises in the second set but insert additional exercises that may be new to your participants. For example, combine two moves to create a new move. This lesson plan combines jumping jacks (see figure 3.5) with kick forward (see figure 3.6), and jumping jacks with skate kick (see figure 3.7). Repeat the second set and insert even more exercises, so that each succeeding set is more complex than the preceding one.

WARM-UP

Instructor's choice

A SET

Jumping jacks
Jumping jacks with elbows bent
Inner-thigh lift
Straddle jog with shoulder blade squeeze
Rocking horse R, travel backward
Rocking horse L, travel forward
Jump backward
Knee-high jog, travel forward
Cross-country ski, travel sideways R and L
Cross-country ski with unison arm swing
Cross-country ski with rotation
Knee-high jog

B SET

Jumping jacks
Jumping jacks, arms cross in front and in back
Jumping jacks, doubles
Jumping jacks 1×, kick forward 1×

Inner-thigh lift
Hopscotch
Straddle jog with shoulder blade squeeze
Rocking horse L, travel backward
Rocking horse R, travel forward
Jump backward
Knee-high jog, travel forward
Jump backward
Leap forward
Cross-country ski, travel backward and forward
Cross-country ski with unison arm swing
Cross-country ski, clap hands
Cross-country ski with rotation, hands together
Knee-high jog

C SET

Jumping jacks
Jumping jacks, palms touch in front and in back
Jumping jacks, doubles
Jumping jacks 2×, jumping jacks doubles 1×
Jumping jacks 1×, kick forward 1×
Jumping jacks 1×, skate kick 1×
Inner-thigh lift 1×, hopscotch 1×
Straddle jog with shoulder blade squeeze
Rocking horse R, travel backward and forward
Rocking horse L, travel backward and forward
Jump backward
Knee-high jog, travel forward
Jump backward
Leap forward

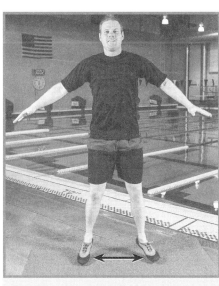

FIGURE 3.5 **Jumping jacks.**

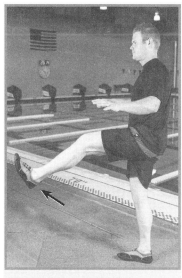

FIGURE 3.6 **Kick forward.**

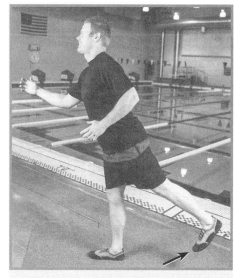

FIGURE 3.7 **Skate kick.**

Jump backward

Skate kick, travel forward

Cross-country ski with quarter turn

Cross-country ski with unison arm swing

Cross-country ski, clap hands

Cross-country ski with forearm press

Cross-country ski with rotation and log jump, forward and back, alternate

Knee-high jog

COOL-DOWN

Jumping jacks

Jumping jacks 1×, kick forward 1×

Jumping jacks 1×, skate kick 1×

Skate kick

Kick forward

Kick and lunge R

Hold lunge position and R bowstring pull

Lunge deeper and return

Warrior III (balance on L leg with R leg extended back)

Kick and lunge L

Hold lunge position and L bowstring pull

Lunge deeper and return

Warrior III (balance on R leg with L leg extended back)

Stretch: hamstrings, outer thigh, quadriceps, hip flexors, gastrocnemius, upper back

▶ Shallow-Water Interval Lesson Plan 3

INTERVAL 60

EQUIPMENT

None

TEACHING TIP

Shallow-water cardio lesson plan 3 is modified to include interval training. Interval 60 in the preseason is 60 seconds of work to 2 minutes of recovery (1:2 ratio). The intensity level is 60 percent.

Level 6 (60 percent HR max)—Moderate

WARM-UP

Instructor's choice

A SET

Jumping jacks

Jumping jacks with elbows bent

Jumping jacks 2×, jumping jacks doubles 1×

Inner-thigh lift

Straddle jog with shoulder blade squeeze

Rocking horse R, travel backward

Rocking horse L, travel forward

Jump backward

Knee-high jog, travel forward

Jump backward

Knee-high jog, travel forward

Knee-high jog

B SET

Jumping jacks

Jumping jacks, arms cross in front and in back

Jumping jacks 1×, kick forward 1×

Hopscotch

Straddle jog with shoulder blade squeeze

Rocking horse L, travel backward

Rocking horse R, travel forward

Jump backward

Knee-high jog, travel forward

Jump backward

Leap forward

Knee-high jog

C SET INTERVALS

Work: Knee lift and lunge R (30 seconds)

Knee lift and lunge L (30 seconds)

Recovery: Kick forward (30 seconds)

Lunge R (30 seconds)

Kick forward (30 seconds)

Lunge L (30 seconds)

Work: Kick side to side, arms and legs opposite (60 seconds)

Recovery: Run tires (30 seconds)

Squat (30 seconds)

Run tires (30 seconds)

Squat (30 seconds)

Work: Inner-thigh lift, full ROM (60 seconds)

Recovery: Straddle jog (30 seconds)

Kick to the corners (30 seconds)

Straddle jog (30 seconds)

Kick to the corners (30 seconds)

Work: Kick and lunge R (30 seconds)

Kick and lunge L (30 seconds)

Recovery: Crossover knees (30 seconds)

Crossover kick (30 seconds)

Crossover knees (30 seconds)

Crossover kick (30 seconds)

Work: Cross-country ski, full ROM (60 seconds)

Recovery: Heel jog (30 seconds)

    Rocking horse R (30 seconds)

    Heel jog (30 seconds)

    Rocking horse L (30 seconds)

Work: Cross-country ski, full ROM, neutral position (60 seconds)

Recovery: Knee-high jog (30 seconds)

    Skateboard R (30 seconds)

    Knee-high jog (30 seconds)

    Skateboard L (30 seconds)

COOL-DOWN

Jumping jacks

Jumping jacks, palms touch in front and in back

Jumping jacks 1×, skate kick 1×

Inner-thigh lift 1×, hopscotch 1×

Straddle jog with shoulder blade squeeze

Rocking horse R, travel backward and forward

Rocking horse L, travel backward and forward

Jump backward

Knee-high jog, travel forward

Kick and lunge R

Hold lunge position and R bowstring pull

Lunge deeper and return

Warrior III (balance on L leg with R leg extended back)

Kick and lunge L

Hold lunge position and L bowstring pull

Lunge deeper and return

Warrior III (balance on R leg with L leg extended back)

Stretch: hamstrings, outer thigh, quadriceps, hip flexors, gastrocnemius, upper back

▶ Shallow-Water Interval Lesson Plan 3

INTERVAL 60

EQUIPMENT

None

TEACHING TIP

Interval 60 in the transition season is 60 seconds of work to 90 seconds of recovery (1:1.5 ratio). The intensity level is 70 percent.

    Level 7 (70 percent HR max)—Somewhat hard

WARM-UP

Instructor's choice

A SET

Jumping jacks

Jumping jacks with elbows bent

Jumping jacks 2×, jumping jacks doubles 1×

Inner-thigh lift

Straddle jog with shoulder blade squeeze

Rocking horse R, travel backward

Rocking horse L, travel forward

Jump backward

Knee-high jog, travel forward

Jump backward

Knee-high jog, travel forward

Knee-high jog

B SET

Jumping jacks

Jumping jacks, arms cross in front and in back

Jumping jacks 1×, kick forward 1×

Hopscotch

Straddle jog with shoulder blade squeeze

Rocking horse L, travel backward

Rocking horse R, travel forward

Jump backward

Knee-high jog, travel forward

Jump backward

Leap forward

Knee-high jog

C SET INTERVALS

Work: Kick forward, faster (60 seconds)

Recovery: Lunge R (30 seconds)

    Kick forward (30 seconds)

    Lunge L (30 seconds)

Work: Kick side to side, faster (60 seconds)

Recovery: Squat (30 seconds)

    Run tires (30 seconds)

    Squat (30 seconds)

Work: Inner-thigh lift, faster (60 seconds)

Recovery: Kick to the corners (30 seconds)

    Straddle jog (30 seconds)

    Kick to the corners (30 seconds)

Work: Skate kick, faster (60 seconds)

Recovery: Skateboard R (30 seconds)

    Tuck ski (30 seconds)

    Skateboard L (30 seconds)

Work: High kick (60 seconds)

Recovery: Crossover kick (30 seconds)

   Crossover knees (30 seconds)

   Crossover kick (30 seconds)

Work: Jumping jacks, faster (60 seconds)

Recovery: Jumping jacks (30 seconds)

   Jacks tuck (30 seconds)

   Jumping jacks (30 seconds)

Work: Cross-country ski, suspended (60 seconds)

Recovery: Rocking horse R (30 seconds)

   Heel jog (30 seconds)

   Rocking horse L (30 seconds)

Work: Cross-country ski, faster, suspended (60 seconds)

Recovery: R leg kicks forward and back, no bounce (30 seconds)

   Tuck ski (30 seconds)

   L leg kicks forward and back, no bounce (30 seconds)

COOL-DOWN

Jumping jacks

Jumping jacks, palms touch in front and in back

Jumping jacks 1×, skate kick 1×

Inner-thigh lift 1×, hopscotch 1×

Straddle jog with shoulder blade squeeze

Rocking horse R

Rocking horse L

Jump backward

Knee-high jog, travel forward

Kick and lunge R

Hold lunge position and R bowstring pull

Warrior III (balance on L leg with R leg extended back)

Kick and lunge L

Hold lunge position and L bowstring pull

Warrior III (balance on R leg with L leg extended back)

Stretch: hamstrings, outer thigh, quadriceps, hip flexors, gastrocnemius, upper back

▶ Shallow-Water Interval Lesson Plan 3

INTERVAL 60

EQUIPMENT

None

TEACHING TIP

Interval 60 in the peak fitness season is 60 seconds of work to 60 seconds of recovery (1:1 ratio). The intensity level is 80 percent. Level 8 is high-intensity interval training (HIIT). For safety's sake, encourage your participants to modify the intensity to a level that is challenging for them rather than try to keep up with other participants.

   Level 8 (80 percent HR max)—Hard

WARM-UP

Instructor's choice

A SET

Jumping jacks

Jumping jacks with elbows bent

Jumping jacks 2×, jumping jacks doubles 1×

Inner-thigh lift

Straddle jog with shoulder blade squeeze

Rocking horse R, travel backward

Rocking horse L, travel forward

Jump backward

Knee-high jog, travel forward

Jump backward

Knee-high jog, travel forward

Knee-high jog

B SET

Jumping jacks

Jumping jacks, arms cross in front and in back

Jumping jacks 1×, kick forward 1×

Hopscotch

Straddle jog with shoulder blade squeeze

Rocking horse L, travel backward

Rocking horse R, travel forward

Jump backward

Knee-high jog, travel forward

Jump backward

Leap forward

Knee-high jog

C SET INTERVALS

Work: High kick, power down (60 seconds)

Recovery: Lunge R (30 seconds)

   Lunge L (30 seconds)

Work: Kick side to side with power, grounded (60 seconds)

Recovery: Squat (30 seconds)

   Run tires (30 seconds)

Work: Inner-thigh lift R with double arms (30 seconds)

Inner-thigh lift L with double arms (30 seconds)

Recovery: Straddle jog (30 seconds)

Kick to the corners (30 seconds)

Work: Cross-country ski with power (60 seconds)

Recovery: Skateboard R (30 seconds)

Skateboard L (30 seconds)

Work: Cross-country ski with rotation (60 seconds)

Recovery: Tuck ski (30 seconds)

Tuck ski with rotation (30 seconds)

Work: Kick and lunge R with double-arm press-down (30 seconds)

Kick and lunge L with double-arm press-down (30 seconds)

Recovery: Crossover knees (30 seconds)

Crossover kick (30 seconds)

Work: Jumping jacks, land feet out only (60 seconds)

Recovery: Jumping jacks (30 seconds)

Jacks tuck (30 seconds)

Work: Cross-country ski with power (60 seconds)

Recovery: Rocking horse R (30 seconds)

Rocking horse L (30 seconds)

Work: Cross-country ski with rotation (60 seconds)

Recovery: Tuck ski (30 seconds)

Tuck ski with rotation (30 seconds)

Work: Cross-country ski with power, neutral position (60 seconds)

Recovery: R leg kicks forward and back, no bounce (30 seconds)

L leg kicks forward and back, no bounce (30 seconds)

COOL-DOWN

Jumping jacks

Jumping jacks, palms touch in front and in back

Jumping jacks 1×, skate kick 1×

Inner-thigh lift 1×, hopscotch 1×

Straddle jog with shoulder blade squeeze

Rocking horse R

Rocking horse L

Jump backward

Knee-high jog, travel forward

Kick and lunge R

Hold lunge position and R bowstring pull

Warrior III (balance on L leg with R leg extended back)

Kick and lunge L

Hold lunge position and L bowstring pull

Warrior III (balance on R leg with L leg extended back)

Stretch: hamstrings, outer thigh, quadriceps, hip flexors, gastrocnemius, upper back

▶ Shallow-Water Cardio Lesson Plan 4

BLOCK CHOREOGRAPHY WITH FIVE MOVES

EQUIPMENT

Noodles

TEACHING TIP

In block choreography you start with a set of basic moves and in each succeeding set you change something about the moves. This lesson plan uses just five moves—knee-high jog (see figure 3.8), kick forward (see figure 3.9), jumping jacks (see figure 3.10), skate kick (see figure 3.11), and cross-country ski (see figure 3.12). It ends with an arm medley.

WARM-UP

Instructor's choice

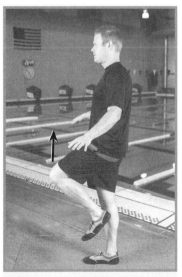 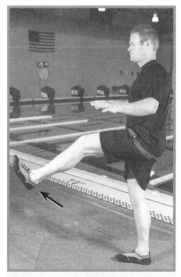

FIGURE 3.8 Knee-high jog.   **FIGURE 3.9 Kick forward.**

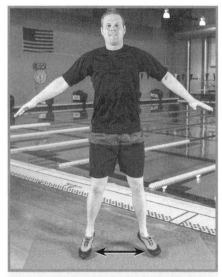

FIGURE 3.10 **Jumping jacks.**

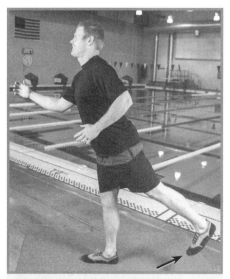

FIGURE 3.11 **Skate kick.**

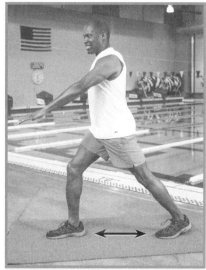

FIGURE 3.12 **Cross-country ski.**

A SET

Knee-high jog

Kick forward

Jumping jacks

In-line skate

Cross-country ski

B SET

Knee-high jog, punch forward and side

Chorus-line kick

Jumping jacks with diagonal turn

Skate kick with pumping arms

Cross-country ski, two easy and one with power

C SET

Knee-high jog, push across and slice back

High kick

Jumping jacks, doubles

Knee lift and lunge R

Knee lift and lunge L

Cross-country ski, four easy and four with power

D SET

Knee-high jog with breaststroke

Kick forward with lat pull-down

Jumping jacks with arms out of the water

Skate kick with pumping arms

Cross-country ski, two easy and one with power

E SET

Knee-high jog, punch across

Crossover kick

Jumping jacks, syncopate

Kick and lunge R

Kick and lunge L

Cross-country ski, four easy and four with power

F SET

Knee-high jog with triceps extension

Crossover kick and sweep out

Jumping jacks squat

Skate kick with pumping arms

Cross-country ski, two easy and one with power

G SET

Knee-high jog

Kick forward, neutral position, travel backward

Jumping jacks, neutral position, travel forward

In-line skate

Skip rope

H SET

Straddle jog, clap hands

Squat, shoulder sweep out R and L, alternate

Squat, shoulder sweep in R and L, alternate

Squat, clap hands with power

Knee-high jog with crawl stroke

L lunge with R bowstring pull

R lunge with L bowstring pull

Lunge with standing row with power

Cross-country ski

Cross-country ski with R arm swing, L hand on hip

Cross-country ski with L arm swing, R hand on hip

Lunge with unison arm swing with power

Straddle jog, open and close doors

Squat, open and close R and L, alternate

Squat, open R, open L, close R, close L with power

Squat with forearm press

COOL-DOWN

(Sit on noodle like a swing)

Seated kick with scull

Pike and scull

Seated jacks

Seated leg press

Seated kick, upper-body twist, arms to sides 70 degrees

Brace core, arms down, turbulent hand movements

Stretch: quadriceps, hip flexors, inner thigh, hamstrings, pectorals, upper back

▶ Shallow-Water Interval Lesson Plan 4

INTERVALS WITH REDUCED RECOVERY TIME 1

EQUIPMENT

None

TEACHING TIP

Shallow-water cardio lesson plan 4 is modified to include interval training. Interval training with reduced recovery time in the preseason is 60 seconds of work to 30 seconds of recovery (2:1 ratio). The intensity level is 60 percent.

Level 6 (60 percent HR max)—Moderate

WARM-UP

Instructor's choice

A SET

Knee-high jog

Kick forward

Jumping jacks

In-line skate

Cross-country ski

Work: Kick side to side, arms and legs opposite (60 seconds)

Recovery: In, in, out, out (30 seconds)

Work: Jacks cross (60 seconds)

Recovery: Run tires (30 seconds)

B SET

Knee-high jog, punch forward and side

Chorus-line kick

Jumping jacks with diagonal turn

Skate kick with pumping arms

Cross-country ski, two easy and one with power

C SET

Knee-high jog, push across and slice back

High kick

Jumping jacks, doubles

Knee lift and lunge R

Knee lift and lunge L

Cross-country ski, four easy and four with power

Work: Inner-thigh lift, full ROM (60 seconds)

Recovery: In, in, out, out (30 seconds)

Work: Hopscotch, full ROM (60 seconds)

Recovery: Run tires (30 seconds)

D SET

Knee-high jog with breaststroke

Kick forward with lat pull-down

Jumping jacks with arms out of the water

Skate kick with pumping arms

Cross-country ski, two easy and one with power

E SET

Knee-high jog, punch across

Crossover kick

Jumping jacks, syncopate

Kick and lunge R

Kick and lunge L

Cross-country ski, four easy and four with power

Work: Rocking horse R with a front kick (60 seconds)

Recovery: In, in, out, out (30 seconds)

Work: Rocking horse L with a front kick (60 seconds)

Recovery: Run tires (30 seconds)

F SET

Knee-high jog

Kick forward, neutral position, travel backward

Jumping jacks, neutral position, travel forward

In-line skate

Skip rope

COOL-DOWN

Straddle jog, clap hands

Squat, shoulder sweep out R and L, alternate

Squat, shoulder sweep in R and L, alternate

Squat, clap hands with power

Knee-high jog with crawl stroke

L lunge with R bowstring pull

R lunge with L bowstring pull

Lunge with standing row with power

Cross-country ski

Cross-country ski with R arm swing, L hand on hip

Cross-country ski with L arm swing, R hand on hip

Lunge with unison arm swing with power

Straddle jog, open and close doors

Squat, open and close R and L, alternate

Squat, open R, open L, close R, close L with power

Squat with forearm press

Squat, travel sideways R and L

Squat with shoulder roll

Stretch: quadriceps, hip flexors, inner thigh, hamstrings, pectorals, upper back

▶ Shallow-Water Interval Lesson Plan 4

INTERVALS WITH REDUCED RECOVERY TIME 1

EQUIPMENT

None

TEACHING TIP

Interval training with reduced recovery time in the transition season is two minutes of work to one minute of recovery (2:1 ratio). The intensity level is 70 percent.

Level 7 (70 percent HR max)—Somewhat hard

WARM-UP

Instructor's choice

A SET

Knee-high jog

Kick forward

Jumping jacks

In-line skate

Cross-country ski

Work: Kick side to side, faster (60 seconds)

Jumping jacks, faster (60 seconds)

Recovery: In, in, out, out (30 seconds)

Run tires (30 seconds)

B SET

Knee-high jog, punch forward and side

Chorus-line kick

Jumping jacks with diagonal turn

Skate kick with pumping arms

Cross-country ski, two easy and one with power

C SET

Knee-high jog, push across and slice back

High kick

Jumping jacks, doubles

Knee lift and lunge R

Knee lift and lunge L

Cross-country ski, four easy and four with power

Work: Inner-thigh lift, faster (60 seconds)

Hopscotch, faster (60 seconds)

Recovery: In, in, out, out (30 seconds)

Run tires (30 seconds)

D SET

Knee-high jog with breaststroke

Kick forward with lat pull-down

Jumping jacks with arms out of the water

Skate kick with pumping arms

Cross-country ski, two easy and one with power

E SET

Knee-high jog, punch across

Crossover kick

Jumping jacks, syncopate

Kick and lunge R

Kick and lunge L

Cross-country ski, four easy and four with power

Work: Jumping jacks, suspended (60 seconds)

Frog, suspended (60 seconds)

Recovery: In, in, out, out (30 seconds)

Run tires (30 seconds)

F SET

Knee-high jog

Kick forward, neutral position, travel backward

Jumping jacks, neutral position, travel forward

In-line skate

Skip rope

COOL-DOWN

Straddle jog, clap hands

Squat, shoulder sweep out R and L, alternate

Squat, shoulder sweep in R and L, alternate

Squat, clap hands with power

Knee-high jog with crawl stroke

L lunge with R bowstring pull

R lunge with L bowstring pull

Lunge with standing row with power

Cross-country ski

Cross-country ski with R arm swing, L hand on hip

Cross-country ski with L arm swing, R hand on hip

Lunge with unison arm swing with power

Straddle jog, open and close doors

Squat, open and close R and L, alternate

Squat, open R, open L, close R, close L with power

Squat with forearm press

Squat, travel sideways R and L

Squat with shoulder roll

Stretch: quadriceps, hip flexors, inner thigh, hamstrings, pectorals, upper back

▶ Shallow-Water Interval Lesson Plan 4

INTERVALS WITH REDUCED RECOVERY TIME 1

PF

EQUIPMENT

None

TEACHING TIP

Interval training with reduced recovery time in the peak fitness season is 3 minutes of work to 90 seconds of recovery (2:1 ratio). The intensity level is 80 percent. Level 8 is high-intensity interval training (HIIT). For safety's sake, encourage your participants to modify the intensity to a level that is challenging for them rather than try to keep up with other participants.

Level 8 (80 percent HR max)—Hard

WARM-UP

Instructor's choice

A SET

Knee-high jog

Kick forward

Jumping jacks

In-line skate

Cross-country ski

B SET

Knee-high jog, punch forward and side

Chorus-line kick

Jumping jacks with diagonal turn

Skate kick with pumping arms

Cross-country ski, two easy and one with power

C SET

Knee-high jog, push across and slice back

High kick

Jumping jacks, doubles

Knee lift and lunge R

Knee lift and lunge L

Cross-country ski, four easy and four with power

D SET INTERVALS

Work: Kick side to side with power, grounded (60 seconds)

Inner-thigh lift with power (60 seconds)

Jacks cross with power, grounded (60 seconds)

Recovery: In, in, out, out (30 seconds)

Run tires (30 seconds)

Knee-high jog (30 seconds)

Work: Squat and power leg (60 seconds)

Hopscotch with power (60 seconds)

Frog jump (60 seconds)

Recovery: In, in, out, out (30 seconds)

Run tires (30 seconds)

Knee-high jog (30 seconds)

E SET

Knee-high jog with breaststroke

Kick forward with lat pull-down

Jumping jacks with arms out of the water

Skate kick with pumping arms

Cross-country ski, two easy and one with power

F SET

Knee-high jog, punch across

Crossover kick

Jacks cross

Kick and lunge R

Kick and lunge L

Cross-country ski, four easy and four with power

G SET

Knee-high jog

Kick forward, neutral position

Jumping jacks, neutral position

In-line skate

Skip rope

COOL-DOWN

Straddle jog, clap hands

Squat, shoulder sweep out R and L, alternate

Squat, shoulder sweep in R and L, alternate

Squat, clap hands with power

Knee-high jog with crawl stroke

L lunge with R bowstring pull

R lunge with L bowstring pull

Lunge with standing row with power

Cross-country ski

Cross-country ski with R arm swing, L hand on hip

Cross-country ski with L arm swing, R hand on hip

Lunge with unison arm swing with power

Straddle jog open and close doors

Squat, open and close R and L, alternate

Squat, open R, open L, close R, close L with power

Squat with forearm press

Squat, travel sideways R and L

Squat with shoulder roll

Stretch: quadriceps, hip flexors, inner thigh, hamstrings, pectorals, upper back

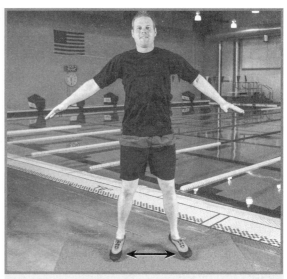

FIGURE 3.13 Jumping jacks.

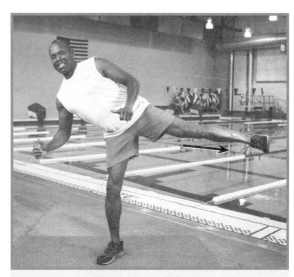

FIGURE 3.14 Side kick (karate).

▶ Shallow-Water Cardio Lesson Plan 5

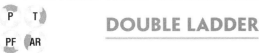

DOUBLE LADDER

EQUIPMENT

Noodles

TEACHING TIP

In a double ladder, two exercises, such as jumping jacks (see figure 3.13) and side kick (karate) (see figure 3.14), are paired. Perform each exercise for 10 seconds, then 20 seconds, and then 30 seconds, as if ascending a ladder. Next, descend the ladder, performing each exercise for 20 seconds and then 10 seconds. The third double ladder pairs rocking horse to the side with kick side to side. Perform the first rocking horse to the right side for 10 seconds, kick side to side for 10 seconds, perform rocking horse to the left side for 20 seconds, and so on, alternating sides. Each double ladder takes 3 minutes. This lesson plan concludes with some modified synchronized swimming just for fun.

WARM-UP

Instructor's choice

A SET

Kick forward

Crossover kick

Kick side to side

Heel jog

Skip rope

Cross-country ski

Double ladder: 10, 20, 30, 20, and 10 seconds
   Jumping jacks
   Side kick (karate)

B SET

Kick forward, doubles
Crossover kick, doubles, one low and one high
Jumping jacks
Hopscotch, doubles
Knee swing forward, back, forward, and down
Cross-country ski, doubles
Double ladder: 10, 20, 30, 20, and 10 seconds
   Front kick (karate)
   Cross-country ski

C SET

High kick
Skate kick, crossover kick, sweep out and center
Jacks cross
Hopscotch
Knee lift and lunge R
Knee lift and lunge L
Cross-country ski with rotation
Double ladder: 10, 20, 30, 20, and 10 seconds
   Rocking horse to the side
   Kick side to side

D SET

R leg kicks forward, neutral position
L leg kicks forward, neutral position
Crossover kick and sweep out, neutral position
Jacks tuck
Kick forward, suspended
Bicycle, suspended
Tuck ski
Walk backward and forward, hands on hips
Walk backward and forward with resistor arms
Knee-high jog in multiple directions, hands on hips

COOL-DOWN: MODIFIED SYNCHRONIZED SWIMMING

(Sit on a noodle as if riding a bicycle. The class is in a big circle. Count off A, B, A, B, and so on. If you have an odd number of class participants, you will need to participate so that no one is left out.)

Bicycle, travel clockwise around the circle
A's stand up and raise arms
Bicycle, travel counterclockwise around the circle

B's stand up and raise arms
Seated kick, travel toward the center of the circle
Seated leg press with propeller scull, travel backward
Seated row, travel toward the center of the circle
Seated flutter kick with propeller scull, travel backward
Bicycle with R hand in the center of the circle, travel clockwise around the circle
Mermaid, circle clockwise
Bicycle with L hand in the center of the circle, travel counterclockwise around the circle
Mermaid, circle counterclockwise
Stretch: hamstrings, outer thigh, quadriceps, hip flexors, gastrocnemius, ankles

▶ **Shallow-Water Interval Lesson Plan 5**

INTERVALS WITH REDUCED RECOVERY TIME 2

EQUIPMENT

Noodles

TEACHING TIP

Shallow-water cardio lesson plan 5 is modified to include interval training. The double ladder is dropped, and intervals using wall exercises are added. This is another lesson plan for intervals with reduced recovery time. In the preseason, this lesson plan involves 60 seconds of work to 30 seconds of recovery (2:1 ratio). Climbing the wall, pushing off the wall, and jumping on the wall for 60 seconds effectively gets the heart rate into the target zone.

WARM-UP

Instructor's choice

A SET

Kick forward
Crossover kick
Kick side to side
Heel jog
Skip rope
Cross-country ski
Intervals (at the wall)
   Work: Climb the wall, one foot on the wall and one on the floor (see figure 3.15)
      (60 seconds)
   Recovery: Knee-high jog (30 seconds)

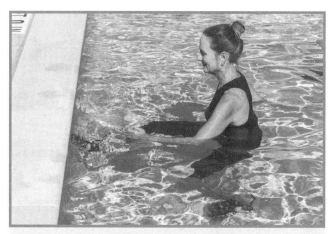

FIGURE 3.15 **One foot on the wall.**

Work: Climb the wall, both feet on the wall and down to the floor (60 seconds)

Recovery: Run tires (30 seconds)

B SET

Kick forward, doubles

Crossover kick, doubles, one low and one high

Jumping jacks

Hopscotch, doubles

Knee swing forward, back, forward and down

Cross-country ski, doubles

Intervals (at the wall)

Work: Push off the wall with both feet (see figure 3.16) and run back (60 seconds)

Recovery: Knee-high jog (30 seconds)

Work: Push off the wall with one foot (see figure 3.17), tuck, and breaststroke back (see figure 3.18) (60 seconds)

Recovery: Run tires (30 seconds)

C SET

High kick

Skate kick, crossover kick, sweep out and center

Jacks cross

Hopscotch

Knee lift and lunge R

Knee lift and lunge L

Cross-country ski with rotation

Intervals (at the wall)

Work: Jump back, jump forward, jump on the wall, and jump down (60 seconds)

Recovery: Knee-high jog (30 seconds)

Work: Jump and jump tuck, hands on the wall (60 seconds)

Recovery: Run tires (30 seconds)

D SET

R leg kicks forward, neutral position

L leg kicks forward, neutral position

Crossover kick and sweep out, neutral position

Jacks tuck

Kick forward, suspended

Bicycle, suspended

Tuck ski

Walk backward and forward, hands on hips

Walk backward and forward with resistor arms

Jog in multiple directions, hands on hips

COOL-DOWN: MODIFIED SYNCHRONIZED SWIMMING

(Sit on a noodle as if riding a bicycle. The class is in a big circle. Count off A, B, A, B, and so on. If you

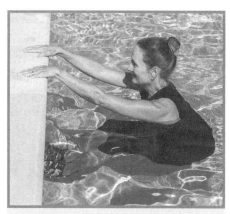

FIGURE 3.16 **Push off the wall with both feet.**

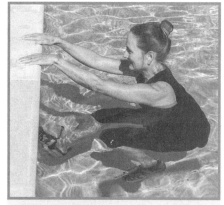

FIGURE 3.17 **Push off the wall with one foot.**

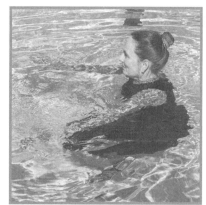

FIGURE 3.18 **Tuck and breaststroke.**

have an odd number of class participants, you will need to participate so that no one is left out.)

Bicycle, travel clockwise around the circle

A's stand up and raise arms

Bicycle, travel counterclockwise around the circle

B's stand up and raise arms

Seated kick, travel toward the center of the circle

Seated leg press with propeller scull, travel backward

Seated row, travel toward the center of the circle

Seated flutter kick with propeller scull, travel backward

Bicycle with R hand in the center of the circle, travel clockwise around the circle

Mermaid, circle clockwise

Bicycle with L hand in the center of the circle, travel counterclockwise around the circle

Mermaid, circle counterclockwise

Stretch: hamstrings, outer thigh, quadriceps, hip flexors, gastrocnemius, ankles

▶ **Shallow-Water Interval Lesson Plan 5**

INTERVALS WITH REDUCED RECOVERY TIME 2

EQUIPMENT
Noodles

TEACHING TIP
The same wall exercises used in the preseason are used in the transition season in this lesson plan, but the duration of the interval doubles from one minute to two minutes. The recovery period is one minute long (2:1 ratio). Climbing the wall, pushing off the wall, and jumping on the wall for two minutes effectively gets the heart rate into the target zone.

WARM-UP
Instructor's choice

A SET
Kick forward

Crossover kick

Kick side to side

Heel jog

Skip rope

Cross-country ski

B SET
Kick forward, doubles

Crossover kick, doubles, one low and one high

Jumping jacks

Hopscotch, doubles

Knee swing forward, back, forward and down

Cross-country ski, doubles

C SET
High kick

Skate kick, crossover kick, sweep out and center

Jacks cross

Hopscotch

Knee lift and lunge R

Knee lift and lunge L

Cross-country ski with rotation

D SET INTERVALS
(At the wall)

Work: Climb the wall, one foot on the wall and one on the floor (60 seconds)

Climb the wall, both feet on the wall and down to the floor (60 seconds)

Recovery: Knee-high jog (30 seconds)

Run tires (30 seconds)

Work: Push off the wall with both feet and run back (60 seconds)

Push off the wall with one foot, tuck, and breaststroke back (60 seconds)

Recovery: Knee-high jog (30 seconds)

Run tires (30 seconds)

Work: Jump back, jump forward, jump on the wall, and jump down
(60 seconds)

Jump and jump tuck, hands on the wall (60 seconds)

Recovery: Knee-high jog (30 seconds)

Run tires (30 seconds)

E SET
R leg kicks forward, neutral position

L leg kicks forward, neutral position

Crossover kick and sweep out, neutral position

Jacks tuck

Kick forward, suspended

Bicycle, suspended

Tuck ski

Walk backward and forward, hands on hips

Walk backward and forward with resistor arms

Jog in multiple directions, hands on hips

COOL-DOWN: MODIFIED SYNCHRONIZED SWIMMING

(Sit on a noodle as if riding a bicycle. The class is in a big circle. Count off A, B, A, B, and so on. If you have an odd number of class participants, you will need to participate so that no one is left out.)

Bicycle, travel clockwise around the circle

A's stand up and raise arms

Bicycle, travel counterclockwise around the circle

B's stand up and raise arms

Seated kick, travel toward the center of the circle

Seated leg press with propeller scull, travel backward

Seated row, travel toward the center of the circle

Seated flutter kick with propeller scull, travel backward

Bicycle with R hand in the center of the circle, travel clockwise around the circle

Mermaid, circle clockwise

Bicycle with L hand in the center of the circle, travel counterclockwise around the circle

Mermaid, circle counterclockwise

Stretch: hamstrings, outer thigh, quadriceps, hip flexors, gastrocnemius, ankles

▶ Shallow-Water Interval Lesson Plan 5

INTERVALS WITH REDUCED RECOVERY TIME 2

EQUIPMENT

Noodles

TEACHING TIP

The same wall exercises used in the preseason are used in the peak fitness season in this lesson plan, but the duration of the interval increases to 3 minutes. The recovery period is 90 seconds long (2:1 ratio). Climbing the wall, pushing off the wall, and jumping on the wall for 3 minutes effectively gets the heart rate into the target zone.

WARM-UP

Instructor's choice

A SET

Kick forward

Crossover kick

Kick side to side

Heel jog

Skip rope

Cross-country ski

B SET

Kick forward, doubles

Crossover kick, doubles, one low and one high

Jumping jacks

Hopscotch, doubles

Knee swing forward, back, forward and down

Cross-country ski, doubles

C SET

High kick

Skate kick, crossover kick, sweep out and center

Jacks cross

Hopscotch

Knee lift and lunge R

Knee lift and lunge L

Cross-country ski with rotation

D SET INTERVALS

(At the wall)

Work: Climb the wall, one foot on the wall and one on the floor (60 seconds)

Climb the wall, both feet on the wall and down to the floor (60 seconds)

Push off the wall with both feet and run back (60 seconds)

Recovery: Knee-high jog (30 seconds)

Run tires (30 seconds)

Heel jog (30 seconds)

Work: Push off the wall with one foot, tuck, and breaststroke back (60 seconds)

Jump back, jump forward, jump on the wall, and jump down (60 seconds)

Jump and jump tuck, hands on the wall (60 seconds)

Recovery: Knee-high jog (30 seconds)

Run tires (30 seconds)

Heel jog (30 seconds)

E SET

R leg kicks forward, neutral position

L leg kicks forward, neutral position

Crossover kick and sweep out, neutral position

Jacks tuck

Kick forward, suspended

Bicycle, suspended

Tuck ski

Walk backward and forward, hands on hips

Walk backward and forward with resistor arms

Jog in multiple directions, hands on hips

COOL-DOWN: MODIFIED SYNCHRONIZED SWIMMING

(Sit on a noodle as if riding a bicycle. The class is in a big circle. Count off A, B, A, B, and so on. If you have an odd number of class participants, you will need to participate so that no one is left out.)

Bicycle, travel clockwise around the circle

A's stand up and raise arms

Bicycle, travel counterclockwise around the circle

B's stand up and raise arms

Seated kick, travel toward the center of the circle

Seated leg press with propeller scull, travel backward

Seated row, travel toward the center of the circle

Seated flutter kick with propeller scull, travel backward

Bicycle with R hand in the center of the circle, travel clockwise around the circle

Mermaid, circle clockwise

Bicycle with L hand in the center of the circle, travel counterclockwise around the circle

Mermaid, circle counterclockwise

Stretch: hamstrings, outer thigh, quadriceps, hip flexors, gastrocnemius, ankles

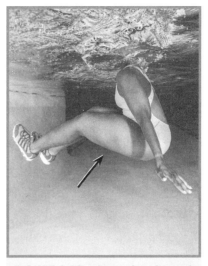

FIGURE 3.19 **Jump backward.**

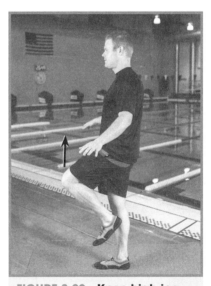

FIGURE 3.20 **Knee-high jog.**

▶ Shallow-Water Cardio Lesson Plan 6

ZIGZAG PATTERN

EQUIPMENT

None

TEACHING TIP

When you jump backward (see figure 3.19) and then knee-high jog (see figure 3.20) and travel forward in a zigzag pattern, you create a lot of turbulence, which adds to the intensity. To travel in a zigzag with jumping jacks in D set, travel sideways toward the left corner 4×, make a quarter turn, and travel sideways toward the right corner 4×.

WARM-UP

Instructor's choice

A SET

In, in, out, out

Jumping jacks

Jumping jacks with diagonal turn

Crossover kick

Tuck and hold with reverse breaststroke, travel backward

Knee-high jog, travel forward

Jump backward

Knee-high jog, travel in a zigzag

Skateboard R

Skateboard L

Kick forward
Kick forward, neutral position
Squat, R shoulder sweep out and in
Squat, L shoulder sweep out and in
Knee-high jog
Crab walk sideways

B SET

In, in, out, out
Jumping jacks
Jumping jacks with diagonal turn
Crossover kick, doubles, one low and one high
Tuck and hold with reverse breaststroke, travel backward
Run 3× and hurdle 1×, travel forward
Jump backward
Cross-country ski, travel in a zigzag
Skate kick
Cross-country ski
Cross-country ski, neutral position
R leg sweeps out and in, neutral position
L leg sweeps out and in, neutral position
Knee-high jog
Rocking horse to R side, travel sideways R
Rocking horse to L side, travel sideways L

C SET

In, in, out, out
Jumping jacks
Jumping jacks with diagonal turn
Crossover kick and sweep out
Tuck and hold with reverse breaststroke, travel backward
Leap forward
Jump backward
Bicycle, suspended, travel in a zigzag
Skateboard jump R
Skateboard jump L
Tuck ski
Cross-country ski, neutral position
Kick forward 3× and hold, one leg sweeps out and in 1×, neutral position
Knee-high jog
Run tires, travel sideways R and L

D SET

In, in, out, out
Jumping jacks

Jumping jacks with diagonal turn
Skate kick, crossover kick, sweep out and center
Tuck and hold with reverse breaststroke, travel backward
Jacks tuck with breaststroke, travel forward
Jump backward
Jumping jacks, travel in a zigzag
Frog jump
Jacks tuck
Jumping jacks, neutral position
Kick forward 3×, crossover kick 1×, neutral position
Knee-high jog
Squat, travel sideways R and L

COOL-DOWN

R leg kicks forward and back
L leg kicks forward and back
R leg kicks side and crosses midline
L leg kicks side and crosses midline
R knee swings forward and back
L knee swings forward and back
Clamshells R
Clamshells L
Lunge position with double-arm press-down
Lunge position with lat pull-down
Brace core, arms down, turbulent hand movements
Stand on R foot, arms sweep side to side
Stand on R foot, arms sweep side to side, eyes closed
Stand on L foot, turn head R and L
Stretch: upper back, lower back, hamstrings, outer thighs, quadriceps, hip flexors

▶ Shallow-Water Interval Lesson Plan 6

ROLLING INTERVALS

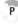

EQUIPMENT

None

TEACHING TIP

Shallow-water cardio lesson plan 6 is modified to include interval training. During rolling intervals an exercise is performed for one minute. It then rolls into a higher intensity level for one minute and finally rolls into an even higher intensity level for another minute. In the preseason, the intensity begins at level 5 and increases up to level 7.

Level 5 (50 percent HR max)—Somewhat easy

Level 6 (60 percent HR max)—Moderate

Level 7 (70 percent HR max)—Somewhat hard

WARM-UP

Instructor's choice

A SET

In, in, out, out

Jumping jacks

Jumping jacks with diagonal turn

Crossover kick

Tuck and hold with reverse breaststroke, travel backward

Knee-high jog, travel forward

Jump backward

Knee-high jog, travel in a zigzag

Work: Knee-high jog 50 percent (1 minute)

Steep climb 60 percent (1 minute)

Steep climb, faster 70 percent (1 minute)

Recovery: Straddle jog (1 minute)

R side quad kick (30 seconds)

L side quad kick (30 seconds)

B SET

In, in, out, out

Jumping jacks

Jumping jacks with diagonal turn

Crossover kick, doubles, one low and one high

Tuck and hold with reverse breaststroke, travel backward

Run 3× and hurdle 1×, travel forward

Jump backward

Cross-country ski, travel in a zigzag

Work: Rocking horse R 50 percent (30 seconds)

Rocking horse L 50 percent (30 seconds)

Cross-country ski, full ROM, neutral position 60 percent (1 minute)

Cross-country ski, suspended 70 percent (1 minute)

Recovery: Heel jog (1 minute)

Skateboard R (30 seconds)

Skateboard L (30 seconds)

C SET

In, in, out, out

Jumping jacks

Jumping jacks with diagonal turn

Crossover kick and sweep out

Tuck and hold with reverse breaststroke, travel backward

Leap forward

Jump backward

Bicycle, suspended, travel in a zigzag

Work: Kick forward 50 percent (1 minute)

Knee lift, straighten and power press-down 60 percent (1 minute)

High kick 70 percent (1 minute)

Recovery: Knee-high jog (1 minute)

R quad kick (30 seconds)

L quad kick (30 seconds)

D SET

In, in, out, out

Jumping jacks

Jumping jacks with diagonal turn

Skate kick, crossover kick, sweep out and center

Tuck and hold with reverse breaststroke, travel backward

Jacks tuck with breaststroke, travel forward

Jump backward

Jumping jacks, travel in a zigzag

Work: Jumping jacks 50 percent (1 minute)

Jacks cross 60 percent (1 minute)

Jumping jacks, suspended 70 percent (1 minute)

Recovery: Run tires (1 minute)

Log jump, side to side, neutral position (1 minute)

COOL-DOWN

R leg kicks forward and back

L leg kicks forward and back

R leg kicks side and crosses midline

L leg kicks side and crosses midline

R knee swings forward and back

L knee swings forward and back

Clamshells R

Clamshells L

Lunge position with double-arm press-down

Lunge position with lat pull-down

Brace core, arms down, turbulent hand movements

Stand on R foot, arms sweep side to side

Stand on R foot, arms sweep side to side, eyes closed

Stand on L foot, turn head R and L

Stretch: upper back, lower back, hamstrings, outer thighs, quadriceps, hip flexors

▶ **Shallow-Water Interval Lesson Plan 6**

ROLLING INTERVALS

EQUIPMENT

None

TEACHING TIP

During rolling intervals an exercise is performed for one minute. Then it rolls into a higher intensity level for one minute and finally rolls into an even higher intensity level for another minute. In the transition season, the intensity begins at level 6 and increases up to level 8. Level 8 is high-intensity interval training (HIIT). For safety's sake, encourage your participants to modify the intensity to a level that is challenging for them rather than try to keep up with other participants.

Level 6 (60 percent HR max)—Moderate

Level 7 (70 percent HR max)—Somewhat hard

Level 8 (80 percent HR max)—Hard

WARM-UP

Instructor's choice

A SET

In, in, out, out

Jumping jacks

Jumping jacks with diagonal turn

Crossover kick

Tuck and hold with reverse breaststroke, travel backward

Knee-high jog, travel forward

Jump backward

Knee-high jog, travel in a zigzag

Work: Steep climb 60 percent (1 minute)

Knee-high jog, faster 70 percent (1 minute)

Steep climb with power 80 percent (1 minute)

Recovery: Straddle jog (1 minute)

R side quad kick (30 seconds)

L side quad kick (30 seconds)

B SET

In, in, out, out

Jumping jacks

Jumping jacks with diagonal turn

Crossover kick, doubles, one low and one high

Tuck and hold with reverse breaststroke, travel backward

Run 3× and hurdle 1×, travel forward

Jump backward

Cross-country ski, travel in a zigzag

Work: Cross-country ski, full ROM, neutral position 60 percent (1 minute)

Cross-country ski, suspended 70 percent (1 minute)

Cross-country ski with power, neutral position 80 percent (1 minute)

Recovery: Heel jog (1 minute)

Rocking horse R (30 seconds)

Rocking horse L (30 seconds)

C SET

In, in, out, out

Jumping jacks

Jumping jacks with diagonal turn

Crossover kick and sweep out

Tuck and hold with reverse breaststroke, travel backward

Leap forward

Jump backward

Bicycle, suspended, travel in a zigzag

Work: Knee lift, straighten and power press-down 60 percent (1 minute)

High kick 70 percent (1 minute)

High kick power down 80 percent (1 minute)

Recovery: Knee-high jog (1 minute)

R quad kick (30 seconds)

L quad kick (30 seconds)

D SET

In, in, out, out

Jumping jacks

Jumping jacks with diagonal turn

Skate kick, crossover kick, sweep out and center

Tuck and hold with reverse breaststroke, travel backward

Jacks tuck with breaststroke, travel forward

Jump backward

Jumping jacks, travel in a zigzag

Work: Jacks cross 60 percent (1 minute)

Jumping jacks, faster 70 percent (1 minute)

Jacks cross with power, grounded 80 percent (1 minute)

Recovery: Run tires (1 minute)

  Log jump, side to side, neutral position (1 minute)

COOL-DOWN

R leg kicks forward and back

L leg kicks forward and back

R leg kicks side and crosses midline

L leg kicks side and crosses midline

R knee swings forward and back

L knee swings forward and back

Clamshells R

Clamshells L

Lunge position with double-arm press-down

Lunge position with lat pull-down

Brace core, arms down, turbulent hand movements

Stand on R foot, arms sweep side to side

Stand on R foot, arms sweep side to side, eyes closed

Stand on L foot, turn head R and L

Stretch: upper back, lower back, hamstrings, outer thighs, quadriceps, hip flexors

▶ Shallow-Water Interval Lesson Plan 6

ROLLING INTERVALS

EQUIPMENT

None

TEACHING TIP

During rolling intervals an exercise is performed for one minute. It then rolls into a higher intensity level for one minute and finally rolls into an even higher intensity level for another minute. In the peak fitness season, the intensity begins at level 7 and increases up to level 9. Levels 8 and 9 are high-intensity interval training (HIIT). For safety's sake, encourage your participants to modify the intensity to a level that is challenging for them rather than try to keep up with other participants.

  Level 7 (70 percent HR max)—Somewhat hard

  Level 8 (80 percent HR max)—Hard

  Level 9 (90 percent HR max)—Very hard

WARM-UP

Instructor's choice

A SET

In, in, out, out

Jumping jacks

Jumping jacks with diagonal turn

Crossover kick

Tuck and hold with reverse breaststroke, travel backward

Knee-high jog, travel forward

Jump backward

Knee-high jog, travel in a zigzag

B SET

In, in, out, out

Jumping jacks

Jumping jacks with diagonal turn

Crossover kick, doubles, one low and one high

Tuck and hold with reverse breaststroke, travel backward

Run 3× and hurdle 1×, travel forward

Jump backward

Cross-country ski, travel in a zigzag

C SET INTERVALS

Work: Knee-high jog, faster 70 percent (1 minute)

  Steep climb with power 80 percent (1 minute)

  Steep climb with power, faster 90 percent (1 minute)

Recovery: Straddle jog (1 minute)

  R side quad kick (30 seconds)

  L side quad kick (30 seconds)

Work: Cross-country ski, suspended 70 percent (1 minute)

  Cross-country ski with power, neutral position 80 percent (1 minute)

  Cross-country ski, arms sweep side to side 90 percent (1 minute)

Recovery: Heel jog (1 minute)

  Rocking horse R (30 seconds)

  Rocking horse L (30 seconds)

Work: High kick 70 percent (1 minute)

  High kick, power down 80 percent (1 minute)

  High kick with lat pull-down 90 percent (1 minute)

Recovery: Knee-high jog (1 minute)

  R quad kick (30 seconds)

  L quad kick (30 seconds)

Work: Jumping jacks, suspended 70 percent (1 minute)

  Jumping jacks with power, neutral position 80 percent (1 minute)

  Jumping jacks, land feet out only 90 percent (1 minute)

Recovery: Run tires (1 minute)

Log jump, side to side, neutral position (1 minute)

D SET

In, in, out, out

Jumping jacks

Jumping jacks with diagonal turn

Crossover kick and sweep out

Tuck and hold with reverse breaststroke, travel backward

Leap forward

Jump backward

Bicycle, suspended, travel in a zigzag

E SET

In, in, out, out

Jumping jacks

Jumping jacks with diagonal turn

Skate kick, crossover kick, sweep out and center

Tuck and hold with reverse breaststroke, travel backward

Jacks tuck with breaststroke, travel forward

Jump backward

Jumping jacks, travel in a zigzag

COOL-DOWN

R leg kicks forward and back

L leg kicks forward and back

R leg kicks side and crosses midline

L leg kicks side and crosses midline

R knee swings forward and back

L knee swings forward and back

Clamshells R

Clamshells L

Lunge position with double-arm press-down

Lunge position with lat pull-down

Brace core, arms down, turbulent hand movements

Stand on R foot, arms sweep side to side

Stand on R foot, arms sweep side to side, eyes closed

Stand on L foot, turn head R and L

Stretch: upper back, lower back, hamstrings, outer thighs, quadriceps, hip flexors

▶ Shallow-Water Cardio Lesson Plan 7

CARDIO WITH WALL EXERCISES

EQUIPMENT

None

TEACHING TIP

Take advantage of the pool wall for some of your exercises. Here are two options:

Climb wall, one foot on wall and one on floor (see figure 3.21)—begin with one foot on the wall and one foot on the floor and then switch feet, hopping from one foot on the wall to the other.

Climb wall, both feet on wall and down to floor (see figure 3.22*a* and *b*)—begin with both feet on the wall. Hop down to the floor, and back up to the wall.

The cool-down includes jumping jacks 2× and warrior II (see figures 3.23 and 3.24). Warrior II is a yoga

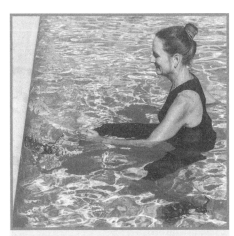

FIGURE 3.21 **One foot on the wall.**

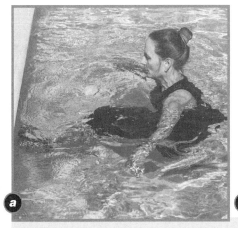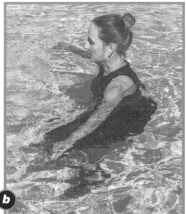

FIGURE 3.22 **(*a*) both feet on the wall, (*b*) down to the floor.**

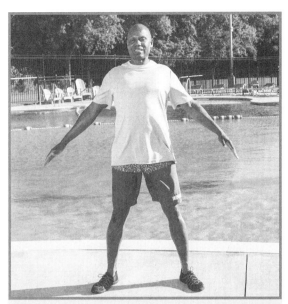

FIGURE 3.23 Jumping jacks.

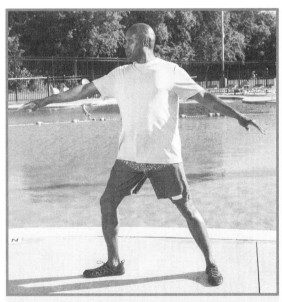

FIGURE 3.24 Warrior II.

pose that may be unfamiliar to some. Lunge to the side with arms extended side to side.

WARM-UP

Instructor's choice

A SET

Straddle jog, clap hands

Jumping jacks, clap hands

Inner-thigh lift

Jacks cross

Run to one side of the pool and back to the wall

Climb wall, one foot on wall and one on floor

Cross-country ski, travel backward

Knee-high jog, travel forward

Kick forward, travel backward

Knee-high jog, travel forward

Crossover kick

B SET

Straddle jog, palms touch in back

Jumping jacks, palms touch in back

Hopscotch

Jacks cross

Run to one side of the pool and back to the wall

Climb wall, both feet on wall and down to floor

Cross-country ski, clap hands, travel backward

Knee-high jog, travel forward

Kick forward, clap hands, travel backward

Knee-high jog, travel forward

Chorus-line kick

C SET

Straddle jog, open and close doors

Jumping jacks, open and close doors

Inner-thigh lift R and hopscotch L, alternate

Jacks cross

Run to one side of the pool and back to the wall

Climb wall, one foot on wall and one on floor

Cross-country ski with unison arm swing, travel backward

Knee-high jog, travel forward

Kick forward with unison arm swing, travel backward

Knee-high jog, travel forward

Crossover kick, doubles, one low and one high

D SET

Straddle jog with forearm press

Jumping jacks with forearm press

Inner-thigh lift L and hopscotch R, alternate

Jacks cross

Run to one side of the pool and back to the wall

Climb wall, both feet on wall and down to floor

Cross-country ski, push forward, travel backward

Knee-high jog, travel forward

Kick forward, push forward, travel backward

Knee-high jog, travel forward

Crossover kick and sweep out

COOL-DOWN

Tuck ski, neutral position

Tuck ski 3×, jumping jacks, suspended 1×

Jumping jacks 1×, kick forward 1×, neutral position

Frog jump, neutral position

Frog jump 2×, side extension 1×, alternate R and L

Side extension, tuck and down, alternate R and L

Side extension, tuck and down 2×, alternate R and L

Jacks tuck, neutral position

Jumping jacks squat

Jumping jacks 2× and warrior II

Stretch: lower back, hamstrings, inner thigh, hip flexors, gastrocnemius, shoulders

▶ Shallow-Water Interval Lesson Plan 7

SURGES 1

EQUIPMENT

None

TEACHING TIP

Shallow-water cardio lesson plan 7 is modified to include interval training. In a surge in the preseason, an interval is performed at level 6 for 45 seconds and then bumped up to level 7 for 15 seconds.

Level 6 (60 percent HR max)—Moderate

Level 7 (70 percent HR max)—Somewhat hard

WARM-UP

Instructor's choice

A SET

Straddle jog, clap hands

Jumping jacks, clap hands

Inner-thigh lift

Jacks cross

Run to one side of the pool and back to the wall

Climb wall, one foot on wall and one on floor

Work: Cross-country ski, full ROM 60 percent (45 seconds)

Cross-country ski, faster 70 percent (15 seconds)

Recovery: Knee-high jog (1 minute)

Work: Knee lift, straighten and power press-down 60 percent (45 seconds)

High kick 70 percent (15 seconds)

Recovery: Knee-high jog (1 minute)

Crossover kick

B SET

Straddle jog, palms touch in back

Jumping jacks, palms touch in back

Hopscotch

Jacks cross

Run to one side of the pool and back to the wall

Climb wall, both feet on wall and down to floor

Work: Run 60 percent (45 seconds)

Sprint 70 percent (15 seconds)

Recovery: Knee-high jog (1 minute)

Work: Bicycle, full ROM, suspended 60 percent (45 seconds)

Bicycle, faster, suspended 70 percent (15 seconds)

Recovery: Knee-high jog (1 minute)

Chorus-line kick

C SET

Straddle jog, open and close doors

Jumping jacks, open and close doors

Inner-thigh lift R and hopscotch L, alternate

Jacks cross

Run to one side of the pool and back to the wall

Climb wall, one foot on wall and one on floor

Work: Cross-country ski, full ROM 60 percent (45 seconds)

Cross-country ski, faster 70 percent (15 seconds)

Recovery: Knee-high jog (1 minute)

Work: Knee lift, straighten and power press-down 60 percent (45 seconds)

High kick 70 percent (15 seconds)

Recovery: Knee-high jog (1 minute)

Crossover kick, doubles, one low and one high

D SET

Straddle jog with forearm press

Jumping jacks with forearm press

Inner-thigh lift L and hopscotch R, alternate

Jacks cross

Run to one side of the pool and back to the wall

Climb wall, both feet on wall and down to floor

Work: Run 60 percent (45 seconds)

Sprint 70 percent (15 seconds)

Recovery: Knee-high jog (1 minute)

Work: Bicycle, full ROM, suspended 60 percent (45 seconds)

Bicycle, faster, suspended 70 percent (15 seconds)

Recovery: Knee-high jog (1 minute)

Crossover kick and sweep out

COOL-DOWN

Tuck ski, neutral position

Tuck ski 3×, jumping jacks, suspended 1×

Jumping jacks 1×, kick forward 1×, neutral position

Frog jump, neutral position

Frog jump 2×, side extension 1×, alternate R and L

Side extension, tuck and down, alternate R and L

Side extension, tuck and down 2×, alternate R and L

Jacks tuck, neutral position

Jumping jacks squat

Jumping jacks 2× and warrior II

Stretch: lower back, hamstrings, inner thigh, hip flexors, gastrocnemius, shoulders

▶ Shallow-Water Interval Lesson Plan 7

SURGES 1

EQUIPMENT

None

TEACHING TIP

In a surge in the transition season, an interval is performed at level 7 for 45 seconds and then bumped up to level 8 for 15 seconds. Level 8 is high-intensity interval training (HIIT). For safety's sake, encourage your participants to modify the intensity to a level that is challenging for them rather than try to keep up with other participants.

Level 7 (70 percent HR max)—Somewhat hard

Level 8 (80 percent HR max)—Hard

WARM-UP

Instructor's choice

A SET

Straddle jog, clap hands

Jumping jacks, clap hands

Inner-thigh lift

Jacks cross

Run to one side of the pool and back to the wall

Climb wall, one foot on wall and one on floor

Work: Cross-country ski, faster 70 percent (45 seconds)

Cross-country ski with rotation 80 percent (15 seconds)

Recovery: Knee-high jog (1 minute)

Work: High kick 70 percent (45 seconds)

High kick with power 80 percent (15 seconds)

Recovery: Knee-high jog (1 minute)

Crossover kick

B SET

Straddle jog, palms touch in back

Jumping jacks, palms touch in back

Hopscotch

Jacks cross

Run to one side of the pool and back to the wall

Climb wall, both feet on wall and down to floor

Work: Sprint 70 percent (45 seconds)

Power run 80 percent (15 seconds)

Recovery: Knee-high jog (1 minute)

Work: Bicycle, faster, suspended 70 percent (45 seconds)

Bicycle with power, suspended 80 percent (15 seconds)

Recovery: Knee-high jog (1 minute)

Chorus-line kick

C SET

Straddle jog, open and close doors

Jumping jacks, open and close doors

Inner-thigh lift R and hopscotch L, alternate

Jacks cross

Run to one side of the pool and back to the wall

Climb wall, one foot on wall and one on floor

Work: Cross-country ski, faster 70 percent (45 seconds)

Cross-country ski with rotation 80 percent (15 seconds)

Recovery: Knee-high jog (1 minute)

Work: High kick 70 percent (45 seconds)

High kick with power 80 percent (15 seconds)

Recovery: Knee-high jog (1 minute)

Crossover kick, doubles, one low and one high

D SET

Straddle jog with forearm press

Jumping jacks with forearm press

Inner-thigh lift L and hopscotch R, alternate

Jacks cross

Run to one side of the pool and back to the wall

Climb wall, both feet on wall and down to floor

Work: Sprint 70 percent (45 seconds)

   Power run 80 percent (15 seconds)

Recovery: Knee-high jog (1 minute)

Work: Bicycle, faster, suspended 70 percent (45 seconds)

   Bicycle with power, suspended 80 percent (15 seconds)

Recovery: Knee-high jog (1 minute)

Crossover kick and sweep out

COOL-DOWN

Tuck ski, neutral position

Tuck ski 3×, jumping jacks, suspended 1×

Jumping jacks 1×, kick forward 1×, neutral position

Frog jump, neutral position

Frog jump 2×, side extension 1×, alternate R and L

Side extension, tuck and down, alternate R and L

Side extension, tuck and down 2×, alternate R and L

Jacks tuck, neutral position

Jumping jacks squat

Jumping jacks 2× and warrior II

Stretch: lower back, hamstrings, inner thigh, hip flexors, gastrocnemius, shoulders

▶ Shallow-Water Interval Lesson Plan 7

SURGES 1

PF

EQUIPMENT

None

TEACHING TIP

In a surge in the peak fitness season, an interval is performed at level 8 for 45 seconds and then bumped up to level 9 for 15 seconds. Levels 8 and 9 are high-intensity interval training (HIIT). For safety's sake, encourage your participants to modify the intensity to a level that is challenging for them rather than try to keep up with other participants.

Level 8 (80 percent HR max)—Hard

Level 9 (90 percent HR max)—Very hard

WARM-UP

Instructor's choice

A SET

Straddle jog, clap hands

Jumping jacks, clap hands

Inner-thigh lift

Jacks cross

Run to one side of the pool and back to the wall

Climb wall, one foot on wall and one on floor

Crossover kick

B SET

Straddle jog, palms touch in back

Jumping jacks, palms touch in back

Hopscotch

Jacks cross

Run to one side of the pool and back to the wall

Climb wall, both feet on wall and down to floor

Chorus-line kick

C SET INTERVALS

Work: Cross-country ski with rotation 80 percent (45 seconds)

   Cross-country ski, arms sweep side to side 90 percent (15 seconds)

Recovery: Knee-high jog (1 minute)

Work: High kick with power 80 percent (45 seconds)

   High kick, clap over and under 90 percent (15 seconds)

Recovery: Knee-high jog (1 minute)

Work: Power run 80 percent (45 seconds)

   Skate kick with power, travel forward 90 percent (15 seconds)

Recovery: Knee-high jog (1 minute)

Work: Bicycle with power, suspended 80 percent (45 seconds)

   Frog jump with hands up 90 percent (15 seconds)

Recovery: Knee-high jog (1 minute)

Work: Cross-country ski with rotation 80 percent (45 seconds)

   Cross-country ski, arms sweep side to side 90 percent (15 seconds)

Recovery: Knee-high jog (1 minute)

Work: High kick with power 80 percent (45 seconds)

   High kick, clap over and under 90 percent (15 seconds)

Recovery: Knee-high jog (1 minute)

Work: Power run 80 percent (45 seconds)

Skate kick with power, travel forward 90 percent (15 seconds)

Recovery: Knee-high jog (1 minute)

Work: Bicycle with power, suspended 80 percent (45 seconds)

Frog jump with hands up 90 percent (15 seconds)

Recovery: Knee-high jog (1 minute)

D SET

Straddle jog, open and close doors

Jumping jacks, open and close doors

Inner-thigh lift R and hopscotch L, alternate

Jacks cross

Run to one side of the pool and back to the wall

Climb wall, one foot on wall and one on floor

Crossover kick, doubles, one low and one high

E SET

Straddle jog with forearm press

Jumping jacks with forearm press

Inner-thigh lift L and hopscotch R, alternate

Jacks cross

Run to one side of the pool and back to the wall

Climb wall, both feet on wall and down to floor

Crossover kick and sweep out

COOL-DOWN

Tuck ski, neutral position

Tuck ski 3×, jumping jacks, suspended 1×

Jumping jacks 1×, kick forward 1×, neutral position

Frog jump, neutral position

Frog jump 2×, side extension 1×, alternate R and L

Side extension, tuck and down, alternate R and L

Side extension, tuck and down 2×, alternate R and L

Jacks tuck, neutral position

Jumping jacks squat

Jumping jacks 2× and warrior II

Stretch: lower back, hamstrings, inner thigh, hip flexors, gastrocnemius, shoulders

▶ **Shallow-Water Cardio Lesson Plan 8**

CHANGES

EQUIPMENT

None

TEACHING TIP

Changes in the flow of exercises challenge core strength. Try performing an exercise 3× and then pausing or bouncing in the center. Use a single, single, double pattern. Perform one exercise 3× and then another exercise 1×. Figure 3.25 shows cross-country ski, tuck, diagonal turn, and center from B set.

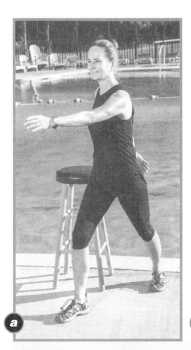 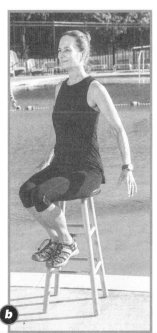 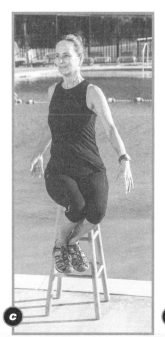 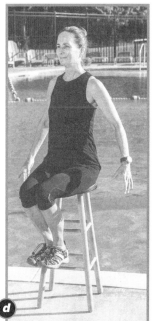

FIGURE 3.25 *(a)* **cross-country ski,** *(b)* **tuck,** *(c)* **diagonal turn,** *(d)* **center.**

WARM-UP

Instructor's choice

A SET

Knee-high jog with jog press

Run tires, reach side to side

Jumping jacks

Squat

Tuck and hold with reverse breaststroke, travel backward

Tuck and hold with breaststroke, travel forward

Cross-country ski, with R arm swing, L hand on hip

Knee-high jog with jog press

Run tires, reach side to side

Jumping jacks

Squat

Tuck and hold with reverse breaststroke, travel backward

Tuck and hold with breaststroke, travel forward

Cross-country ski with L arm swing, R hand on hip

Cross-country ski 3× and hold

Cross-country ski 3× and bounce center

Cross-country ski, neutral position

Tuck ski

Jacks tuck

Knee-high jog

B SET

Knee-high jog, punch forward and side

Run tires with hand waves

Jumping jacks with diagonal turn

Kick and squat

Jump backward

Frog jump, travel forward

Cross-country ski single, single, double

Knee-high jog, punch forward and side

Run tires with hand waves

Jumping jacks with diagonal turn

Kick and squat

Jump backward

Frog jump, travel forward

Cross-country ski single, single, double

Cross-country ski with rotation

Tuck ski with rotation

Cross-country ski, tuck, diagonal turn, and center

Jacks tuck

Knee-high jog

C SET

Knee-high jog with R bowstring pull

Run tires, clap hands

Jumping jacks with arms out of the water

Inner-thigh lift and squat

Jacks tuck with reverse breaststroke, travel backward

Jacks tuck with breaststroke, travel forward

Knee-high jog with L bowstring pull

Run tires, clap hands

Jumping jacks with arms out of the water

Inner-thigh lift and squat

Jacks tuck with reverse breaststroke, travel backward

Jacks tuck with breaststroke, travel forward

Cross-country ski, slow

Cross-country ski, slower

Cross-country ski, slowest with power

Cross-country ski 3×, suspended and touch center

Tuck ski 3×, jumping jacks, suspended 1×

Jacks tuck

Knee-high jog

COOL-DOWN

Skateboard R, hands on hips

Skateboard L, hands on hips

Tuck, mermaid, tuck, down and tuck, unison kick to the corners, tuck, down

Jumping jacks, neutral position

R side extension, tuck and down

L side extension, tuck and down

Fall forward, tuck, and stand

Stretch: hamstrings, hip flexors, quadriceps, gastrocnemius, outer thigh, shoulders

▶ **Shallow-Water Interval Lesson Plan 8**

SURGES 2

EQUIPMENT

None

TEACHING TIP

Shallow-water cardio lesson plan 8 is modified to include interval training. This is another lesson plan for intervals with surges. In a surge in the preseason, an interval is performed at level 6 for 45 seconds and then bumped up to level 7 for 15 seconds.

Level 6 (60 percent HR max)—Moderate

Level 7 (70 percent HR max)—Hard

WARM-UP

Instructor's choice

A SET

Knee-high jog with jog press

Run tires, reach side to side

Jumping jacks

Squat

Tuck and hold with reverse breaststroke, travel backward

Tuck and hold with breaststroke, travel forward

Cross-country ski with R arm swing, L hand on hip

Cross-country ski with L arm swing, R hand on hip

Cross-country ski 3× and hold

Cross-country ski 3× and bounce center

Cross-country ski, neutral position

Tuck ski

Jacks tuck

Knee-high jog

B SET INTERVALS

Work: Steep climb 60 percent (45 seconds)

Steep climb, faster 70 percent (15 seconds)

Recovery: Lunge position with standing row (45 seconds)

Deep lunge R (15 seconds)

Work: Cross-country ski, full ROM 60 percent (45 seconds)

Cross-country ski, faster 70 percent (15 seconds)

Recovery: Lunge position, clap hands (45 seconds)

Deep lunge L (15 seconds)

Work: Knee lift, straighten and power press-down 60 percent (45 seconds)

High kick 70 percent (15 seconds)

Recovery: Lunge position with lat pull-down (45 seconds)

Deep lunge R (15 seconds)

Work: Steep climb 60 percent (45 seconds)

Steep climb, faster 70 percent (15 seconds)

Recovery: Lunge position with arm curl (45 seconds)

Deep lunge L (15 seconds)

Work: Cross-country ski, full ROM 60 percent (45 seconds)

Cross-country ski, faster 70 percent (15 seconds)

Recovery: Lunge position with triceps extension (45 seconds)

Deep lunge R (15 seconds)

Work: Knee-lift, straighten and power press-down 60 percent (45 seconds)

High kick 70 percent (15 seconds)

Recovery: Lunge position with forearm press (45 seconds)

Deep lunge L (15 seconds)

C SET

Knee-high jog, punch forward and side

Run tires with hand waves

Jumping jacks with diagonal turn

Kick and squat

Jump backward

Frog jump, travel forward

Cross-country ski single, single, double

Cross-country ski with rotation

Tuck ski with rotation

Cross-country ski, tuck, diagonal turn, and center

Jacks tuck

Knee-high jog

D SET

Knee-high jog with R bowstring pull

Knee-high jog with L bowstring pull

Run tires, clap hands

Jumping jacks with arms out of the water

Inner-thigh lift and squat

Jacks tuck with reverse breaststroke, travel backward

Jacks tuck, with breaststroke travel forward

Cross-country ski, slow

Cross-country ski, slower

Cross-country ski, slowest with power

Cross-country ski 3×, suspended and touch center

Tuck ski 3×, jumping jacks, suspended 1×

Jacks tuck

Knee-high jog

COOL-DOWN

Skateboard R, hands on hips

Skateboard L, hands on hips

Tuck, mermaid, tuck, down and tuck, unison kick to the corners, tuck, down

Jumping jacks, neutral position

R side extension, tuck and down

L side extension, tuck and down

Fall forward, tuck, and stand

Stretch: hamstrings, hip flexors, quadriceps, gastrocnemius, outer thigh, shoulders

▶ Shallow-Water Interval Lesson Plan 8

SURGES 2

EQUIPMENT
None

TEACHING TIP
In a surge in the transition season, an interval is performed at level 7 for 45 seconds and then bumped up to level 8 for 15 seconds. Level 8 is high-intensity interval training (HIIT). For safety's sake, encourage your participants to modify the intensity to a level that is challenging for them rather than try to keep up with other participants.

Level 7 (70 percent HR max)—Somewhat hard

Level 8 (80 percent HR max)—Hard.

WARM-UP
Instructor's choice

A SET
Knee-high jog with jog press

Run tires, reach side to side

Jumping jacks

Squat

Tuck and hold with reverse breaststroke, travel backward

Tuck and hold with breaststroke, travel forward

Cross-country ski with R arm swing, L hand on hip

Cross-country ski with L arm swing, R hand on hip

Cross-country ski 3× and hold

Cross-country ski 3× and bounce center

Cross-country ski, neutral position

Tuck ski

Jacks tuck

Knee-high jog

B SET INTERVALS
Work: Steep climb, faster 70 percent (45 seconds)

Steep climb with power 80 percent (15 seconds)

Recovery: Lunge position with standing row (45 seconds)

Deep lunge R (15 seconds)

Work: Cross-country ski, faster 70 percent (45 seconds)

Cross-country ski with rotation 80 percent (15 seconds)

Recovery: Lunge position, clap hands (45 seconds)

Deep lunge L (15 seconds)

Work: High kick 70 percent (45 seconds)

Front kick (karate) 80 percent (15 seconds)

Recovery: Lunge position with lat pull-down (45 seconds)

Deep lunge R (15 seconds)

Work: Steep climb, faster 70 percent (45 seconds)

Steep climb with power 80 percent (15 seconds)

Recovery: Lunge position with arm curl (45 seconds)

Deep lunge L (15 seconds)

Work: Cross-country ski, faster 70 percent (45 seconds)

Cross-country ski with rotation 80 percent (15 seconds)

Recovery: Lunge position with triceps extension (45 seconds)

Deep lunge R (15 seconds)

Work: High kick 70 percent (45 seconds)

Front kick (karate) 80 percent (15 seconds)

Recovery: Lunge position with forearm press (45 seconds)

Deep lunge L (15 seconds)

C SET

Knee-high jog, punch forward and side

Run tires with hand waves

Jumping jacks with diagonal turn

Kick and squat

Jump backward

Frog jump, travel forward

Cross-country ski single, single, double

Cross-country ski with rotation

Tuck ski with rotation

Cross-country ski, tuck, diagonal turn, and center

Jacks tuck

Knee-high jog

D SET

Knee-high jog with R bowstring pull

Knee-high jog with L bowstring pull

Run tires, clap hands

Jumping jacks with arms out of the water

Inner-thigh lift and squat

Jacks tuck with reverse breaststroke, travel backward

Jacks tuck with breaststroke, travel forward

Cross-country ski, slow

Cross-country ski, slower

Cross-country ski, slowest with power

Cross-country ski 3×, suspended and touch center

Tuck ski 3×, jumping jacks, suspended 1×

Jacks tuck

Knee-high jog

COOL-DOWN

Skateboard R, hands on hips

Skateboard L, hands on hips

Tuck, mermaid, tuck, down and tuck, unison kick to the corners, tuck, down

Jumping jacks, neutral position

R side extension, tuck and down

L side extension, tuck and down

Fall forward, tuck, and stand

Stretch: hamstrings, hip flexors, quadriceps, gastrocnemius, outer thigh, shoulders

▶ Shallow-Water Interval Lesson Plan 8

SURGES 2

PF

EQUIPMENT

None

TEACHING TIP

In a surge in the peak fitness season, an interval is performed at level 8 for 45 seconds and then bumped up to level 9 for 15 seconds. Levels 8 and 9 are high-intensity interval training (HIIT). For safety's sake, encourage your participants to modify the intensity to a level that is challenging for them rather than try to keep up with other participants.

Level 8 (80 percent HR max)—Hard

Level 9 (90 percent HR max)—Very hard.

WARM-UP

Instructor's choice

A SET

Knee-high jog with jog press

Run tires, reach side to side

Jumping jacks

Squat

Tuck and hold with reverse breaststroke, travel backward

Tuck and hold with breaststroke, travel forward

Cross-country ski with R arm swing, L hand on hip

Cross-country ski with L arm swing, R hand on hip

Cross-country ski 3× and hold

Cross-country ski 3× and bounce center

Cross-country ski, neutral position

Tuck ski

Jacks tuck

Knee-high jog

B SET INTERVALS

Work: Steep climb with power 80 percent (45 seconds)

Steep climb with power, faster 90 percent (15 seconds)

Recovery: Lunge position with standing row (45 seconds)

Deep lunge R (15 seconds)

Work: Cross-country ski with rotation 80 percent (45 seconds)

Cross-country ski with rotation, hands together 90 percent (15 seconds)

Recovery: Lunge position, clap hands (45 seconds)

Deep lunge L (15 seconds)

Work: Front kick (karate) 80 percent (45 seconds)

Front kick (karate), faster 90 percent (15 seconds)

Recovery: Lunge position with lat pull-down (45 seconds)

Deep lunge R (15 seconds)

Work: Steep climb with power 80 percent (45 seconds)

Steep climb with power, faster 90 percent (15 seconds)

Recovery: Lunge position with arm curl (45 seconds)

Deep lunge L (15 seconds)

Work: Cross-country ski with rotation 80 percent (45 seconds)

Cross-country ski with rotation, hands together 90 percent (15 seconds)

Recovery: Lunge position with triceps extension (45 seconds)

Deep lunge R (15 seconds)

Work: Front kick (karate) 80 percent (45 seconds)

Front kick (karate), faster 90 percent (15 seconds)

Recovery: Lunge position with forearm press (45 seconds)

Deep lunge L (15 seconds)

C SET

Knee-high jog, punch forward and side

Run tires with hand waves

Jumping jacks with diagonal turn

Kick and squat

Jump backward

Frog jump, travel forward

Cross-country ski single, single, double

Cross-country ski with rotation

Tuck ski with rotation

Cross-country ski, tuck, diagonal turn, and center

Jacks tuck

Knee-high jog

D SET

Knee-high jog with R bowstring pull

Knee-high jog with L bowstring pull

Run tires, clap hands

Jumping jacks with arms out of the water

Inner-thigh lift and squat

Jacks tuck with reverse breaststroke, travel backward

Jacks tuck with breaststroke, travel forward

Cross-country ski, slow

Cross-country ski, slower

Cross-country ski, slowest with power

Cross-country ski 3×, suspended and touch center

Tuck ski 3×, jumping jacks, suspended 1×

Jacks tuck

Knee-high jog

COOL-DOWN

Skateboard R, hands on hips

Skateboard L, hands on hips

Tuck, mermaid, tuck, down and tuck, unison kick to the corners, tuck, down

Jumping jacks, neutral position

R side extension, tuck and down

L side extension, tuck and down

Fall forward, tuck, and stand

Stretch: hamstrings, hip flexors, quadriceps, gastrocnemius, outer thigh, shoulders

▶ Shallow-Water Cardio Lesson Plan 9

BLOCK CARDIO WITH SIX MOVES

EQUIPMENT

Noodles

TEACHING TIP

In block choreography you start with a set of basic moves and in each succeeding set you change something about each move. This lesson plan uses six basic moves—knee-high jog (see figure 3.26), run tires (see figure 3.27), jumping jacks (see figure 3.28), cross-country ski (see figure 3.29), kick forward (see figure 3.30), and heel jog (see figure 3.31). The moves are modified by adding arm exercises, traveling, alternating intensity variables, going into the neutral position

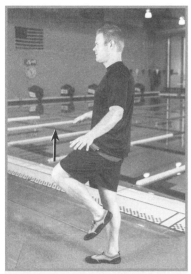

FIGURE 3.26 **Knee-high jog.**

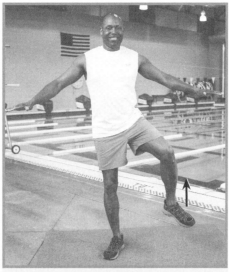

FIGURE 3.27 **Run tires.**

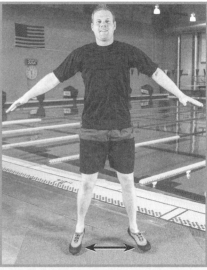

FIGURE 3.28 **Jumping jacks.**

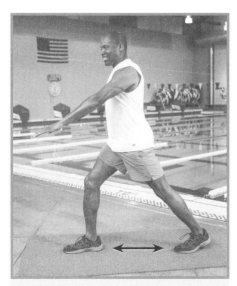

FIGURE 3.29 **Cross-country ski.**

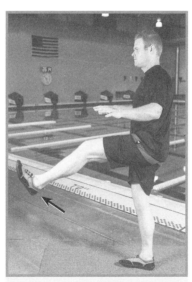

FIGURE 3.30 **Kick forward.**

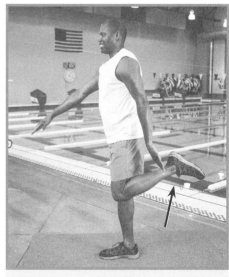

FIGURE 3.31 **Heel jog.**

or suspended, increasing the range of motion, crossing the midline, and combining the moves.

WARM-UP

Instructor's choice

A SET

Knee-high jog

Run tires

Jumping jacks

Cross-country ski

Kick forward

Heel jog

B SET

Knee-high jog with pumping arms

Run tires with shoulder blade squeeze

Jumping jacks, clap hands

Cross-country ski with windshield wiper arms

Kick forward with triceps extension

Heel jog with forearm press

C SET

Knee-high jog, travel backward

Run tires, travel forward

Jumping jacks, travel backward

Cross-country ski, travel forward

Kick forward, travel backward

Heel jog, travel forward

D SET

Knee-high jog, faster and knee-high jog, alternate

Run tires, faster and run tires, alternate

Jumping jacks with power, neutral position and jumping jacks, neutral position, alternate

Cross-country ski with power and cross-country ski, alternate

Kick and lunge R and kick forward, alternate

Kick and lunge L and kick forward, alternate

Knee lift and lunge R and heel jog, alternate

Knee lift and lunge L and heel jog, alternate

E SET

Hip curl, suspended

Frog jump, neutral position

Jumping jacks, suspended

Tuck ski, neutral position

Kick forward, suspended, emphasize quadriceps

Kick forward, suspended, emphasize hamstrings

F SET

Leap forward

Leap sideways

Jumping jacks with arms out of the water

Cross-country ski, full ROM

High kick

Skate kick

G SET

Crossover knees

Inner-thigh lift

Jacks cross

Cross-country ski with rotation

Crossover kick

Hopscotch

H SET

In, in, out, out

Cross-country ski 1×, jumping jacks 1×

R leg kicks forward and back

In, in, out, out

Cross-country ski 1×, jumping jacks 1×

L leg kicks forward and back

COOL-DOWN

(Sit on noodle like a swing)

Seated kick, arms to sides 70 degrees

Bicycle R leg

Bicycle L leg

Seated jacks, arms to sides 70 degrees

Point and flex feet

Seated kick, R shoulder sweep out, circle counterclockwise

Seated kick, L shoulder sweep out, circle clockwise

Hip hike

Stretch: quadriceps, hip flexors, hamstrings, outer thigh, inner thigh, pectorals

▶ Shallow-Water Interval Lesson Plan 9

RANDOM INTERVALS

EQUIPMENT

Noodles

TEACHING TIP

Shallow-water cardio lesson plan 9 is modified to include interval training. In random intervals, the timing and duration varies so that the exercise session seems unpredictable to the participant. This example features two sets of 30-second intervals, two sets of 45-second intervals, and a set of rolling intervals in which the intensity increases every 15 seconds from level 5 to level 8. Level 8 is high-intensity interval training (HIIT). For safety's sake, encourage your participants to modify the intensity to a level that is challenging for them rather than try to keep up with other participants.

Level 5 (50 percent HR max)—Somewhat easy

Level 6 (60 percent HR max)—Moderate

Level 7 (70 percent HR max)—Somewhat hard

Level 8 (80 percent HR max)—Hard

WARM-UP

Instructor's choice

A SET

Knee-high jog

Run tires

Jumping jacks

Cross-country ski

Kick forward

Heel jog

B SET

Knee-high jog with pumping arms

Run tires with shoulder blade squeeze

Jumping jacks, clap hands

Cross-country ski with windshield wiper arms

Kick forward with triceps extension

Heel jog with forearm press

C SET

Knee-high jog, travel backward

Run tires, travel forward

Jumping jacks, travel backward

Cross-country ski, travel forward

Kick forward, travel backward

Heel jog, travel forward

D SET INTERVALS

Work: Run 60 percent (30 seconds)

Recovery: Knee-high jog (30 seconds)

Work: Kick and lunge R 60 percent (45 seconds)

Recovery: Kick forward (45 seconds)

Rolling interval:

Work: Cross-country ski 50 percent (15 seconds)

Cross-country ski, full ROM 60 percent (15 seconds)

Cross-country ski, faster 70 percent (15 seconds)

Cross-country ski with rotation 80 percent (15 seconds)

Recovery: Heel jog (1 minute)

Work: Kick and lunge L 60 percent (45 seconds)

Recovery: Kick forward (45 seconds)

Work: Run 60 percent (30 seconds)

Recovery: Knee-high jog (30 seconds)

E SET

Hip curl, suspended

Frog jump, neutral position

Jumping jacks, suspended

Tuck ski, neutral position

Kick forward, suspended, emphasize quadriceps

Kick forward, suspended, emphasize hamstrings

F SET

Leap forward

Leap sideways

Jumping jacks with arms out of the water

Cross-country ski, full ROM

High kick

Skate kick

G SET

Crossover knees

Inner-thigh lift

Jacks cross

Cross-country ski with rotation

Crossover kick

Hopscotch

H SET

In, in, out, out

Cross-country ski 1×, jumping jacks 1×

R leg kicks forward and back

In, in, out, out

Cross-country ski 1×, jumping jacks 1×

L leg kicks forward and back

COOL-DOWN

(Sit on noodle like a swing)

Seated kick, arms to sides 70 degrees

Bicycle R leg

Bicycle L leg

Seated jacks, arms to sides 70 degrees

Point and flex feet

Seated kick, R shoulder sweep out, circle counterclockwise

Seated kick, L shoulder sweep out, circle clockwise

Hip hike

Stretch: quadriceps, hip flexors, hamstrings, outer thigh, inner thigh, pectorals

▶ Shallow-Water Interval Lesson Plan 9

RANDOM INTERVALS

EQUIPMENT

Noodles

TEACHING TIP

In random intervals, the timing and duration varies so that the exercise session seems unpredictable to the participant. This example features two sets of rolling intervals. In the first set the intensity increases every 15 seconds, and in the second set the intensity increases every 30 seconds from level 6 to level 9. The rolling intervals are separated by a three-set cycle of 30-second intervals and a four-set cycle of 15-second intervals. Levels 8 and 9 are high-intensity interval training (HIIT). For safety's sake, encourage your participants to modify the intensity to a level that is challenging for them rather than try to keep up with other participants.

    Level 6 (60 percent HR max)—Moderate
    Level 7 (70 percent HR max)—Somewhat hard
    Level 8 (80 percent HR max)—Hard.
    Level 9 (90 percent HR max)—Very hard

WARM-UP

Instructor's choice

A SET

    Knee-high jog
    Run tires
    Jumping jacks
    Cross-country ski
    Kick forward
    Heel jog

B SET

    Knee-high jog with pumping arms
    Run tires with shoulder blade squeeze
    Jumping jacks, clap hands
    Cross-country ski with windshield wiper arms
    Kick forward with triceps extension
    Heel jog with forearm press

C SET

    Knee-high jog, travel backward
    Run tires, travel forward
    Jumping jacks, travel backward
    Cross-country ski, travel forward
    Kick forward, travel backward
    Heel jog, travel forward

D SET INTERVALS

Rolling interval:
    Work: Run 60 percent (15 seconds)
        Sprint 70 percent (15 seconds)
        Power run 80 percent (15 seconds)
        Cross-country ski with power, travel forward 90 percent (15 seconds)
    Recovery: Knee-high jog (1 minute)

3 sets:
Work: Jumping jacks, suspended 70 percent (30 seconds)
Recovery: Jumping jacks, neutral position (30 seconds)
4 sets:
Work: High kick 70 percent (15 seconds)
Recovery: Kick forward (15 seconds)
Rolling interval:
    Work: Cross-country ski, full ROM 60 percent (30 seconds)
        Cross-country ski, faster 70 percent (30 seconds)
        Cross-country ski with rotation 80 percent (30 seconds)
        Cross-country ski with rotation, hands together 90 percent (30 seconds)
    Recovery: Heel jog (1 minute)

E SET

    Hip curl, suspended
    Frog jump, neutral position
    Jumping jacks, suspended
    Tuck ski, neutral position
    Kick forward, suspended, emphasize quadriceps
    Kick forward, suspended, emphasize hamstrings

F SET

    Leap forward
    Leap sideways
    Jumping jacks with arms out of the water
    Cross-country ski, full ROM
    High kick
    Skate kick

G SET

    Crossover knees
    Inner-thigh lift
    Jacks cross
    Cross-country ski with rotation
    Crossover kick
    Hopscotch

H SET

    In, in, out, out
    Cross-country ski 1×, jumping jacks 1×
    R leg kicks forward and back
    In, in, out, out

Cross-country ski 1×, jumping jacks 1×

L leg kicks forward and back

COOL-DOWN

(Sit on noodle like a swing)

Seated kick, arms to sides 70 degrees

Bicycle R leg

Bicycle L leg

Seated jacks, arms to sides 70 degrees

Point and flex feet

Seated kick, R shoulder sweep out, circle counterclockwise

Seated kick, L shoulder sweep out, circle clockwise

Hip hike

Stretch: quadriceps, hip flexors, hamstrings, outer thigh, inner thigh, pectorals

▶ Shallow-Water Interval Lesson Plan 9

RANDOM INTERVALS

EQUIPMENT

Noodles

TEACHING TIP

In random intervals, the timing and duration varies so that the exercise session seems unpredictable to the participant. This example features two sets of rolling intervals back to back. In the first set the intensity increases every 30 seconds, and in the second set the intensity increases every 15 seconds from level 6 to level 9. Next is a four-set cycle of 30-second intervals. Finish with a Tabata cycle. Levels 8 and 9 are high-intensity interval training (HIIT). For safety's sake, encourage your participants to modify the intensity to a level that is challenging for them rather than try to keep up with other participants.

Level 6 (60 percent HR max)—Moderate

Level 7 (70 percent HR max)—Somewhat hard

Level 8 (80 percent HR max)—Hard

Level 9 (90 percent HR max)—Very hard

WARM-UP

Instructor's choice

A SET

Knee-high jog

Run tires

Jumping jacks

Cross-country ski

Kick forward

Heel jog

B SET

Knee-high jog with pumping arms

Run tires with shoulder blade squeeze

Jumping jacks, clap hands

Cross-country ski with windshield wiper arms

Kick forward with triceps extension

Heel jog with forearm press

C SET

Knee-high jog, travel backward

Run tires, travel forward

Jumping jacks, travel backward

Cross-country ski, travel forward

Kick forward, travel backward

Heel jog, travel forward

D SET INTERVALS

Rolling interval:

Work: Cross-country ski, full ROM 60 percent (30 seconds)

Cross-country ski, faster 70 percent (30 seconds)

Cross-country ski with rotation 80 percent (30 seconds)

Cross-country ski with rotation, hands together 90 percent (30 seconds)

Recovery: Heel jog (1 minute)

Rolling interval:

Work: Run 60 percent (15 seconds)

Sprint 70 percent (15 seconds)

Power run 80 percent (15 seconds)

Cross-country ski with power, travel forward 90 percent (15 seconds)

Recovery: Rocking horse R (30 seconds)

Rocking horse L (30 seconds)

4 sets:

Work: Frog jump 80 percent (30 seconds)

Recovery: Jumping jacks (30 seconds)

Tabata 8 sets (4 minutes):

Work: High kick, clap over and under 90 percent (20 seconds)

Recovery: Rest

E SET

Hip curl, suspended

Frog jump, neutral position

Jumping jacks, suspended

Tuck ski, neutral position

Kick forward, suspended, emphasize quadriceps

Kick forward, suspended, emphasize hamstrings

F SET

Leap forward

Leap sideways

Jumping jacks with arms out of the water

Cross-country ski, full ROM

High kick

Skate kick

G SET

Crossover knees

Inner-thigh lift

Jacks cross

Cross-country ski with rotation

Crossover kick

Hopscotch

H SET

In, in, out, out

Cross-country ski 1×, jumping jacks 1×

R leg kicks forward and back

In, in, out, out

Cross-country ski 1×, jumping jacks 1×

L leg kicks forward and back

COOL-DOWN

(Sit on noodle like a swing)

Seated kick, arms to sides 70 degrees

Bicycle R leg

Bicycle L leg

Seated jacks, arms to sides 70 degrees

Point and flex feet

Seated kick, R shoulder sweep out, circle counterclockwise

Seated kick, L shoulder sweep out, circle clockwise

Hip hike

Stretch: quadriceps, hip flexors, hamstrings, outer thigh, inner thigh, pectorals

▶ Shallow-Water Cardio Lesson Plan 10

LAYER TECHNIQUE

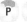

EQUIPMENT

Noodles

TEACHING TIP

The layer technique is a type of choreography in which you start with base moves and then repeat all the moves except one. That move is replaced with a different exercise. This lesson plan accelerates the layering process. The base moves are introduced in the warm-up. The first set repeats all of the base moves and then adds a variation. The second set repeats the variations, adds a new variation, and so on. Each succeeding variation is a little more complex than the previous one. Jumping jacks squat, hopscotch, and heel jog do not get new variations because they are transition moves that allow you to move smoothly from the previous exercise to the succeeding one. Two moves that may be new to participants are kayak row (see figure 3.32) and a suspended move, in which you hold one leg up and the other leg kicks forward and sweeps out (see figure 3.33).

WARM-UP

Jumping jacks squat

Jumping jacks

Inner-thigh lift

Hopscotch

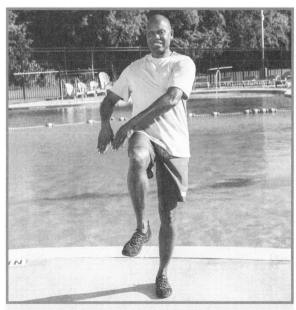

FIGURE 3.32 **Kayak row.**

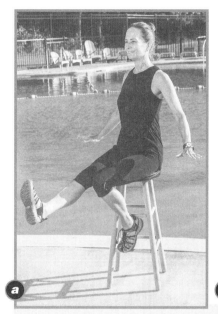 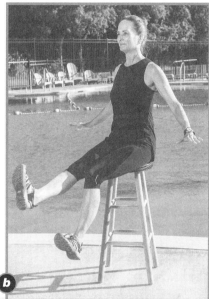 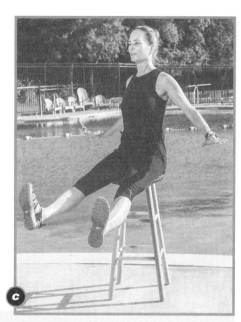

FIGURE 3.33 (*a*) hold R leg up, (*b*) L leg kicks forward and (*c*) sweeps out, suspended.

Heel jog
Cross-country ski
Knee-high jog
Kick forward

A SET

Jumping jacks squat
Jumping jacks
Jumping jacks 1×, kick forward 1×
Inner-thigh lift
Inner-thigh lift R
Inner-thigh lift L
Hopscotch
Heel jog
Cross-country ski
Cross-country ski 3× and hold
Knee-high jog
Knee-high jog 3× and hold
Kick forward
Kick forward, neutral position

B SET

Jumping jacks squat
Jumping jacks 1×, kick forward 1×
Jumping jacks 1×, skate kick 1×
Inner-thigh lift R
Inner-thigh lift L

Inner-thigh lift, doubles
Hopscotch
Heel jog
Cross-country ski 3× and hold
Cross-country ski 2× and cross-country ski with
    power 1×
Knee-high jog 3× and hold
Knee-high jog 3× and hold with kayak row
Kick forward, neutral position
Hold R leg up, L leg kicks forward, suspended
Hold L leg up, R leg kicks forward, suspended

C SET

Jumping jacks squat
Jumping jacks 1×, skate kick 1×
Jumping jacks 2×, jumping jacks, doubles 1×
Inner-thigh lift, doubles
Inner-thigh lift R and hopscotch L, alternate
Inner-thigh lift L and hopscotch R, alternate
Hopscotch
Heel jog
Cross-country ski 2× and cross-country ski with
    power 1×
Cross-country ski with lat pull-down
Knee-high jog 3× and hold with kayak row
Tuck and down
Hold R leg up, L leg kicks forward, suspended

Hold L leg up, R leg kicks forward, suspended

Hold R leg up, L leg kicks forward 3× suspended and down

Hold L leg up, R leg kicks forward 3× suspended and down

D SET

Jumping jacks squat

Jumping jacks 2×, jumping jacks doubles 1×

Jumping jacks 2×, warrior II

Inner-thigh lift R and hopscotch L, alternate

Inner-thigh lift L and hopscotch R, alternate

Inner-thigh lift 1×, hopscotch 1×

Hopscotch

Heel jog

Cross-country ski with lat pull-down

Cross-country ski, tuck, diagonal turn, and center

Tuck and down

Tuck and down 2× and tuck and pike 2×

Hold R leg up, L leg kicks forward 3× suspended and down

Hold L leg up, R leg kicks forward 3× suspended and down

Hold R leg up, L leg kicks forward and sweeps out, suspended

Hold L leg up, R leg kicks forward and sweeps out, suspended

COOL-DOWN

(Noodle in hands)

Rocking horse R, plunge noodle in front

Rocking horse to R side, scoop noodle out, L hand on hip

Lateral flexion R

Rocking horse L, plunge noodle in front

Rocking horse to L side, scoop noodle out, R hand on hip

Lateral flexion L

Lower-body twist

Knee lift and lunge R

Knee lift and lunge L

Cross-country ski, noodle in R hand

Cross-country ski, noodle in L hand

(Foot on a noodle)

Standing leg press R

Standing leg press to R side

Standing leg press L

Standing leg press to L side

(Noodle in hands)

Stand on one foot, hold noodle overhead in a rainbow

Stretch: latissimus dorsi, upper back, hip flexors, gastrocnemius, hamstrings, inner thigh

▶ Shallow-Water Interval Lesson Plan 10

PYRAMID

EQUIPMENT

Noodles

TEACHING TIP

Shallow-water cardio lesson plan 10 is modified to include interval training. In pyramid intervals in the preseason, the work time increases by 5 seconds in each set, but the recovery time stays at 45 seconds. The intensity level is 60 percent.

Level 6 (60 percent HR max)—Moderate

WARM-UP

Jumping jacks squat

Jumping jacks

Inner-thigh lift

Hopscotch

Heel jog

Cross-country ski

Knee-high jog

Kick forward

A SET

Jumping jacks squat

Jumping jacks

Jumping jacks 1×, kick forward 1×

Inner-thigh lift

Inner-thigh lift R

Inner-thigh lift L

Hopscotch

Heel jog

Cross-country ski

Cross-country ski 3× and hold

Knee-high jog

Knee-high jog 3× and hold

Kick forward

Kick forward, neutral position

B SET INTERVALS

Work: Kick side to side, arms and legs opposite (15 seconds)

Recovery: Knee-high jog (45 seconds)

Work: Kick side to side, arms and legs opposite (20 seconds)

Recovery: Straddle jog (45 seconds)

Work: Kick side to side, arms and legs opposite (25 seconds)

Recovery: Run tires (45 seconds)

Work: Kick side to side, arms and legs opposite (30 seconds)

Recovery: Heel jog (45 seconds)

C SET

Jumping jacks squat

Jumping jacks 1×, kick forward 1×

Jumping jacks 1×, skate kick 1×

Inner-thigh lift R

Inner-thigh lift L

Inner-thigh lift, doubles

Hopscotch

Heel jog

Cross-country ski 3× and hold

Cross-country ski 2× and cross-country ski with power 1×

Knee-high jog 3× and hold

Knee-high jog 3× and hold with kayak row

Kick forward, neutral position

Hold R leg up, L leg kicks forward, suspended

Hold L leg up, R leg kicks forward, suspended

D SET INTERVALS

Work: Jacks cross (15 seconds)

Recovery: Knee-high jog (45 seconds)

Work: Jacks cross (20 seconds)

Recovery: Straddle jog (45 seconds)

Work: Jacks cross (25 seconds)

Recovery: Run tires (45 seconds)

Work: Jacks cross (30 seconds)

Recovery: Heel jog (45 seconds)

E SET

Jumping jacks squat

Jumping jacks 1×, skate kick 1×

Jumping jacks 2×, jumping jacks, doubles 1×

Inner-thigh lift, doubles

Inner-thigh lift R and hopscotch L, alternate

Inner-thigh lift L and hopscotch R, alternate

Hopscotch

Heel jog

Cross-country ski 2× and cross-country ski with power 1×

Cross-country ski with lat pull-down

Knee-high jog 3× and hold with kayak row

Tuck and hold

Hold R leg up, L leg kicks forward, suspended

Hold L leg up, R leg kicks forward, suspended

Hold R leg up, L leg kicks forward 3× suspended and down

Hold L leg up, R leg kicks forward 3× suspended and down

COOL-DOWN

(Noodle in hands)

Rocking horse R, plunge noodle in front

Rocking horse to R side, scoop noodle out, L hand on hip

Lateral flexion R

Rocking horse L, plunge noodle in front

Rocking horse to L side, scoop noodle out, R hand on hip

Lateral flexion L

Lower-body twist

Knee lift and lunge R

Knee lift and lunge L

Cross-country ski, noodle in R hand

Cross-country ski, noodle in L hand

(Foot on a noodle)

Standing leg press R

Standing leg press to R side

Standing leg press L

Standing leg press to L side

(Noodle in hands)

Stand on one foot, hold noodle overhead in a rainbow

Stretch: latissimus dorsi, upper back, hip flexors, gastrocnemius, hamstrings, inner thigh

▶ **Shallow-Water Interval Lesson Plan 10**

PYRAMID

EQUIPMENT

Noodles

TEACHING TIP

In pyramid intervals in the transition season, the work time increases by 5 seconds in each set, but the recovery time stays at 30 seconds. The intensity level is 70 percent.

Level 7 (70 percent HR max)—Somewhat hard

WARM-UP

Jumping jacks squat
Jumping jacks
Inner-thigh lift
Hopscotch
Heel jog
Cross-country ski
Knee-high jog
Kick forward

A SET

Jumping jacks squat
Jumping jacks
Jumping jacks 1×, kick forward 1×
Inner-thigh lift
Inner-thigh lift R
Inner-thigh lift L
Hopscotch
Heel jog
Cross-country ski
Cross-country ski 3× and hold
Knee-high jog
Knee-high jog 3× and hold
Kick forward
Kick forward, neutral position

B SET INTERVALS

Work: Kick side to side, faster (15 seconds)
Recovery: Knee-high jog (30 seconds)
Work: Kick side to side, faster (20 seconds)
Recovery: Straddle jog (30 seconds)
Work: Kick side to side, faster (25 seconds)
Recovery: Run tires (30 seconds)
Work: Kick side to side, faster (30 seconds)
Recovery: Heel jog (30 seconds)

C SET

Jumping jacks squat
Jumping jacks 1×, kick forward 1×
Jumping jacks 1×, skate kick 1×
Inner-thigh lift R

Inner-thigh lift L
Inner-thigh lift, doubles
Hopscotch
Heel jog
Cross-country ski 3× and hold
Cross-country ski 2× and cross-country ski with power 1×
Knee-high jog 3× and hold
Knee-high jog 3× and hold with kayak row
Kick forward, neutral position
Hold R leg up, L leg kicks forward, suspended
Hold L leg up, R leg kicks forward, suspended

D SET INTERVALS

Work: Frog, suspended (15 seconds)
Recovery: Knee-high jog (30 seconds)
Work: Frog, suspended (20 seconds)
Recovery: Straddle jog (30 seconds)
Work: Frog, suspended (25 seconds)
Recovery: Run tires (30 seconds)
Work: Frog, suspended (30 seconds)
Recovery: Heel jog (30 seconds)

E SET

Jumping jacks squat
Jumping jacks 1×, skate kick 1×
Jumping jacks 2×, jumping jacks doubles 1×
Inner-thigh lift, doubles
Inner-thigh lift R and hopscotch L, alternate
Inner-thigh lift L and hopscotch R, alternate
Hopscotch
Heel jog
Cross-country ski 2× and cross-country ski with power 1×
Cross-country ski with lat pull-down
Knee-high jog 3× and hold with kayak row
Tuck and hold
Hold R leg up, L leg kicks forward, suspended
Hold L leg up, R leg kicks forward, suspended
Hold R leg up, L leg kicks forward 3× suspended and down
Hold L leg up, R leg kicks forward 3× suspended and down

F SET INTERVALS

Work: Jumping jacks, suspended (15 seconds)
Recovery: Knee-high jog (30 seconds)

Work: Jumping jacks, suspended (20 seconds)

Recovery: Straddle jog (30 seconds)

Work: Jumping jacks, suspended (25 seconds)

Recovery: Run tires (30 seconds)

Work: Jumping jacks, suspended (30 seconds)

Recovery: Heel jog (30 seconds)

COOL-DOWN

(Noodle in hands)

Rocking horse R, plunge noodle in front

Rocking horse to R side, scoop noodle out, L hand on hip

Lateral flexion R

Rocking horse L, plunge noodle in front

Rocking horse to L side, scoop noodle out, R hand on hip

Lateral flexion L

Lower-body twist

Knee lift and lunge R

Knee lift and lunge L

Cross-country ski, noodle in R hand

Cross-country ski, noodle in L hand

(Foot on a noodle)

Standing leg press R

Standing leg press to R side

Standing leg press L

Standing leg press to L side

(Noodle in hands)

Stand on one foot, hold noodle overhead in a rainbow

Stretch: latissimus dorsi, upper back, hip flexors, gastrocnemius, hamstrings, inner thigh

▶ Shallow-Water Interval Lesson Plan 10

PYRAMID

EQUIPMENT

Noodles

TEACHING TIP

In pyramid intervals in the peak fitness season, the work time increases by 5 seconds in each set, but the recovery time stays at 15 seconds. The intensity level is 80 percent. Level 8 is high-intensity interval training (HIIT). For safety's sake, encourage your participants to modify the intensity to a level that is challenging for them rather than try to keep up with other participants.

Level 8 (80 percent HR max)—Hard

WARM-UP

Jumping jacks squat

Jumping jacks

Inner-thigh lift

Hopscotch

Heel jog

Cross-country ski

Knee-high jog

Kick forward

A SET

Jumping jacks squat

Jumping jacks

Jumping jacks 1×, kick forward 1×

Inner-thigh lift

Inner-thigh lift R

Inner-thigh lift L

Hopscotch

Heel jog

Cross-country ski

Cross-country ski 3× and hold

Knee-high jog

Knee-high jog 3× and hold

Kick forward

Kick forward, neutral position

B SET INTERVALS

Work: Kick side to side with power, grounded (15 seconds)

Recovery: Knee-high jog (15 seconds)

Work: Kick side to side with power, grounded (20 seconds)

Recovery: Straddle jog (15 seconds)

Work: Kick side to side with power, grounded (25 seconds)

Recovery: Run tires (15 seconds)

Work: Kick side to side with power, grounded (30 seconds)

Recovery: Heel jog (15 seconds)

Work: Squat and power leg (15 seconds)

Recovery: Knee-high jog (15 seconds)

Work: Squat and power leg (20 seconds)

Recovery: Straddle jog (15 seconds)

Work: Squat and power leg (25 seconds)

Recovery: Run tires (15 seconds)

Work: Squat and power leg (30 seconds)

Recovery: Heel jog (15 seconds)

C SET

Jumping jacks squat

Jumping jacks 1×, kick forward 1×

Jumping jacks 1×, skate kick 1×

Inner-thigh lift R

Inner-thigh lift L

Inner-thigh lift, doubles

Hopscotch

Heel jog

Cross-country ski 3× and hold

Cross-country ski 2× and cross-country ski with power 1×

Knee-high jog 3× and hold

Knee-high jog 3× and hold with kayak row

Kick forward, neutral position

Hold R leg up, L leg kicks forward, suspended

Hold L leg up, R leg kicks forward, suspended

D SET INTERVALS

Work: Jacks cross with power, grounded (15 seconds)

Recovery: Knee-high jog (15 seconds)

Work: Jacks cross with power, grounded (20 seconds)

Recovery: Straddle jog (15 seconds)

Work: Jacks cross with power, grounded (25 seconds)

Recovery: Run tires (15 seconds)

Work: Jacks cross with power, grounded (30 seconds)

Recovery: Heel jog (15 seconds)

Work: R side kick (karate) (15 seconds)

Recovery: Knee-high jog (15 seconds)

Work: L side kick (karate) (20 seconds)

Recovery: Straddle jog (15 seconds)

Work: L side kick (karate) (25 seconds)

Recovery: Run tires (15 seconds)

Work: R side kick (karate) (30 seconds)

Recovery: Heel jog (15 seconds)

E SET

Jumping jacks squat

Jumping jacks 1×, skate kick 1×

Jumping jacks 2×, jumping jacks, doubles 1×

Inner-thigh lift, doubles

Inner-thigh lift R and hopscotch L, alternate

Inner-thigh lift L and hopscotch R, alternate

Hopscotch

Heel jog

Cross-country ski 2× and cross-country ski with power 1×

Cross-country ski with lat pull-down

Knee-high jog 3× and hold with kayak row

Tuck and hold

Hold R leg up, L leg kicks forward, suspended

Hold L leg up, R leg kicks forward, suspended

Hold R leg up, L leg kicks forward 3× suspended and down

Hold L leg up, R leg kicks forward 3× suspended and down

COOL-DOWN

(Noodle in hands)

Rocking horse R, plunge noodle in front

Rocking horse to R side, scoop noodle out, L hand on hip

Lateral flexion R

Rocking horse L, plunge noodle in front

Rocking horse to L side, scoop noodle out, R hand on hip

Lateral flexion L

Lower-body twist

Knee lift and lunge R

Knee lift and lunge L

Cross-country ski, noodle in R hand

Cross-country ski, noodle in L hand

(Foot on a noodle)

Standing leg press R

Standing leg press to R side

Standing leg press L

Standing leg press to L side

(Noodle in hands)

Stand on one foot, hold noodle overhead in a rainbow

Stretch: latissimus dorsi, upper back, hip flexors, gastrocnemius, hamstrings, inner thigh

▶ Shallow-Water Cardio Lesson Plan 11

TABATA TIMING 1   P   T

                                  PF AR

EQUIPMENT

None

TEACHING TIP

This lesson plan uses Tabata Timing for cardiorespiratory training. Each set begins with some basic exercises, knee-high jog (see figure 3.34), straddle jog (see figure 3.35), rocking horse (see figure 3.36), and heel jog (see figure 3.37), using a variety of arm moves. Travel and stationary exercises alternate. At the end of each set is a Tabata Timing cycle in which two exercises are paired. One is more difficult because it is a longer-lever move or because it is performed faster. Have the participants do this exercise for 20 seconds and the easier exercise for 10 seconds, repeating the set eight times. This lesson plan concludes with a game called You Be the Teacher just for fun.

WARM-UP

Instructor's choice

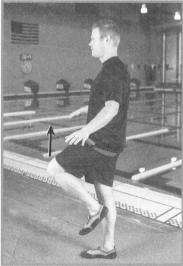

FIGURE 3.34 **Knee-high jog.**

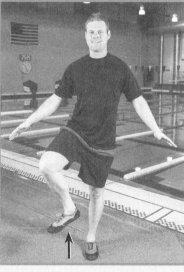

FIGURE 3.35 **Straddle jog.**

FIGURE 3.36 **Rocking horse.**

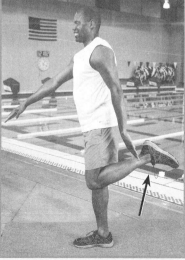

FIGURE 3.37 **Heel jog.**

A SET

Knee-high jog, push forward, travel backward

Straddle jog, clap hands

Knee-high jog, hands cupped, travel forward

Straddle jog with shoulder blade squeeze

Knee-high jog, push forward, travel backward

Straddle jog, clap hands

Knee-high jog, hands cupped, travel forward

Straddle jog with shoulder blade squeeze

Tabata 8 sets (4 minutes):

Cross-country ski (20 seconds)

In-line skate (10 seconds)

B SET

Straddle jog with reverse breaststroke, travel backward

Rocking horse R with shoulder blade squeeze

Straddle jog with breaststroke, travel forward

Rocking horse L with arm curl

Straddle jog with reverse breaststroke, travel backward

Rocking horse L with shoulder blade squeeze

Straddle jog with breaststroke, travel forward

Rocking horse R with arm curl

Tabata 8 sets (4 minutes):

Kick forward (20 seconds)

Squat (10 seconds)

C SET

Heel jog with unison arm swing, travel backward

Jumping jacks with bowstring pull to R side

Heel jog with triceps kick back, travel forward

Jumping jacks with bowstring pull to L side

Heel jog with unison arm swing, travel backward

Jumping jacks with bowstring pull to R side

Heel jog with triceps kick back, travel forward

Jumping jacks with bowstring pull to L side

Tabata 8 sets (4 minutes):

    Jacks tuck (20 seconds)

    Run tires (10 seconds)

D SET

    Rocking horse R, travel backward

    Heel jog with forearm press

    Rocking horse L, travel forward

    Hitchhike

    Rocking horse L, travel backward

    Heel jog with forearm press

    Rocking horse R, travel forward

    Hitchhike

Tabata 8 sets (4 minutes):

    Cross-country ski (20 seconds)

    In-line skate (10 seconds)

COOL-DOWN: YOU BE THE TEACHER

(The class is in a big circle)

Ask one participant to lead the class in his or her favorite exercise. Then go around the circle until everyone has had a turn. Allow any participant who does not wish to lead an exercise to pass.

    Stretch: hip flexors, quadriceps, gastrocnemius, outer thigh, hamstrings, lower back

▶ Shallow-Water Interval Lesson Plan 11

TABATA TIMING 1

EQUIPMENT

None

TEACHING TIP

Shallow-water cardio lesson plan 11 is modified to include interval training. In Tabata Timing during the preseason, the work phase is performed at level 7. During the recovery, the participant stands in place for 10 seconds to rest.

    Level 7 (70 percent HR max)—Somewhat hard

WARM-UP

Instructor's choice

A SET

    Knee-high jog, push forward, travel backward

    Straddle jog, clap hands

    Knee-high jog, hands cupped, travel forward

    Straddle jog with shoulder blade squeeze

    Knee-high jog, push forward, travel backward

    Straddle jog, clap hands

    Knee-high jog, hands cupped, travel forward

    Straddle jog with shoulder blade squeeze

Tabata 8 sets (4 minutes):

    Work: Mini ski, faster 70 percent (20 seconds)

    Recovery: Rest (10 seconds)

B SET

    Straddle jog with reverse breaststroke, travel backward

    Rocking horse R with shoulder blade squeeze

    Straddle jog with breaststroke, travel forward

    Rocking horse L with arm curl

    Straddle jog with reverse breaststroke, travel backward

    Rocking horse L with shoulder blade squeeze

    Straddle jog with breaststroke, travel forward

    Rocking horse R with arm curl

Tabata 8 sets (4 minutes):

    Work: Knee-high jog, faster 70 percent (20 seconds)

    Recovery: Rest (10 seconds)

C SET

    Heel jog with unison arm swing, travel backward

    Jumping jacks with bowstring pull to R side

    Heel jog with triceps kick back, travel forward

    Jumping jacks with bowstring pull to L side

    Heel jog with unison arm swing, travel backward

    Jumping jacks with bowstring pull to R side

    Heel jog with triceps kick back, travel forward

    Jumping jacks with bowstring pull to L side

Tabata 8 sets (4 minutes):

    Work: Mini jacks, faster 70 percent (20 seconds)

    Recovery: Rest (10 seconds)

D SET

    Rocking horse R, travel backward

    Heel jog with forearm press

    Rocking horse L, travel forward

    Hitchhike

    Rocking horse L, travel backward

    Heel jog with forearm press

    Rocking horse R, travel forward

    Hitchhike

Tabata 8 sets (4 minutes):

    Work: Mini ski, faster 70 percent (20 seconds)

    Recovery: Rest (10 seconds)

COOL-DOWN: YOU BE THE TEACHER

(The class is in a big circle)

Ask one participant to lead the class in his or her favorite exercise. Then go around the circle until everyone has had a turn. Allow any participant who does not wish to lead an exercise to pass.

Stretch: hip flexors, quadriceps, gastrocnemius, outer thigh, hamstrings, lower back

▶ Shallow-Water Interval Lesson Plan 11

TABATA TYPE 1

EQUIPMENT

None

TEACHING TIP

In Tabata intervals during the transition season, the work phase is performed at level 8. During the recovery, the participant stands in place for 10 seconds to rest. Level 8 is high-intensity interval training (HIIT), so you are doing Tabata Type rather than Tabata Timing. For safety's sake, encourage your participants to modify the intensity to a level that is challenging for them rather than try to keep up with other participants.

Level 8 (80 percent HR max)—Hard

WARM-UP

Instructor's choice

A SET

Knee-high jog, push forward, travel backward
Straddle jog, clap hands
Knee-high jog, hands cupped, travel forward
Straddle jog with shoulder blade squeeze
Knee-high jog, push forward, travel backward
Straddle jog, clap hands
Knee-high jog, hands cupped, travel forward
Straddle jog with shoulder blade squeeze

Tabata 8 sets (4 minutes):

Work: Cross-country ski with power 80 percent (20 seconds)

Recovery: Rest (10 seconds)

B SET

Straddle jog with reverse breaststroke, travel backward
Rocking horse R with shoulder blade squeeze
Straddle jog with breaststroke, travel forward
Rocking horse L with arm curl

Straddle jog with reverse breaststroke, travel backward
Rocking horse L with shoulder blade squeeze
Straddle jog with breaststroke, travel forward
Rocking horse R with arm curl

Tabata repeat 4× (4 minutes):

Work: Skateboard jump R 80 percent (20 seconds)

Recovery: Rest (10 seconds)

Work: Skateboard jump L 80 percent (20 seconds)

Recovery: Rest (10 seconds)

C SET

Heel jog with unison arm swing, travel backward
Jumping jacks with bowstring pull to R side
Heel jog with triceps kick back, travel forward
Jumping jacks with bowstring pull to L side
Heel jog with unison arm swing, travel backward
Jumping jacks with bowstring pull to R side
Heel jog with triceps kick back, travel forward
Jumping jacks with bowstring pull to L side

Tabata 8 sets (4 minutes):

Work: Jumping jacks with power, neutral position 80 percent (20 seconds)

Recovery: Rest (10 seconds)

D SET

Rocking horse R, travel backward
Heel jog with forearm press
Rocking horse L, travel forward
Hitchhike
Rocking horse L, travel backward
Heel jog with forearm press
Rocking horse R, travel forward
Hitchhike

Tabata 8 sets (4 minutes):

Work: Cross-country ski with rotation 80 percent (20 seconds)

Recovery: Rest (10 seconds)

COOL-DOWN: YOU BE THE TEACHER

(The class is in a big circle)

Ask one participant to lead the class in his or her favorite exercise. Then go around the circle until everyone has had a turn. Allow any participant who does not wish to lead an exercise to pass.

Stretch: hip flexors, quadriceps, gastrocnemius, outer thigh, hamstrings, lower back

▶ Shallow-Water Interval Lesson Plan 11

PF

TABATA TYPE 1

EQUIPMENT
None

TEACHING TIP
In Tabata intervals during the peak fitness season, the work phase is performed at level 9. During the recovery, the participant stands in place for 10 seconds to rest. Level 9 is high-intensity interval training (HIIT), so you are doing Tabata Type rather than Tabata Timing. For safety's sake, encourage your participants to modify the intensity to a level that is challenging for them rather than try to keep up with other participants.
Level 9 (90 percent HR max)—Very hard

WARM-UP
Instructor's choice

A SET
Knee-high, jog push forward, travel backward
Straddle jog, clap hands
Knee-high jog, hands cupped, travel forward
Straddle jog with shoulder blade squeeze
Knee-high jog, push forward, travel backward
Straddle jog, clap hands
Knee-high jog, hands cupped, travel forward
Straddle jog with shoulder blade squeeze
Tabata 8 sets (4 minutes):
> *Work*: Cross-country ski, arms sweep side to side 90 percent (20 seconds)
> *Recovery*: Rest (10 seconds)

B SET
Straddle jog with reverse breaststroke, travel backward
Rocking horse R with shoulder blade squeeze
Straddle jog with breaststroke, travel forward
Rocking horse L with arm curl
Straddle jog with reverse breaststroke, travel backward
Rocking horse L with shoulder blade squeeze
Straddle jog with breaststroke, travel forward
Rocking horse R with arm curl
Tabata 8 sets (4 minutes):
> *Work*: Front kick (karate), faster 90 percent (20 seconds)
> *Recovery*: Rest (10 seconds)

C SET
Heel jog with unison arm swing, travel backward
Jumping jacks with bowstring pull to R side
Heel jog with triceps kick back, travel forward
Jumping jacks with bowstring pull to L side
Heel jog with unison arm swing, travel backward
Jumping jacks with bowstring pull to R side
Heel jog with triceps kick back, travel forward
Jumping jacks with bowstring pull to L side
Tabata 8 sets (4 minutes):
> *Work*: Frog jump with double-arm press-down 90 percent (20 seconds)
> *Recovery*: Rest (10 seconds)

D SET
Rocking horse R, travel backward
Heel jog with forearm press
Rocking horse L, travel forward
Hitchhike
Rocking horse L, travel backward
Heel jog with forearm press
Rocking horse R, travel forward
Hitchhike
Tabata 8 sets (4 minutes):
> *Work*: Cross-country ski with rotation, hands together 90 percent (20 seconds)
> *Recovery*: Rest (10 seconds)

COOL-DOWN: YOU BE THE TEACHER
(The class is in a big circle)
Ask one participant to lead the class in his or her favorite exercise. Then go around the circle until everyone has had a turn. Allow any participant who does not wish to lead an exercise to pass.
> Stretch: hip flexors, quadriceps, gastrocnemius, outer thigh, hamstrings, lower back

▶ Shallow-Water Cardio Lesson Plan 12

TABATA TIMING 2

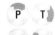

EQUIPMENT
None

TEACHING TIP
This lesson plan uses Tabata Timing all the way through except for the warm-up and the stretches. Sets A through F are cardiorespiratory training. Sets

G and H are training for the upper body. Sets I and J are core strength training. One core exercise is performed in a tandem stance, which means that one foot is directly in front of the other foot. Tabata cycles are four minutes long, and breaks after each cycle are one minute long, which means that the timing is specific. Instructors may wish to use a deck timer to help them manage the time.

Two exercises in this lesson plan use the variation in tempo called syncopate—knee-high jog (see figure 3.38) and jumping jacks (see figure 3.39). Syncopate means slow, slow, quick, quick, quick.

WARM-UP

Instructor's choice

A SET

Tabata repeat 4× (4 minutes):

Knee lift, doubles (20 seconds)

Knee-high jog (10 seconds)

Knee-high jog, syncopate (20 seconds)

Knee-high jog (10 seconds)

One-minute break:

Walk backward (30 seconds)

Walk forward (30 seconds)

B SET

Tabata repeat 4× (4 minutes):

R quad kick (20 seconds)

Kick forward (10 seconds)

L quad kick (20 seconds)

Kick forward (10 seconds)

One-minute break:

Walk backward, big steps (30 seconds)

Walk forward, big steps (30 seconds)

C SET

Tabata repeat 4× (4 minutes):

Kick side to side, doubles (20 seconds)

Straddle jog (10 seconds)

Kick side to side (20 seconds)

Straddle jog (10 seconds)

One-minute break:

Step sideways R (30 seconds)

Step sideways L (30 seconds)

D SET

Tabata repeat 4× (4 minutes):

Hopscotch (20 seconds)

Heel jog (10 seconds)

In-line skate (20 seconds)

Heel jog (10 seconds)

One-minute break:

Knee-high jog, travel backward (30 seconds)

Lunge walk (30 seconds)

E SET

Tabata repeat 4× (4 minutes):

Tuck ski, doubles (20 seconds)

Lunge R (10 seconds)

Tuck ski (20 seconds)

Lunge L (10 seconds)

One-minute break:

Knee-high jog, travel backward (30 seconds)

Crossover step, travel forward (30 seconds)

F SET

Tabata repeat 4× (4 minutes):

Jumping jacks (20 seconds)

Run tires (10 seconds)

Jumping jacks, syncopate (20 seconds)

Run tires (10 seconds)

One-minute break:

Step sideways R (30 seconds)

Step sideways L (30 seconds)

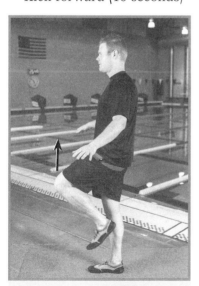

FIGURE 3.38 **Knee-high jog.**

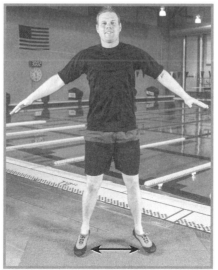

FIGURE 3.39 **Jumping jacks.**

G SET

Tabata repeat 2× (4 minutes):

Clap hands, lunge position (20 seconds)

Skip rope (10 seconds)

Standing row, lunge position (20 seconds)

Rocking horse R (10 seconds)

Lat pull-down, lunge position (20 seconds)

Skip rope (10 seconds)

Arm lift to sides, lunge position (20 seconds)

Rocking horse L (10 seconds)

One-minute break:

Knee-high jog, travel backward (30 seconds)

Walk on a tightrope, travel forward (30 seconds)

H SET

Tabata repeat 2× (4 minutes):

Push forward, squat position (20 seconds)

Inner-thigh lift (10 seconds)

Push across, squat position (20 seconds)

Jumping jacks squat (10 seconds)

Open and close doors, squat position (20 seconds)

Inner-thigh lift (10 seconds)

Forearm press, squat position (20 seconds)

Jumping jacks squat (10 seconds)

One-minute break:

Crab walk sideways R (30 seconds)

Crab walk sideways L (30 seconds)

I SET

Tabata repeat 2× (4 minutes):

Log jump, forward and back (20 seconds)

Stand on R foot (10 seconds)

Log jump, side to side (20 seconds)

Stand on L foot (10 seconds)

Arms sweep side to side, tandem stance (20 seconds)

Stand on R foot (10 seconds)

Brace core, arms down, turbulent hand movements (20 seconds)

Stand on L foot (10 seconds)

One-minute break:

Fall forward, tuck, and stand (1 minute)

J SET

Tabata repeat 2× (4 minutes):

Upper-body twist, slow (20 seconds)

Yoga tree pose R (10 seconds)

Hula-hoop (20 seconds)

Yoga tree pose L (10 seconds)

Hip hike (20 seconds)

Yoga tree pose R (10 seconds)

Climb a rope (20 seconds)

Yoga tree pose L (10 seconds)

One-minute break:

Fall sideways R, tuck, and stand (30 seconds)

Fall sideways L, tuck, and stand (30 seconds)

Stretch: quadriceps, gastrocnemius, hamstrings, outer thigh, pectorals, upper back

▶ Shallow-Water Interval Lesson Plan 12

TABATA TIMING 2

EQUIPMENT

None

TEACHING TIP

Shallow-water cardio lesson plan 12 is modified to include interval training. Set A is a cardiorespiratory transition into the Tabata intervals in sets B through F. Sets G and H are training for the upper body, and sets I and J are core strength training.

In Tabata intervals during the preseason, the work phase is performed at level 7. During the recovery, the participant stands in place for 10 seconds to rest.

Level 7 (70 percent HR max)—Somewhat hard

Tabata cycles are four minutes long, and breaks after each cycle are one minute long, which means that the timing is specific. Instructors may wish to use a deck timer to help them manage the time.

WARM-UP

Instructor's choice

A SET

Tabata repeat 4× (4 minutes):

Knee lift, doubles (20 seconds)

Knee-high jog (10 seconds)

Knee-high jog, syncopate (20 seconds)

Knee-high jog (10 seconds)

One-minute break:

Walk backward (30 seconds)

Walk forward (30 seconds)

B SET

Tabata repeat 4× (4 minutes):

Work: Knee-high jog, faster 70 percent (20 seconds)

Recovery: Rest (10 seconds)

Work: Steep climb, faster 70 percent (20 seconds)

Recovery: Rest (10 seconds)

One-minute break:

Walk backward, big steps (30 seconds)

Walk forward, big steps (30 seconds)

C SET

Tabata repeat 4× (4 minutes):

Work: Kick side to side, faster 70 percent (20 seconds)

Recovery: Rest (10 seconds)

Work: Jumping jacks, faster, suspended 70 percent (20 seconds)

Recovery: Rest (10 seconds)

One-minute break:

Step sideways R (30 seconds)

Step sideways L (30 seconds)

D SET

Tabata repeat 4× (4 minutes):

Work: Inner-thigh lift, faster 70 percent (20 seconds)

Recovery: Rest (10 seconds)

Work: Hopscotch, faster 70 percent (20 seconds)

Recovery: Rest (10 seconds)

One-minute break:

Knee-high jog, travel backward (30 seconds)

Lunge walk (30 seconds)

E SET

Tabata repeat 4× (4 minutes):

Work: Cross-country ski, suspended 70 percent (20 seconds)

Recovery: Rest (10 seconds)

Work: Cross-country ski, faster, suspended 70 percent (20 seconds)

Recovery: Rest (10 seconds)

One-minute break:

Knee-high jog, travel backward (30 seconds)

Crossover step, travel forward (30 seconds)

F SET

Tabata repeat 4× (4 minutes):

Work: Mini jacks, faster 70 percent (20 seconds)

Recovery: Rest (10 seconds)

Work: Jumping jacks, faster 70 percent (20 seconds)

Recovery: Rest (10 seconds)

Repeat 4× (4 minutes)

One-minute break:

Step sideways R (30 seconds)

Step sideways L (30 seconds)

G SET

Tabata repeat 2× (4 minutes):

Clap hands, lunge position (20 seconds)

Skip rope (10 seconds)

Standing row, lunge position (20 seconds)

Rocking horse R (10 seconds)

Lat pull-down, lunge position (20 seconds)

Skip rope (10 seconds)

Arm lift to sides, lunge position (20 seconds)

Rocking horse L (10 seconds)

One-minute break:

Knee-high jog, travel backward (30 seconds)

Walk on a tightrope, travel forward (30 seconds)

H SET

Tabata repeat 2× (4 minutes):

Push forward, squat position (20 seconds)

Inner-thigh lift (10 seconds)

Push across, squat position (20 seconds)

Jumping jacks squat (10 seconds)

Open and close doors, squat position (20 seconds)

Inner-thigh lift (10 seconds)

Forearm press, squat position (20 seconds)

Jumping jacks squat (10 seconds)

One-minute break:

Crab walk sideways R (30 seconds)

Crab walk sideways L (30 seconds)

I SET

Tabata repeat 2× (4 minutes):

Log jump, forward and back (20 seconds)

Stand on R foot (10 seconds)

Log jump, side to side (20 seconds)

Stand on L foot (10 seconds)

Arms sweep side to side, tandem stance (20 seconds)

Stand on R foot (10 seconds)

Brace core, arms down, turbulent hand movements (20 seconds)

Stand on L foot (10 seconds)

One-minute break:

Fall forward, tuck, and stand (1 minute)

J SET

Tabata repeat 4× (4 minutes):

Upper-body twist, slow (20 seconds)

Yoga tree pose R (10 seconds)

Hula-hoop (20 seconds)

Yoga tree pose L (10 seconds)

Hip hike (20 seconds)

Yoga tree pose R (10 seconds)

Climb a rope (20 seconds)

Yoga tree pose L (10 seconds)

One-minute break:

Fall sideways R, tuck, and stand (30 seconds)

Fall sideways L, tuck, and stand (30 seconds)

Stretch: quadriceps, gastrocnemius, hamstrings, outer thigh, pectorals, upper back

▶ Shallow-Water Interval Lesson Plan 12

TABATA TYPE 2

EQUIPMENT

None

TEACHING TIP

Set A is a cardiorespiratory transition into the Tabata intervals in sets B through F. Sets G and H are training for the upper body, and sets I and J are core strength training.

In Tabata intervals during the transition season, the work phase is performed at level 8. Level 8 is high-intensity interval training (HIIT), so you are doing Tabata Type rather than Tabata Timing. During the recovery, the participant stands in place for 10 seconds to rest. For safety's sake, encourage your participants to modify the intensity to a level that is challenging for them rather than try to keep up with other participants.

Level 8 (80 percent HR max)—Hard

Tabata cycles are four minutes long, and breaks after each cycle are one minute long, which means that the timing is specific. Instructors may wish to use a deck timer to help them manage the time.

WARM-UP

Instructor's choice

A SET

Tabata repeat 4× (4 minutes):

Knee lift, doubles (20 seconds)

Knee-high jog (10 seconds)

Knee-high jog, syncopate (20 seconds)

Knee-high jog (10 seconds)

One-minute break:

Walk backward (30 seconds)

Walk forward (30 seconds)

B SET

Tabata repeat 4× (4 minutes):

Work: High kick, power down 80 percent (20 seconds)

Recovery: Rest (10 seconds)

Work: Front kick (karate) 80 percent (20 seconds)

Recovery: Rest (10 seconds)

One-minute break:

Walk backward, big steps (30 seconds)

Walk forward, big steps (30 seconds)

C SET

Tabata repeat 4× (4 minutes):

Work: R side kick (karate) 80 percent (20 seconds)

Recovery: Rest (10 seconds)

Work: L side kick (karate) 80 percent (20 seconds)

Recovery: Rest (10 seconds)

One-minute break:

Step sideways R (30 seconds)

Step sideways L (30 seconds)

D SET

Tabata repeat 4× (4 minutes):

Work: Inner-thigh lift with power 80 percent (20 seconds)

Recovery: Rest (10 seconds)

Work: Hopscotch with power 80 percent (20 seconds)

Recovery: Rest (10 seconds)

One-minute break:

Knee-high jog, travel backward (30 seconds)

Lunge walk (30 seconds)

E SET

Tabata repeat 4× (4 minutes):

Work: Cross-country ski with power 80 percent (20 seconds)

Recovery: Rest (10 seconds)

Work: Cross-country ski with power, neutral position 80 percent (20 seconds)

Recovery: Rest (10 seconds)

One-minute break:

    Knee-high jog, travel backward (30 seconds)

    Crossover step, travel forward (30 seconds)

F SET

Tabata repeat 4× (4 minutes):

    Work: Frog jump 80 percent (20 seconds)

    Recovery: Rest (10 seconds)

    Work: Squat and jump 80 percent (20 seconds)

    Recovery: Rest (10 seconds)

One-minute break:

    Step sideways R (30 seconds)

    Step sideways L (30 seconds)

G SET

Tabata repeat 2× (4 minutes):

    Clap hands, lunge position (20 seconds)

    Skip rope (10 seconds)

    Standing row, lunge position (20 seconds)

    Rocking horse R (10 seconds)

    Lat pull-down, lunge position (20 seconds)

    Skip rope (10 seconds)

    Arm lift to sides, lunge position (20 seconds)

    Rocking horse L (10 seconds)

One-minute break:

    Knee-high jog, travel backward (30 seconds)

    Walk on a tightrope, travel forward (30 seconds)

H SET

Tabata repeat 2× (4 minutes):

    Push forward, squat position (20 seconds)

    Inner-thigh lift (10 seconds)

    Push across, squat position (20 seconds)

    Jumping jacks squat (10 seconds)

    Open and close doors, squat position (20 seconds)

    Inner-thigh lift (10 seconds)

    Forearm press, squat position (20 seconds)

    Jumping jacks squat (10 seconds)

One-minute break:

    Crab walk sideways R (30 seconds)

    Crab walk sideways L (30 seconds)

I SET

Tabata repeat 2× (4 minutes):

    Log jump, forward and back (20 seconds)

    Stand on R foot (10 seconds)

    Log jump, side to side (20 seconds)

    Stand on L foot (10 seconds)

    Arms sweep side to side, tandem stance (20 seconds)

    Stand on R foot (10 seconds)

    Brace core, arms down, turbulent hand movements (20 seconds)

    Stand on L foot (10 seconds)

One-minute break:

    Fall forward, tuck, and stand (1 minute)

J SET

Tabata repeat 2× (4 minutes):

    Upper-body twist slow (20 seconds)

    Yoga tree pose R (10 seconds)

    Hula-hoop (20 seconds)

    Yoga tree pose L (10 seconds)

    Hip hike (20 seconds)

    Yoga tree pose R (10 seconds)

    Climb a rope (20 seconds)

    Yoga tree pose L (10 seconds)

One-minute break:

    Fall sideways R, tuck, and stand (30 seconds)

    Fall sideways L, tuck, and stand (30 seconds)

    Stretch: quadriceps, gastrocnemius, hamstrings, outer thigh, pectorals, upper back

▶ Shallow-Water Interval Lesson Plan 12

TABATA TYPE 2

PF

EQUIPMENT

None

TEACHING TIP

Set A is a cardiorespiratory transition into the Tabata intervals in sets B through F. Sets G and H are training for the upper body, and sets I and J are core strength training.

In Tabata intervals during the peak fitness season, the work phase is performed at level 9. Level 9 is high-intensity interval training (HIIT), so you are doing Tabata Type rather than Tabata Timing. For safety's sake, encourage your participants to modify the intensity to a level that is challenging for them rather than try to keep up with other participants. During the recovery, the participant stands in place for 10 seconds to rest.

Level 9 (90 percent HR max)—Very Hard

Tabata cycles are four minutes long, and breaks after each cycle are one minute long, which means that the timing is specific. Instructors may wish to use a deck timer to help them manage the time.

WARM-UP

Instructor's choice

A SET

Tabata repeat 4× (4 minutes):

Knee lift, doubles (20 seconds)

Knee-high jog (10 seconds)

Knee-high jog, syncopate (20 seconds)

Knee-high jog (10 seconds)

One-minute break:

Walk backward (30 seconds)

Walk forward (30 seconds)

B SET

Tabata repeat 4× (4 minutes):

Work: High kick with lat pull-down 90 percent (20 seconds)

Recovery: Rest (10 seconds)

Work: High kick, clap over and under 90 percent (20 seconds)

Recovery: Rest (10 seconds)

One-minute break:

Walk backward, big steps (30 seconds)

Walk forward, big steps (30 seconds)

C SET

Tabata repeat 4× (4 minutes):

Work: Kick side to side, arms sweep side to side 90 percent (20 seconds)

Recovery: Rest (10 seconds)

Work: Side kick (karate), faster 90 percent (20 seconds)

Recovery: Rest (10 seconds)

One-minute break:

Step sideways R (30 seconds)

Step sideways L (30 seconds)

D SET

Tabata repeat 4× (4 minutes):

Work: Inner-thigh lift 1×, jumping jacks 1×, faster 90 percent (20 seconds)

Recovery: Rest (10 seconds)

Work: Hopscotch 1×, jumping jacks 1×, faster 90 percent (20 seconds)

Recovery: Rest (10 seconds)

One-minute break:

Knee-high jog, travel backward (30 seconds)

Lunge walk (30 seconds)

E SET

Tabata repeat 4× (4 minutes):

Work: Cross-country ski with rotation and power 90 percent (20 seconds)

Recovery: Rest (10 seconds)

Work: Cross-country ski with rotation, hands together 90 percent (20 seconds)

Recovery: Rest (10 seconds)

One-minute break:

Knee-high jog, travel backward (30 seconds)

Crossover step, travel forward (30 seconds)

F SET

Tabata repeat 4× (4 minutes):

Work: Jumping jacks, feet land out only 90 percent (20 seconds)

Recovery: Rest (10 seconds)

Work: Frog jump 1×, tuck ski 1× 90 percent (20 seconds)

Recovery: Rest (10 seconds)

One-minute break:

Step sideways R (30 seconds)

Step sideways L (30 seconds)

G SET

Tabata repeat 2× (4 minutes):

Clap hands, lunge position (20 seconds)

Skip rope (10 seconds)

Standing row, lunge position (20 seconds)

Rocking horse R (10 seconds)

Lat pull-down, lunge position (20 seconds)

Skip rope (10 seconds)

Arm lift to sides, lunge position (20 seconds)

Rocking horse L (10 seconds)

One-minute break:

Knee-high jog, travel backward (30 seconds)

Walk on a tightrope, travel forward (30 seconds)

H SET

Tabata repeat 2× (4 minutes):

Push forward, squat position (20 seconds)

Inner-thigh lift (10 seconds)

Push across, squat position (20 seconds)

Jumping jacks squat (10 seconds)

Open and close doors, squat position (20 seconds)

Inner-thigh lift (10 seconds)

Forearm press, squat position (20 seconds)

Jumping jacks squat (10 seconds)

One-minute break:

    Crab walk sideways R (30 seconds)

    Crab walk sideways L (30 seconds)

I SET

Tabata repeat 2× (4 minutes):

    Log jump, forward and back (20 seconds)

    Stand on R foot (10 seconds)

    Log jump, side to side (20 seconds)

    Stand on L foot (10 seconds)

    Arms sweep side to side, tandem stance (20 seconds)

    Stand on R foot (10 seconds)

    Brace core, arms down, turbulent hand movements (20 seconds)

    Stand on L foot (10 seconds)

One-minute break:

    Fall forward, tuck, and stand (1 minute)

J SET

Tabata repeat 2× (4 minutes):

    Upper-body twist, slow (20 seconds)

    Yoga tree pose R (10 seconds)

    Hula-hoop (20 seconds)

    Yoga tree pose L (10 seconds)

    Hip hike (20 seconds)

    Yoga tree pose R (10 seconds)

    Climb a rope (20 seconds)

    Yoga tree pose L (10 seconds)

One-minute break:

    Fall sideways R, tuck, and stand (30 seconds)

    Fall sideways L, tuck, and stand (30 seconds)

    Stretch: quadriceps, gastrocnemius, hamstrings, outer thigh, pectorals, upper back

SECTION 2: STRENGTH TRAINING

▶ Shallow-Water Strength Training 1

HAND POSITIONS AND LEVER LENGTH

P

EQUIPMENT

None

TEACHING TIP

In the preseason you want your participants to become aware that how they move their limbs through the water can increase or decrease the water's resistance. A hand sliced sideways through the water (see figure 3.40*a*) encounters minimal resistance. A closed fist (see figure 3.40*b*) encounters more resistance. But an open hand or a cupped hand position with the fingers relaxed and slightly apart (see figure 3.40*c*) will pull water more effectively and encounter the most resistance. In addition, a longer lever length will have more drag resistance and require more force than a shorter lever.

WARM-UP

    Knee-high jog

    Run tires

    In, in, out, out

    Jumping jacks

    Jumping jacks 1×, kick forward 1×

    Kick forward, travel backward and forward

    Knee-high jog, travel backward

    Rocking horse R, travel forward

    Knee-high jog, travel backward

    Rocking horse L, travel forward

    Skip rope

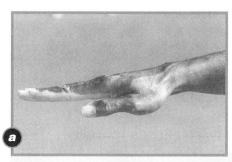 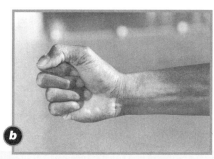 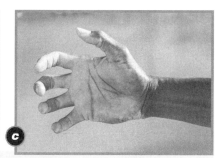

FIGURE 3.40 (*a*) hand slicing, (*b*) closed fist, (*c*) cupped hand.

A SET

R shoulder sweep in, hand slicing, squat position

L shoulder sweep in, hand slicing, squat position

Clamshells R

Clamshells L

R shoulder sweep in, hand cupped, squat position

L shoulder sweep in, hand cupped, squat position

R leg kicks side

L leg kicks side

Knee-high jog with hands fisted, one lap

B SET

R shoulder sweep out, hand slicing, squat position

L shoulder sweep out, hand slicing, squat position

Squat

R shoulder sweep out, hand open, squat position

L shoulder sweep out, hand open, squat position

Squat and jump

Knee-high jog with hands cupped, one lap

C SET

R bowstring pull, hand fisted, lunge position

L bowstring pull, hand fisted, lunge position

R quad kick

L quad kick

R bowstring pull, hand cupped, lunge position

L bowstring pull, hand cupped, lunge position

Kick and lunge R

Kick and lunge L

Knee-high jog with resistor arms, one lap

D SET

R arm curl, hand slicing, lunge position

L arm curl, hand slicing, lunge position

R hamstring curl

L hamstring curl

R arm curl, palm faces direction of motion, lunge position

L arm curl, palm faces direction of motion, lunge position

R leg kicks back

L leg kicks back

Knee-high jog, faster, with hands cupped, one lap

E SET

R forearm press, palm up, hand slicing, squat position

L forearm press, palm up, hand slicing, squat position

Up on toes and down

R forearm press, hand open, squat position

L forearm press, hand open, squat position

Jump and land toe-ball-heel

Knee-high jog with hands cupped, one lap

F SET

Stir the soup, hands fisted

Upper-body twist

Crossover knees

Pelvic circles

Upper-body twist with resistor arms

Log jump, side to side

Crossover step

Walk on a tightrope

Crossover step with hands on hips

Walk three steps and pause, stand on one foot

Crossover step 3× and half turn

Stretch: pectorals, upper back, latissimus dorsi, hip flexors, hamstrings, outer thigh

▶ Shallow-Water Strength Training 2

INERTIA AND FRONTAL RESISTANCE

P

EQUIPMENT

None

TEACHING TIP

Changing movement or direction frequently is harder than continuing with the same move. This lesson plan pairs two upper-body exercises, such as breaststroke and reverse breaststroke, alternating back and forth between them to increase resistance. It does the same with two lower-body exercises, such as kick forward (see figure 3.41) and skate kick (see figure 3.42). In a pyramid, you perform one exercise 8× and then its pair 8×, then 4×, then 2×, and you finally alternate one of each exercise. At the end of each set, the exerciser travels either backward and forward or sideways, whichever uses the most frontal resistance with that exercise.

WARM-UP

Instructor's choice

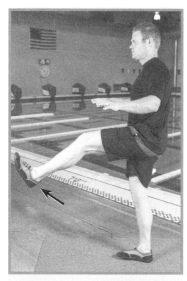

FIGURE 3.41 **Kick forward.**

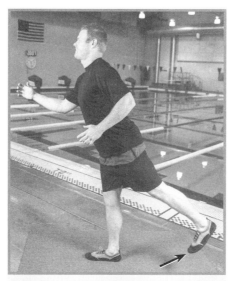

FIGURE 3.42 **Skate kick.**

A SET

Breaststroke, lunge position

Reverse breaststroke, lunge position

Kick forward

Skate kick

Breaststroke and reverse breaststroke, pyramid 8×, 4×, 2×, 1×, lunge position

Kick forward and skate kick, pyramid 8×, 4×, 2×, 1×

Breaststroke 4× and quarter turn, squat position

Reverse breaststroke 4× and quarter turn, squat position

Kick forward 4× and quarter turn

Skate kick 4× and quarter turn

Breaststroke, step sideways

Reverse breaststroke, step sideways

Kick forward, travel backward and forward

Skate kick, travel backward and forward

B SET

Double-arm press-down, lunge position

Lat pull-down, lunge position

Cross-country ski

Jumping jacks

Double-arm press-down and lat pull-down, pyramid 8×, 4×, 2×, 1×, lunge position

Cross-country ski and jumping jacks, pyramid 8×, 4×, 2×, 1×

Double-arm press-down 4× and quarter turn, squat position

Lat pull-down 4× and quarter turn, squat position

Cross-country ski 4× and quarter turn

Jumping jacks 4× and quarter turn

Double-arm press-down, walk backward

Lat pull-down, walk forward

Cross-country ski, travel sideways R and L

Jumping jacks, travel backward and forward

C SET

Standing row, lunge position

Unison push forward, lunge position

Inner-thigh lift

Hopscotch

Standing row and unison push forward, pyramid 8×, 4×, 2×, 1×, lunge position

Inner-thigh lift and hopscotch, pyramid 8×, 4×, 2×, 1×

Standing row 4× and quarter turn, squat position

Unison push forward 4× and quarter turn, squat position

Inner-thigh lift 4× and quarter turn

Hopscotch 4× and quarter turn

Standing row, walk backward

Unison push forward, walk forward

Inner-thigh lift, travel backward and forward

Hopscotch, travel backward and forward

D SET

Triceps extension, lunge position

Arm curl, lunge position

R quad kick

L quad kick

Skateboard R

Skateboard L

Triceps extension and arm curl, pyramid 8×, 4×, 2×, 1×, lunge position

R quad kick and skateboard R, pyramid 8×, 4×, 2×, 1×

L quad kick and skateboard L, pyramid 8×, 4×, 2×, 1×

Triceps extension 4× and quarter turn, squat position

Arm curl 4× and quarter turn, squat position

R quad kick 4× and quarter turn

Skateboard R

L quad kick 4× and quarter turn

Skateboard L

Triceps extension, walk backward

Arm curl, walk forward

E SET

Knee-high jog with R foot forward

Knee-high jog with R foot forward 3× and hold

Knee-high jog with L foot forward

Knee-high jog with L foot forward 3× and hold

Log jump forward and back

Hop forward and back on R foot

Hop forward and back on L foot

R leg kicks forward and back, no bounce

L leg kicks forward and back, no bounce

R leg kicks side, crosses front, kicks side, crosses back, no bounce

L leg kicks side, crosses front, kicks side, crosses back, no bounce

Upper-body twist, slow

Stretch: shoulders, pectorals, latissimus dorsi, quadriceps, gastrocnemius, hamstrings

▶ Shallow-Water Strength Training 3

ACCELERATION

EQUIPMENT

None

TEACHING TIP

Acceleration, the primary means for overloading the muscles in the water, means pushing or pulling hard or applying force against the water's resistance. For example, reach forward and then pull hard in a standing row (see figure 3.43). Apply force when the leg kicks forward (see figure 3.44). Remind your participants to maintain their range of motion as they accelerate with their arms or legs and then to pause briefly before returning to the starting position.

WARM-UP

Instructor's choice

A SET

Shoulder blade squeeze, lunge position

Standing row, lunge position

Breaststroke, lunge position

Arm lift to sides with elbows bent, lunge position

Unison arm swing, lunge position

Knee-high jog, one lap

B SET

R shoulder sweep out, squat position

L shoulder sweep out, squat position

R shoulder sweep in, squat position

L shoulder sweep in, squat position

Lat pull-down, lunge position

Palms touch in back, lunge position

Chest press, lunge position

Clap hands, lunge position

Knee-high jog, one lap

C SET

Forearm press, squat position

Forearm press side to side, squat position

Arm curl, squat position

Open and close doors, squat position

Unison jog press, squat position

Push forward, squat position

Knee-high jog, one lap

D SET

Wall push-ups

Knee-high jog, one lap

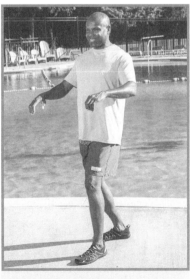

FIGURE 3.43 **Standing row.**

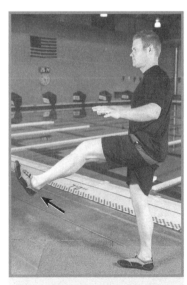

FIGURE 3.44 **Kick forward.**

Climb the wall, one foot on the wall and one on the floor

Knee-high jog, one lap

E SET

R leg kicks forward

L leg kicks forward

Knee lift and lunge R

Knee lift and lunge L

R leg kicks forward and back

L leg kicks forward and back

Cross-country ski

Knee-high jog, one lap

F SET

R leg kicks side

L leg kicks side

R side kick (karate)

L side kick (karate)

R leg kicks side, crosses front, kicks side, crosses back

L leg kicks side, crosses front, kicks side, crosses back

Jacks cross

Knee-high jog, one lap

G SET

R hamstring curl

L hamstring curl

Skateboard R

Skateboard L

R quad kick

L quad kick

Rocking horse R

Rocking horse L

Knee-high jog, one lap

H SET

Climb the wall, both feet on the wall and down to the floor

Knee-high jog, one lap

Push off the wall with both feet and run back

Knee-high jog, one lap

I SET

Kick and lunge R with double-arm press-down

Kick and lunge L with double-arm press-down

Kick and lunge R, arms sweep R

Kick and lunge L, arms sweep L

Inner-thigh lift R with double arms

Inner-thigh lift L with double arms

R knee lift and kick back with double-arm press-down

L knee lift and kick back with double-arm press-down

Upper-body twist

Lower-body twist

Lateral flexion

Stand on R foot

Stand on L foot

Stretch: pectorals, upper back, triceps, lower back, hamstrings, outer thigh, hip flexors

▶ Shallow-Water Strength Training 4

ACTION AND REACTION

P

EQUIPMENT

None

TEACHING TIP

Take advantage of the law of action and reaction by using arm or leg movements that propel the body forward while traveling backward. For example, use a breaststroke while traveling backward (see figure 3.45). You can also use arm or leg movements that propel the body backward while traveling forward. For example, use a reverse breaststroke while traveling forward (see figure 3.46). This action can cause a

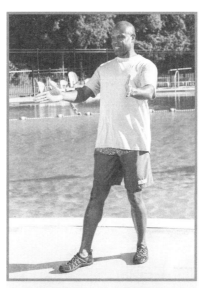

FIGURE 3.45 Breaststroke, travel backward.

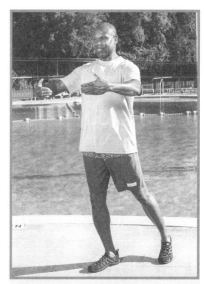

FIGURE 3.46 Reverse breast- stroke, travel forward.

surprising increase in resistance. To walk in a bowtie pattern in I set, first walk backward and then walk diagonally to the front R corner; walk backward again and then walk diagonally to the front L corner.

WARM-UP

Instructor's choice

A SET

Knee-high jog with jog press

Straddle jog with shoulder blade squeeze

Run tires, reach side to side

Inner-thigh lift

Hopscotch

Jumping jacks

Jacks tuck

Tuck ski

Cross-country ski

B SET

Knee-high jog with standing row, travel backward

Knee-high jog, travel forward

Knee-high jog with breaststroke, travel backward

Knee-high jog, travel forward

Knee-high jog with arm lift to sides, travel sideways R and L

Lat pull-down with deep lunge

C SET

Knee-high jog with double-arm press-down, travel backward

Knee-high jog with double-arm lift, travel forward

Knee-high jog with shoulder sweep out, travel backward

Knee-high jog with shoulder sweep in, travel forward

Knee-high jog, travel backward

Knee-high jog with reverse breaststroke, travel forward

Lat pull-down, palms touch in back with deep lunge

D SET

Knee-high jog with forearm press, travel backward

Knee-high jog, travel forward

Knee-high jog with L side arm curl, travel sideways R

Knee-high jog with R side arm curl, travel sideways L

Knee-high jog with triceps kick back, travel backward

Knee-high jog, push forward, travel forward

Lat pull-down with deep lunge

E SET

Knee lift, straighten and power press-down, travel backward

High kick, travel forward

Cross-country ski, travel backward and forward

Kick side to side, travel sideways R and L

F SET

Jumping jacks, travel sideways R and L

Jumping jacks, neutral position, travel backward and forward

Heel jog, travel backward

Kick forward, neutral position, travel forward

G SET

Walk on toes

Walk on heels

Lunge walk backward

Lunge walk forward

Squat, travel sideways R and L

H SET

Cross-country ski

Tuck ski

Jacks tuck

Jumping jacks

Hopscotch

Inner-thigh lift

Run tires, reach side to side

Straddle jog with shoulder blade squeeze

Knee-high jog with jog press

I SET

Crossover step

Walk on a tightrope

Step sideways, hands up

Fall forward, tuck, and stand

Side fall, tuck, and stand

Walk in a bowtie pattern

Walk in a circle clockwise, look L

Walk in a circle counterclockwise, look R

Stretch: pectorals, upper back, triceps, lower back, hamstrings, outer thigh, hip flexors

▶ Shallow-Water Strength Training 5

ᵀ BUOYANT EQUIPMENT—NOODLES
ᴾᶠ

TEACHING TIP

Many instructors are familiar with using the noodle (see figure 3.47) to support the body while performing suspended leg or abdominal exercises. But a noodle can also be used as a piece of resistance equipment, either held in the hands or placed under the foot. Perform 8 to 15 reps of each exercise, depending on the fitness level of your class. Use the noodle for support while performing the plank and side plank. In plank scissors, one leg is hyperextended and held for a few seconds. In side plank pliers, the top leg is abducted and held for a few seconds. You can also use the noodles to assist with stretches at the end of class. If participants have shoulder issues, offer them the option to perform the exercises without equipment. These noodle exercises are a sampling, not a complete list of every possible noodle exercise.

WARM-UP

Knee-high jog with jog press

Run tires

Jumping jacks

Jumping jacks squat

Squat

Knee-high jog, travel backward

Lunge walk

A SET

Knee-high jog with shoulder blade squeeze

Knee-high jog with breaststroke, palms flat

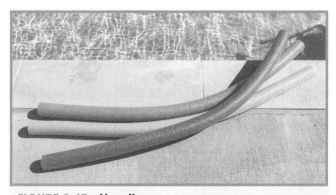

FIGURE 3.47 **Noodles.**

Knee-high jog with reverse breaststroke, palms flat

Cross-country ski

Jumping jacks

Knee-high jog with jog press

B SET

Crawl stroke, lunge position

Standing row, lunge position

Breaststroke, lunge position

Reverse breaststroke, lunge position

Double-arm press-down, lunge position

Double-arm lift, lunge position

Lat pull-down, lunge position

Arm lift to sides with elbows bent, lunge position

Arm curl, lunge position

Triceps extension, lunge position

Jab, squat position

Cross, squat position

Hook, squat position

Upper cut, squat position

Jab, cross, hook and upper cut, squat position

C SET

Tuck ski

Skateboard jump R

Skateboard jump L

Jacks tuck with reverse breaststroke, travel backward

Frog jump, travel forward

Jumping jacks, neutral position, travel backward and forward

Kick forward, neutral position, travel backward and forward

D SET

(Noodle in hands)

Rocking horse R, plunge noodle in front

Rocking horse L, pull noodle toward chest

Jumping jacks with double-arm press-down

Cross-country ski, noodle in R hand

Cross-country ski, noodle in L hand

Jumping jacks, noodle in R hand

Jumping jacks, noodle in L hand

Jumping jacks, touch ends in front

Jumping jacks with forearm press, noodle in
  back

Cross-country ski, push ends forward

Run tires with triceps extension

Knee-high jog, plunge R

Knee-high jog, plunge L

E SET

(Foot on a noodle)

Hip extension R

Hip extension L

Standing leg press R

Standing leg press L

Standing leg press to R side

Standing leg press to L side

F SET

(Sit on noodle like a swing)

Seated jacks

Seated kick

Seated kick with L shoulder sweep out, circle
  clockwise

Seated kick with R shoulder sweep out, circle
  counterclockwise

Point and flex feet

Hip hike

(Noodle in posterior sling)

Lower-body twist

Crunch, V-position

(Noodle in hands under shoulder)

Plank

Plank scissors

Side plank R, noodle in R hand

Side plank pliers R

Side plank L, noodle in L hand

Side plank pliers L

(Noodle in hands)

Stand on R foot, noodle overhead like a rainbow

Stand on L foot, noodle overhead like a rainbow

STRETCH

Upper-body twist, noodle on surface of water

Lateral flexion, noodle overhead like a rainbow

Hamstring stretch, noodle under knee

Lateral hip stretch, noodle under knee

Quad stretch, noodle on surface of water

Gastrocnemius stretch, noodle on surface of
  water

▶ Shallow-Water Strength Training 6

BUOYANT EQUIPMENT— DUMBBELLS

T

PF

TEACHING TIP

Buoyant dumbbells come in a variety of sizes (figure 3.48). The bigger the dumbbell is, the greater the resistance is. Start with the smaller size first. Make sure that participants are able to perform the exercises with the spine in neutral alignment before progressing to the next larger size. If participants have shoulder issues, offer them the option to perform the exercises without dumbbells. This lesson plan has three sets of strength-training exercises for the major muscle groups. Participants perform the first set slowly, the second set with power (acceleration), and the third set with buoyant dumbbells. Have them relax the shoulders and stretch the fingers after each dumbbell set. They should perform 8 to 15 reps of each exercise, depending on their fitness. Dumbbells work well for upper-body exercises, for lunges, and in support of the plank position, but not for most leg exercises. Therefore, use acceleration to increase the intensity of the leg exercises. These dumbbell exercises are a sampling, not a complete list of every possible dumbbell exercise.

WARM-UP

Instructor's choice

A SET

Clap hands, slow, lunge position

Knee-high jog

Clap hands with power, lunge position

Knee-high jog

(With dumbbells) chest fly at 45-degree angle,
  lunge position

Walk, one lap

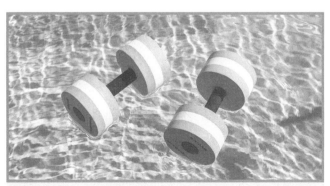

FIGURE 3.48 Dumbbells.

B SET

Arm swing, slow, lunge position

Knee-high jog

Unison arm swing with power, lunge position

Knee-high jog

(With dumbbells) cross-country ski

Step sideways R and L

C SET

Lat pull-down, slow, lunge position

Knee-high jog

Lat pull-down with power, lunge position

Knee-high jog

(With dumbbells) lat pull-down, lunge position

Knee-high jog, one lap

D SET

Triceps extension, slow, lunge position

Knee-high jog

Triceps extension with power, lunge position

Knee-high jog

(With dumbbells) triceps extension, lunge position

Knee-high jog, travel sideways R and L

E SET

Lunge forward and return to center, alternating sides

Knee-high jog

Lunge walk

Knee-high jog

(With dumbbells) lunge walk, hold dumbbells down at sides

Power run, one lap

F SET

Clamshells R, slow

Clamshells L, slow

Knee-high jog

Jumping jacks with power, neutral position

Knee-high jog

Jumping jacks with power, suspended

Knee-high jog, travel sideways R and L

G SET

Dog hike R

Dog hike L

Knee-high jog

R leg kicks side with power

L leg kicks side with power

Knee-high jog

Jacks cross

Knee-high jog, one lap

H SET

Pelvic tilt

Knee-high jog

(With dumbbells) fall forward, tuck, and stand with dumbbells on surface of water

Knee-high jog

(With dumbbells) plank

Step sideways, travel R and L

I SET

Hip hike

Knee-high jog

(With dumbbells) side fall, tuck, and stand with dumbbells on surface of water

Knee-high jog

(With dumbbells) side plank R, side plank L

Walk, one lap

J SET

R leg lift front with double-arm lift and balance

L leg lift front with double-arm lift and balance

R leg lift side with arm lift to sides and balance

L leg lift side with arm lift to sides and balance

Clamshells R with shoulder sweep out and balance

Clamshells L with shoulder sweep out and balance

R hamstring curl with arm curl and balance

L hamstring curl with arm curl and balance

R knee lift, look L

L knee lift, look R

Stretch: pectorals, triceps, lower back, hamstrings, inner thigh, outer thigh

▶ **Shallow-Water Strength Training 7**

BUOYANT EQUIPMENT— DUMBBELLS (CONCENTRIC AND ECCENTRIC CONTRACTIONS

PF

TEACHING TIP

Buoyant equipment can be used to target eccentric contractions by slowing down the dumbbells' return to the surface of the water. The muscles have to maintain their tension as they lengthen. In this lesson plan, three sets using dumbbells are performed for the targeted muscle groups. Participants perform the first set at a steady pace, the second set faster, and the third set fast during the concentric phase and slow during the eccentric phase. Have them relax the shoulders and stretch the fingers after each dumbbell set. They should perform 8 to 15 reps of each exercise, depending on their fitness. If participants have shoulder issues, offer them the option to perform the exercises without dumbbells. The upper-body sets are separated by leg exercises, using the dumbbells as stabilizers. Participants let them float on the surface of the water, keeping a loose grip on the bars and the shoulders relaxed. The last leg exercise is performed suspended without dumbbells. Cross the dumbbells and let them float on the water during this exercise. Dumbbells should not be used continuously for an entire class, so schedule a short break after the first two dumbbell sets and a long break after the fourth dumbbell set. Participants then pick up the dumbbells again for the abdominal exercises. These dumbbell exercises are a sampling, not a complete list of every possible dumbbell exercise.

WARM-UP
Instructor's choice

A SET
(With dumbbells)

Chest fly at 45-degree angle, lunge position

Cross-country ski with dumbbells as stabilizers

Chest fly at 45-degree angle, faster, lunge position

Cross-country ski, faster with dumbbells as stabilizers

Chest fly at 45-degree angle, fast concentric and slow eccentric, lunge position

Cross-country ski, suspended, no dumbbells

B SET
(With dumbbells)

Lat pull-down, lunge position

Jumping jacks, neutral position, with dumbbells as stabilizers

Lat pull-down, faster, lunge position

Jumping jacks, faster, neutral position, with dumbbells as stabilizers

Lat pull-down, fast concentric and slow eccentric, lunge position

Jumping jacks, suspended, no dumbbells

C SET
Walk, one lap

Knee-high jog, one lap

Power run, one lap

Leap, one lap

Lunge walk, one lap

D SET
(With dumbbells)

Double-arm press-down, lunge position

Kick forward, neutral position, with dumbbells as stabilizers

Double-arm press-down, faster, lunge position

Kick forward, faster, neutral position, with dumbbells as stabilizers

Double-arm press-down, fast concentric and slow eccentric, lunge position

Mermaid, suspended, no dumbbells

E SET
(With dumbbells)

Triceps extension, lunge position

Jumping jacks with dumbbells as stabilizers

Triceps extension, faster, lunge position

Jumping jacks, faster, with dumbbells as stabilizers

Triceps extension, fast concentric and slow eccentric, lunge position

Frog, suspended, no dumbbells

F SET
Walk, one lap

Knee-high jog, one lap

Power run, one lap

Leap, one lap

Lunge walk, one lap

G SET
Cross-country ski

Cross-country ski, neutral position

Cross-country ski, suspended

Jumping jacks

Jumping jacks, neutral position

Jumping jacks, suspended

Kick forward

Kick forward, neutral position

Mermaid, suspended

Frog jump

Frog jump, neutral position

Frog, suspended

H SET

Walk, one lap

Knee-high jog, one lap

Power run, one lap

Leap, one lap

Lunge walk, one lap

I SET

(With dumbbells)

Lateral flexion, R and L alternate

Plank

Side plank R

Side plank L

Stretch: pectorals, latissimus dorsi, triceps, hamstrings, outer thigh, quadriceps

▶ Shallow-Water Strength Training 8

T

PF

DRAG EQUIPMENT—
WEBBED GLOVES OR PADDLES

TEACHING TIP

Webbed gloves are one of the most popular pieces of resistance equipment (see figure 3.49). Participants are able to adjust the resistance by slicing through

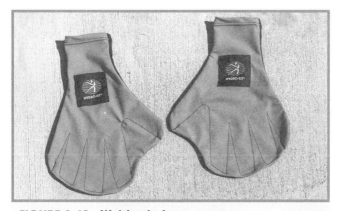

FIGURE 3.49 Webbed gloves.

the water (see figure 3.50a), making a fist (see figure 3.50b), or opening out the hands (see figure 3.50c). They can focus on individual muscles by opening up the hand when the targeted muscle is contracting and then slicing to return to the starting position. When greater resistance is desired, paddles can be used in A through D sets. Paddles can be held in either the free-hold or hand brace position (see figures 3.51a and b).

Select the position that feels most comfortable for any particular exercise. The resistance can be increased or decreased by closing or opening the fans. Between the arm exercises, perform some leg exercises while holding the paddles down at the sides to allow the upper-body muscles to rest between sets. If participants have shoulder issues, offer them the option to perform the exercises without webbed gloves or paddles. This lesson plan concludes with some modified square dance moves just for fun. These webbed glove or paddle exercises are a sampling, not a complete list of every possible exercise with this equipment.

WARM-UP

Instructor's choice

A SET

R shoulder sweep out and slice in, lunge position

L shoulder sweep out and slice in, lunge position

Kick forward

R shoulder sweep in and slice out, lunge position

L shoulder sweep in and slice out, lunge position

Kick forward

Clap hands, faster, lunge position

Kick forward

B SET

R arm press-down and slice up, lunge position

L arm press-down and slice up, lunge position

Kick side to side

R arm lift and slice down, lunge position

L arm lift and slice down, lunge position

Kick side to side

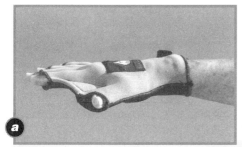
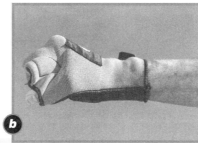
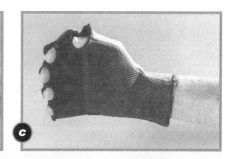

FIGURE 3.50 (a) slice, (b) fist, (c) open hand.

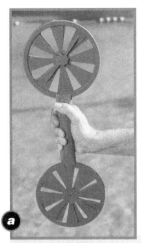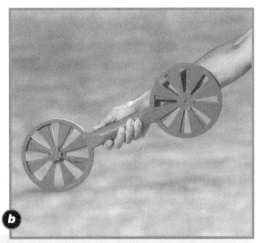

FIGURE 3.51 Paddles: (*a*) freehold position and (*b*) hand brace position.

Unison arm swing, faster, lunge position
Kick side to side

C SET

R lat pull-down and slice up, lunge position
L lat pull-down and slice up, lunge position
Heel jog
R arm lift to side and slice down, lunge position
L arm lift to side and slice down, lunge position
Heel jog
Lat pull-down and lift, faster, lunge position
Heel jog

D SET

R triceps extension and slice up, lunge position
L triceps extension and slice up, lunge position
Rocking horse R
R arm curl and slice down, lunge position
L arm curl and slice down, lunge position
Rocking horse L
Arm curl, palms or paddles face direction of motion, faster, lunge position
Rocking horse R
Rocking horse L

E SET

Clamshells R
Kick forward
Clamshells L
Kick forward
Jumping jacks, faster, neutral position
Kick forward

F SET

R leg kicks forward and back
Kick side to side
L leg kicks forward and back
Kick side to side
Cross-country ski, faster
Kick side to side

G SET

Jumping jacks, emphasize abduction
Heel jog
Jumping jacks, emphasize adduction
Heel jog
Jacks cross, faster
Heel jog

H SET

R quad kick
Rocking horse R
L quad kick
Rocking horse L
Kick forward, faster, neutral position
Rocking horse R
Rocking horse L

I SET

Stand on R foot, up on toes and down
Squat
Stand on L foot, up on toes and down
Squat
Up on toes and down, faster
Squat

J SET

(Square dance: Divide class into two lines facing each other. If you have an odd number of class participants, you will need to participate so that no one is left out.)

Partners run forward, shake R hands, and return
Partners run forward, shake L hands, and return
Partners run forward, do sa do, and return
Partners run forward, high-five, and return
Partners run forward, swing their partner R, and return
Partners run forward, swing their partner L, and return
Promenade—partners at the head of the two lines run forward and then run through the lines to the end; the other partners follow

Stretch: pectorals, upper back, latissimus dorsi, outer thigh, hamstrings, hip flexors

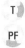

▶ Shallow-Water Strength Training 9

DRAG EQUIPMENT—PADDLES

TEACHING TIP

Paddles can be held in the freehold or hand brace position. The fans can be closed for more resistance or opened for less resistance. In addition, the exercises can be changed by the position of the feet. A squat or lunge position is stable and allows the participant to focus on the targeted muscle. A tandem position with one foot directly in front of the other creates a narrow base of support to challenge core strength and balance. Standing on one foot challenges core strength and balance further. Usually, we think of strength training in terms of flexion and extension in the sagittal plane or abduction and adduction in the frontal plane. Including some exercises in diagonal patterns as well is beneficial (see figure 3.52). For fun, you can add some sport-specific moves, like the ones in G set. If participants have shoulder issues, offer them the option to perform the exercises without paddles. These paddle exercises are a sampling, not a complete list of every possible exercise with paddles.

WARM-UP

Instructor's choice

A SET

Knee-high jog with jog press

Run tires with scull

Inner-thigh lift

Hopscotch

Jumping jacks

Jumping jacks with diagonal turn

Cross-country ski

Cross-country ski with rotation

B SET

(With paddles held in hand brace position)

Breaststroke, lunge position

Cross-country ski, slice

Chest fly, lunge position

Cross-country ski, paddle face against water

Crossovers, lunge position

Jumping jacks, paddles cross in front, slicing

Lat pull-down, lunge position

R shoulder sweep in and slice out, squat position

L shoulder sweep in and slice out, squat position

R shoulder sweep out and slice in, squat position

L shoulder sweep out and slice in, squat position

C SET

Knee-high jog with jog press

Run tires with scull

Inner-thigh lift

Hopscotch

Jumping jacks

Jumping jacks with diagonal turn

Cross-country ski

Cross-country ski with rotation

D SET

(With paddles held in freehold position)

Push forward R arm, squat position

Push forward L arm, squat position

Push forward R arm and L arm, alternate, squat position

Unison push forward, squat position

Pronate and supinate

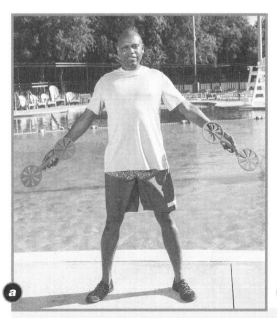
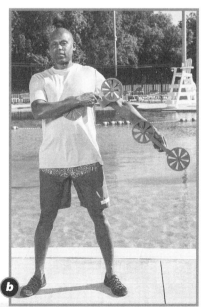

FIGURE 3.52 **Bring arm across to opposite shoulder: (*a*) start and (*b*) finish.**

E SET

(With paddles held in hand brace position)

Arms down at sides, bring R arm across to L shoulder, squat position

Arms down at sides, bring L arm across to R shoulder, squat position

Arms to sides 70 degrees, bring R arm down to L hip, squat position

Arms to sides 70 degrees, bring L arm down to R hip, squat position

Arm curl, lunge position

Rocking horse with triceps extension, hold paddles palms down

Forearm press, squat position

Arms sweep side to side, squat position

Arms sweep side to side, tandem stance (one foot in front of the other)

F SET

Knee-high jog with jog press

Run tires with scull

Inner-thigh lift

Hopscotch

Jumping jacks

Jumping jacks with diagonal turn

Cross-country ski

Cross-country ski with rotation

G SET

(With one paddle)

Glide to the side, hold in both hands like a fishing pole

R tennis backhand

L tennis backhand

R tennis forehand

L tennis forehand

Jog backward and forward, hold both ends of paddle

Baseball swing

Golf swing

H SET

Knee-high jog with jog press

Run tires with scull

Inner-thigh lift

Hopscotch

Jumping jacks

Jumping jacks with diagonal turn

Cross-country ski

Cross-country ski with rotation

I SET

(With paddles held in hand brace position)

Lat pull-down, slice, stand on L foot

R lat pull-down, slice, stand on L foot

L lat pull-down, slice, stand on L foot

(With paddles held in freehold position)

Triceps extension, stand on R foot

R triceps extension, stand on R foot

L triceps extension, stand on R foot

(With paddles held in hand brace position)

Walk backward and forward with resistor arms

Upper-body twist, paddles together

Upper-body twist, paddles extended to sides

Stretch: pectorals, upper back, latissimus dorsi, triceps, shoulders, gastrocnemius

▶ Shallow-Water Strength Training 10

RUBBERIZED EQUIPMENT— BANDS (CONCENTRIC AND ECCENTRIC CONTRACTIONS

PF

TEACHING TIP

Rubberized equipment is popular in land-based training and is now being used in the pool as well. The rubberized equipment used in the gym deteriorates quickly in chlorine, but manufacturers now make chlorine-resistant bands and loops specifically for use in the pool (see figure 3.53). The bands must be anchored to something, usually another body part, and the resistance is in the direction away from the anchor. Although stepping on a band or wrapping a

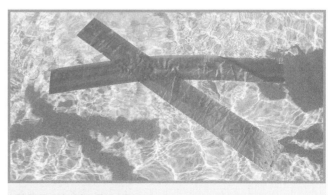

FIGURE 3.53 Bands.

loop around the ankles is possible, some participants may find it difficult or impossible to do that underwater. The exercises in this lesson plan anchor the bands in ways that most participants are able to accomplish, such as bowstring pull (see figure 3.54), single arm press-down (see figure 3.55), arm lift to sides (see figure 3.56), and elbow sweep out (see figure 3.57). The lesson plan includes three sets of exercises for each muscle group. The first set is without equipment. The second set uses the bands. The third set adds a pause and a slow return to focus on eccentric muscle actions. If participants have shoulder issues, offer them the option to perform the exercises without bands. These band exercises are a sampling, not a complete list of every possible exercise with rubberized equipment.

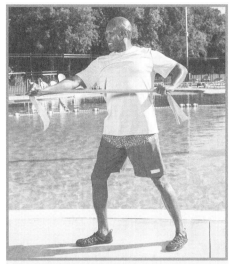

FIGURE 3.54   Bowstring pull.

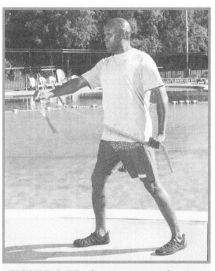

FIGURE 3.55   L arm press-down.

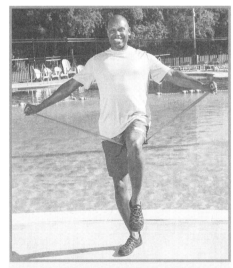

FIGURE 3.56   Arm lift to sides.

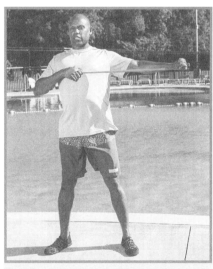

FIGURE 3.57   L elbow sweep out.

WARM-UP

Knee-high jog

Jumping jacks

Rocking horse R

Skip rope

Rocking horse L

Kick forward

Jumping jacks, neutral position

A SET

Cross-country ski with R bowstring pull

Cross-country ski with L bowstring pull

Jumping jacks with double-arm press-down

Cross-country ski, push forward

Jumping jacks with power arms

Cross-country ski with alternating arm curl

Jumping jacks, open and close doors

Cross-country ski with forearm press side to side

B SET

Knee-high jog with propeller scull, travel backward and forward

Jumping jacks, clap hands, travel backward and forward

Cross-country ski, travel backward and forward

Kick forward, neutral position, travel backward and forward

Clamshells R

Clamshells L

C SET

(With band)

R bowstring pull, lunge position

L bowstring pull, lunge position

R arm press-down, lunge position

L arm press-down, lunge position

Chest press, band behind back, lunge position

Arm lift to sides, band under knee

Arm curl, band under knee

R elbow sweep out, squat position

L elbow sweep out, squat position

Forearm press out, squat position

D SET

Knee-high jog, travel sideways R and L

Jumping jacks, travel sideways R and L

Cross-country ski, travel sideways R and L

R side quad kick, travel sideways R

L side quad kick, travel sideways L

Clamshells R

Clamshells L

E SET

(With band, pause at the end range of motion, slow return)

R bowstring pull, lunge position

L bowstring pull, lunge position

R arm press-down, lunge position

L arm press-down, lunge position

Chest press, band behind back, lunge position

Arm lift to sides, band under knee

Arm curl, band under knee

R elbow sweep out, squat position

L elbow sweep out, squat position

Forearm press out, squat position

F SET

Knee-high jog with quarter turn

Jacks tuck with quarter turn

Tuck ski with quarter turn

Mermaid, suspended, circle clockwise

Jumping jacks, neutral position, circle counter-clockwise

G SET

Walk backward with hands on hips

Walk forward with hands on hip

R kick 7× and lunge

L kick 7× and lunge

Walk backward with hands on hips

Lunge walk

Kick and lunge R

Kick and lunge L

Stretch: pectorals, upper back, latissimus dorsi, triceps, shoulders, hamstrings, hip flexors

▶ Shallow-Water Strength Training 11

CIRCUIT CLASS 1

T

PF

EQUIPMENT

Kickboards (figure 3.58), paddles (figure 3.59), dumbbells (figure 3.60), noodles (figure 3.61)

TEACHING TIP

This circuit class gives participants the opportunity to use a variety of equipment. Have the participants do three sets of strength-training exercises for each targeted muscle group. Participants perform the first set slowly, the second set with power (acceleration), and the third set with equipment. Figure 3.62 shows a standing row with the kickboard. Kickboards have a large surface area, so they have a lot of drag resistance. If the drag resistance is too great for some participants, let them substitute paddles instead. If participants have shoulder issues, offer them the option to perform the exercises without equipment.

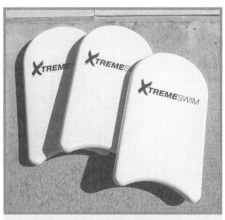

FIGURE 3.58 Kickboards.

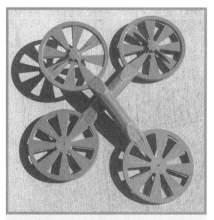

FIGURE 3.59 Paddles.

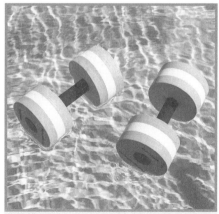

FIGURE 3.60 Dumbbells.

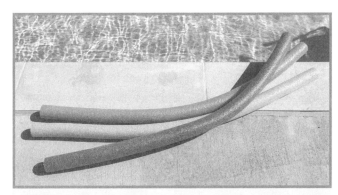

FIGURE 3.61 **Noodles.**

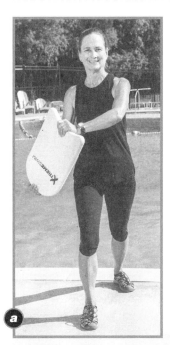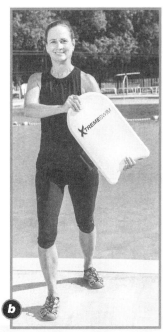

FIGURE 3.62 (*a*) standing row R and (*b*) standing row L.

WARM-UP

Instructor's choice

A SET

Standing row, slow, lunge position

Knee-high jog

Standing row with power, lunge position

Knee-high jog

(With kickboard) standing row, lunge position

Walk, one lap

B SET

Lat pull-down, slow, lunge position

Knee-high jog

Lat pull-down with power, lunge position

Knee-high jog

(With paddles held in hand brace position) lat pull-down, lunge position

Step sideways, travel sideways R and L

C SET

Forearm press, slow, lunge position

Knee-high jog

Forearm press with power, lunge position

Knee-high jog

(With paddles held in freehold position) forearm press, lunge position

Knee-high jog, one lap

D SET

Squat, slow

Knee-high jog

Squat and power leg

Knee-high jog

(With dumbbells down at sides) squat

Knee-high jog, travel sideways R and L

E SET

R quad kick, slow

L quad kick, slow

Knee-high jog

R quad kick with power

L quad kick with power

Knee-high jog

(Sit on noodle like a swing) seated kick

Power run, one lap

F SET

Clamshells R, slow

Clamshells L, slow

Knee-high jog

Clamshells R with power

Clamshells L with power

Knee-high jog

(Foot on a noodle) standing leg press to R side

(Foot on a noodle) standing leg press to L side

Knee-high jog, travel sideways R and L

G SET

Up on toes and down, slow

Knee-high jog

Up on toes and down with power

Knee-high jog

(With dumbbells down at sides) up on toes and down

Knee-high jog, one lap

H SET

(Noodle in posterior sling) crunch, V-position, slow Knee-high jog

(Noodle in posterior sling) crunch, V-position, slower Knee-high jog

(Noodle in hands on surface of water) fall forward, tuck, and stand

Step sideways, travel sideways R and L

I SET

Upper-body twist

Knee-high jog

Upper-body twist, pulse R 2× and L 2×

Knee-high jog

(With kickboard held upright between palms) upper-body twist

Walk, one lap

J SET

Walk three steps, pause, and stand on one foot

Step sideways with hands up

Crossover step

Stand on R foot, raise R arm and then L arm, and balance

Stand on L foot, raise L arm and then R arm, and balance

Stand on R foot, raise R arm and then L arm, close eyes

Stand on L foot, raise L arm and then R arm, close eyes

Stretch: upper back, latissimus dorsi, hamstrings, outer thigh, quadriceps, gastrocnemius

▶ **Shallow-Water Strength Training 12**

CIRCUIT CLASS 2

T
PF

EQUIPMENT

Paddles, multiplane drag equipment, aquatic steps

TEACHING TIP

This circuit class uses two types of drag equipment for the upper body, paddles (figure 3.63) and multiplane drag equipment (figure 3.64). Multiplane drag equipment comes in a variety of sizes. The larger the equipment is, the greater the drag forces and turbulence created are. If the multiplane drag equipment available to you is too large for some participants, let them use the paddles instead. If participants have shoulder issues, offer them the option to perform the exercises without equipment. Aquatic steps are used for the lower body (figure 3.65). Standing on an aquatic step increases the effects of gravity. Stepping down from the step allows a deeper lunge. Participants who do not wish to use the aquatic step can perform the same exercises on the pool floor.

WARM-UP

Knee-high jog

Rocking horse R

Knee-high jog

Rocking horse L

Kick forward

In-line skate

Jumping jacks

Jumping jacks squat

Rocking horse R, travel backward

Rocking horse L, travel forward

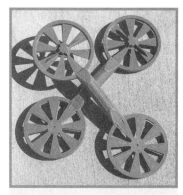

FIGURE 3.63 Paddles.

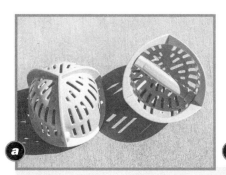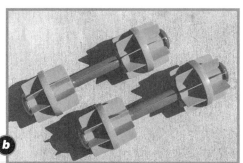

FIGURE 3.64 (a) multiplane hand bells (b) multiplane drag dumbbells.

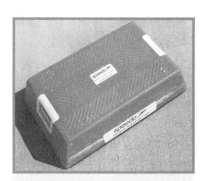

FIGURE 3.65 Aquatic step.

A SET

(On aquatic step or floor)

Knee lift and lunge R, L foot on step

Knee lift and lunge L, R foot on step

Rocking horse R, R foot on step

Rocking horse L, L foot on step

Kick and lunge R, L foot on step

Kick and lunge L, R foot on step

Jumping jacks, land out on floor, land center on step

Squat on step

Skateboard R, L foot on step

Skateboard L, R foot on step

B SET

(With paddles)

Standing row, freehold, lunge position

Double-arm press-down, hand brace, lunge position

Lat pull-down, hand brace, lunge position

Chest fly, hand brace, lunge position

R shoulder sweep in and slice out, hand brace, squat position

L shoulder sweep in and slice out, hand brace, squat position

R shoulder sweep out and slice in, hand brace, squat position

L shoulder sweep out and slice in, hand brace, squat position

Forearm press, freehold, squat position

Open and close doors, freehold, squat position

Arm curl, freehold, squat position

C SET

(On aquatic step or floor)

Knee lift and lunge R, L foot on step

Knee lift and lunge L, R foot on step

Rocking horse R, R foot on step

Rocking horse L, L foot on step

Kick and lunge R, L foot on step

Kick and lunge L, R foot on step

Jumping jacks, land out on floor, land center on step

Squat on step

Skateboard R, L foot on step

Skateboard L, R foot on step

D SET

(With multiplane drag equipment)

Standing row, lunge position

Double-arm press-down, lunge position

Arm swing, lunge position

Lat pull-down, lunge position

Chest fly, lunge position

R shoulder sweep out, squat position

L shoulder sweep out, squat position

R shoulder sweep in, squat position

L shoulder sweep in, squat position

Forearm press, squat position

Arm curl, squat position

Open and close doors, squat position

Triceps extension, squat position

Push forward, lunge position

Plunge down at sides, lunge position

E SET

(On aquatic step or floor)

Knee lift and lunge R, L foot on step

Knee lift and lunge L, R foot on step

Rocking horse R, R foot on step

Rocking horse L, L foot on step

Kick and lunge R, L foot on step

Kick and lunge L, R foot on step

Jumping jacks, land out on floor, land center on step

Squat on step

Skateboard R, L foot on step

Skateboard L, R foot on step

F SET

(With paddles)

Upper-body twist, arms extended to sides, hand brace

Upper-body twist, hands together, freehold

Stir the soup, freehold

Arms sweep side to side, hand brace, squat position

Arms sweep side to side, hand brace, feet tandem

Lat pull-down, hand brace, stand on R foot

Lat pull-down, hand brace, stand on L foot

Lat pull-down, R arm, hand brace, stand on L foot

Lat pull-down, L arm, hand brace, stand on R foot

Triceps extension, freehold, stand on R foot

Triceps extension, freehold, stand on L foot

Triceps extension, R arm, freehold, stand on R foot

Triceps extension, L arm, freehold, stand on L foot

Stretch: pectorals, shoulders, upper back, latissimus dorsi, triceps, hamstrings, hip flexors

▶ **Shallow-Water Strength Training 13**

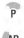

FUNCTIONAL CORE STRENGTH

EQUIPMENT

None

TEACHING TIP

Functional core training involves practicing movements that allow people to perform the activities of daily life more easily. The exercises are designed to challenge the core in multiple planes to improve stability. This lesson plan challenges the core with pauses, one-arm moves, using no arms, and crossing the midline (see figure 3.66 and figure 3.67). Try traveling on a diagonal. Turning to a corner and walking forward is not the same as traveling on a diagonal. Instead, continue to face forward while moving diagonally toward the corner. Use diagonal travel in a bowtie pattern: First, travel backward, then travel diagonally to the R corner, travel backward again, and then travel diagonally to the L corner. The pattern can also be reversed: First, travel forward, then travel diagonally backward to the back R corner, travel forward again, and then travel diagonally backward to the back L corner. Standing on one foot and closing the eyes can make it difficult to balance, but encourage participants to keep trying.

WARM-UP

Instructor's choice

A SET

Walk backward with hands on hips

Walk forward with hands on hips

Walk three steps and pause, stand on one foot

Walk forward, R foot first, with L bowstring pull, R hand on hip

Walk forward, L foot first, with R bowstring pull, L hand on hip

Walk backward with resistor arms

Walk forward with resistor arms

Step sideways with arms to sides 70 degrees

Knee lift, straighten and step

Walk on toes

Lunge walk

Crossover step

B SET

Run tires, travel backward and forward

Knee-high jog with toes in 3× and hold

Knee-high jog with toes out 3× and hold

Knee-high jog with hands on hips, travel in a bowtie pattern

Knee-high jog 3× and pause, stand on one foot, travel sideways R and L

Knee-high jog, travel backward and forward

Brace core, arms down, turbulent hand movements

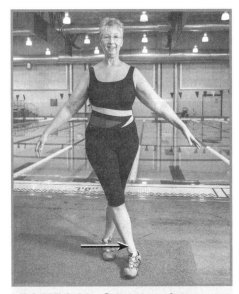

FIGURE 3.66 Crossover step.

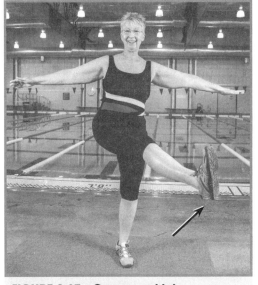

FIGURE 3.67 Crossover kick.

C SET

Rocking horse R, 3× and hold

Rocking horse L, 3× and hold

Cross-country ski

Cross-country ski with R arm swing, L hand on hip

Cross-country ski with L arm swing, R hand on hip

Cross-country ski with feet wide, travel backward and forward

Cross-country ski, travel sideways R and L

Cross-country ski with rotation

Cross-country ski, travel in a bowtie pattern

Cross-country ski, pause in center on toes, neutral position

D SET

Jumping jacks, heels out and toes in center, neutral position

Jumping jacks, neutral position

Jumping jacks squat

Jumping jacks

Jumping jacks, L hand on hip

Jumping jacks, R hand on hip

Jumping jacks with toes in

Jumping jacks with toes out

Jumping jacks, travel in a bowtie pattern

Jumping jacks, circle clockwise

Jumping jacks, circle counterclockwise

E SET

Kick forward with hands on hips

Crossover kick

Crossover kick and sweep out

Skate kick, crossover kick, sweep out and center

Kick and lunge R

Kick and lunge L

Inner-thigh lift

Kick side to side

Kick side to side with hands on hips

Hopscotch

Heel jog

Heel jog 3× and hold

Stand on R foot, arms sweep side to side

Stand on R foot, arms sweep side to side, eyes closed

Stand on L foot, turn head R and L

Stretch: pectorals, upper back, lower back, hamstrings, hip flexors, neck

▶ Shallow-Water Strength Training 14

BALANCE

EQUIPMENT

Paddles

TEACHING TIP

One technique for improving balance is the unpredictable command. When your cues are unexpected, you help your participants learn to react. Quick reactions reduce the risk of falling. Unpredictable commands include performing an exercise with one arm and a different exercise with the other, using arm patterns that are not typical with a specific leg move such as jumping jacks with arm swing (see figure 3.68), changing direction at odd intervals, and traveling in one direction while looking in the opposite direction. You can increase the challenge by asking participants to do something mentally demanding while they exercise, such as counting or spelling backward or creating lists aloud. Exercises with paddles, while standing in unstable positions (see figure 3.69), are included at the end.

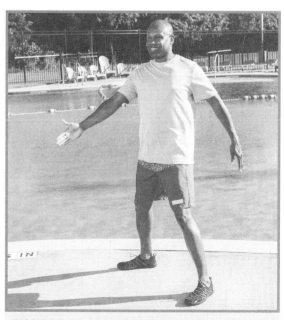

FIGURE 3.68 **Jumping jacks with arm swing.**

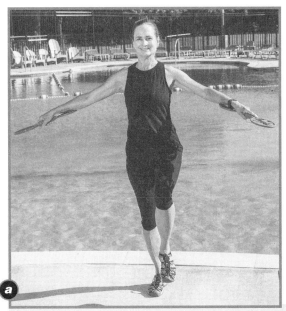
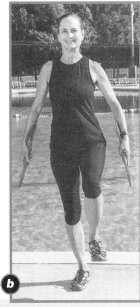

FIGURE 3.69 **Lat pull-down with paddles, standing on one foot: (a) start and (b) finish.**

Walk forward with L arm breast-stroke and R arm crawl stroke

Step sideways, R arm crosses in front and L arm crosses in back

Step sideways, L arm crosses in front and R arm crosses in back

Jumping jacks with arm swing

Cross-country ski with lat pull-down

Knee-high jog travel backward, forward, and sideways with quick change of direction

Step sideways R, look L

Step sideways L, look R

R leg kicks side and crosses midline

L leg kicks side and crosses midline

Clamshells R

Clamshells L

WARM-UP

Walk backward and forward

Step sideways R and L

Jumping jacks

Cross-country ski

Knee-high jog

Squat on R foot

Squat on L foot

A SET

Walk backward

Walk forward on a balance beam

Step sideways R 3× and L 1×

Step sideways L 3× and R 1×

Jumping jacks with R hand behind back

Jumping jacks with L hand behind back

Cross-country ski with R hand behind back

Cross-country ski with L hand behind back

Knee-high jog 3× and hold

Heel jog 3× and hold

R leg kicks forward and back

L leg kicks forward and back

B SET

Walk backward

Walk forward with R arm breaststroke and L arm crawl stroke

Walk backward

C SET

(Travel in a bowtie pattern)

Walk backward

Walk diagonally to front R corner, look L

Walk backward

Walk diagonally to front L corner, look R

Jumping jacks, travel backward

Cross-country ski, travel diagonally to front R corner

Jumping jacks, travel backward

Cross-country ski, travel diagonally to front L corner

Knee-high jog, travel diagonally to back R corner

Knee-high jog, travel forward

Knee-high jog, travel diagonally to back L corner

Knee-high jog, travel forward

D SET

Walk backward

Walk forward, circle both thumbs clockwise

Walk backward

Walk forward, circle both thumbs counterclock-wise

Step sideways R 3× and squat

Step sideways L 3× and squat

Jumping jacks 1×, inner-thigh lift 1×

Cross-country ski and cross-country ski, neutral position, alternate

Knee-high jog, travel in a circle clockwise, look L

Knee-high jog, travel in a circle counterclockwise, look R

Stand on R foot, turn head R and L

Stand on L foot, turn head R and L

E SET

(With paddles)

Arms sweep side to side, hand brace, squat position

Double-arm press-down, hand brace, lunge position

Lat pull-down, hand brace, lunge position

Triceps extension, freehold, lunge position

Forearm press, freehold, lunge position

Arms sweep side to side, hand brace, tandem stance

Lat pull-down, hand brace, tandem stance

Triceps extension, freehold, tandem stance

Lat pull-down R, hand brace, stand on L foot

Lat pull-down L, hand brace, stand on R foot

Triceps extension R, freehold, stand on L foot

Triceps extension L, freehold, stand on R foot

Stretch: shoulders, upper back, lower back, outer thigh, quadriceps, gastrocnemius

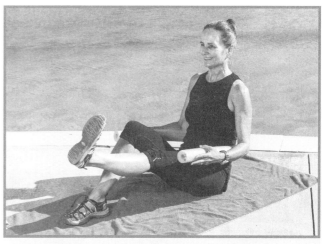

FIGURE 3.70 **Pull R knee toward chest, lift and lower L leg.**

▶ Shallow-Water Strength Training 15

PILATES FUSION

EQUIPMENT

Noodles, dumbbells

TEACHING TIP

Joseph Pilates created the fitness regime named after him to develop deep torso strength and flexibility. Many of his exercises can be adapted for use in the water. When you combine these with other core strength exercises and alternate them with travel to keep participants from getting chilled, you have a Pilates fusion class. Perform the Pilates exercises slowly. Use a noodle for support with some exercises, such as pull R knee toward chest, lift and lower L leg (see figure 3.70). Use dumbbells for support with other exercises such as plank and side plank (see figure 3.71). In plank scissors, one leg is hyperextended and held for a few seconds. In side plank pliers, the top leg is abducted and held for a few seconds.

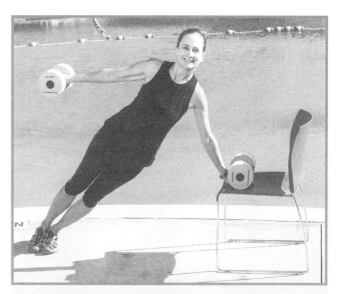

FIGURE 3.71 **Side plank.**

WARM-UP

Knee-high jog

Jumping jacks squat

Straddle jog

Heel jog

Knee-high jog, travel backward and forward

Straddle jog, travel sideways R and L

Heel jog, travel backward and forward

A SET

Tilt pelvis forward and backward to find neutral

Rock pelvis side to side to find neutral

Brace core

Reach side to side, keep feet on floor

Lateral flexion

B SET

Tap R heel in front and toe in back

Tap L heel in front and toe in back

Knee lift and lunge R, pause on knee lift

Knee lift and lunge L, pause on knee lift

R leg kicks forward and back

L leg kicks forward and back

Kick and lunge R with double-arm press-down

Kick and lunge L with double-arm press-down

Kick and lunge R, arms sweep side to side

Kick and lunge L, arms sweep side to side

Knee-high jog, travel backward and forward

Straddle jog, travel sideways R and L

Heel jog, travel backward and forward

C SET

(Sit on noodle like a swing)

Seated kick, arms to sides 70 degrees

Seated jacks, arms to sides 70 degrees

Seated kick, R shoulder sweep out, circle counterclockwise

Seated kick, L shoulder sweep out, circle clockwise

Hip hike

D SET

(Noodle in posterior sling)

Lower-body twist

Pike and hold

Pull R knee toward chest, lift and lower L leg

Pull L knee toward chest, lift and lower R leg

Pull R knee toward chest, hip roll

Pull L knee toward chest, hip roll

Flex R foot and lower, point R foot and lift

Flex L foot and lower, point L foot and lift

E SET

High kick and return

High kick and return, travel backward and forward

Skate kick and return

Skate kick and return, travel backward and forward

R leg kicks side and crosses midline

L leg kicks side and crosses midline

Jacks cross with power, grounded

Inner-thigh lift

Hopscotch

Inner-thigh lift R and hopscotch R, alternate

Inner-thigh lift L and hopscotch L, alternate

Knee-high jog, travel backward and forward

Straddle jog, travel sideways R and L

Heel jog, travel backward and forward

F SET

(One dumbbell)

Lunge R, sweep dumbbell L to center, hands on top of dumbbell

Lunge L, sweep dumbbell R to center, hands on top of dumbbell

Cross-country ski, sweep dumbbell side to side, hands on top of dumbbell

Side fall, tuck, and stand R, dumbbell in R hand

Side fall, tuck, and stand L, dumbbell in L hand

G SET

(Two dumbbells)

Squat, slow, hold dumbbells down at sides

R knee lift, extend knee, flex knee and lower, dumbbells on surface of water

L knee lift, extend knee, flex knee and lower, dumbbells on surface of water

Crossover kick toward opposite dumbbell

Ankle circles to R side, dumbbells on surface of water

Ankle circles to L side, dumbbells on surface of water

Lat pull-down, slow return, squat position

Alternating triceps extension, dumbbells upright, squat position

Fall forward, tuck, and stand

Fall forward and hold position, then pull back

Stand on one foot and gently pulse dumbbells down

Plank

Plank scissors

Side plank R

Side plank pliers R

Side plank L

Side plank pliers L

STRETCH:

Double-arm lift, sweep out, lat pull-down and reverse, squat position

Squat, slow

Upper-body twist with arms to sides 70 degrees

Upper-body twist with palms together, keep hips stable

Lunge R, hands forward, L hip hyperextension and balance

Lunge L, hands forward, R hip hyperextension and balance

Round out back and stretch chest, squat position

Shoulder shrug

Look R and L

SECTION 3: FUN ACTIVITIES

Additional fun activities are described in chapter 4, Shallow-Water Lesson Plans for Classes With Two Objectives.

▶ Shallow-Water Fun Activities

(AR) CIRCUIT CLASS WITH PARTNERS

EQUIPMENT

Noodles, dumbbells, kickboards, aquatic steps

TEACHING TIP

The season for active recovery is a good time to try a circuit class with partners. These stations allow partners to cooperate on some activities and engage in a little friendly competition with others. Set up the equipment stations before class with one of the four types of equipment pictured in figures 3.72 through 3.75 at each station. Participants do two exercises at each station. After your warm-up and a short cardio section, let the participants choose their partners. If you have an odd number of participants, you will need to get in the pool and be someone's partner so that no one is left out. Spend two minutes at each station doing the first of the two exercises. Then go through the stations again doing the second exercise. Two exercises are called see saw, which are squats in which one partner squats down as the other rises. At one station the partners work against buoyancy, and at the other they work against gravity. After the participants have completed the circuit, bring the class together for a second cardio set. Then ask everyone to choose a new partner and work through the stations again, spending one minute at each station instead of two. Before you know it, class time will be up and it will be time for stretching.

WARM-UP

Instructor's choice

A SET

Knee-high jog

Skip rope

In-line skate

Kick forward

Crossover kick

Crossover kick and sweep out

Kick forward, neutral position

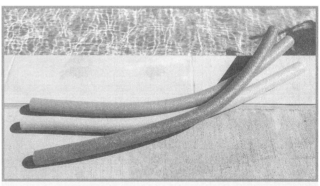

FIGURE 3.72 **Noodles.**

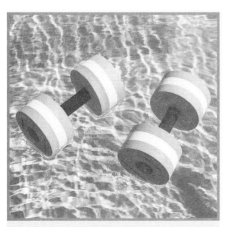

FIGURE 3.73 **Dumbbells.**

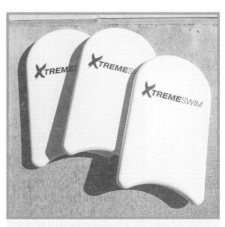

FIGURE 3.74 **Kickboards.**

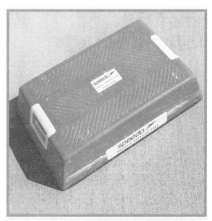

FIGURE 3.75 **Aquatic step.**

Jacks tuck

Frog jump

Frog suspended

Run tires

B SET

Knee-high jog

Skip rope

In-line skate

Kick forward

Crossover kick

Crossover kick and sweep out, doubles

Kick forward, neutral position

Jacks tuck

Surfboard jump R

Surfboard jump L

Bicycle, suspended

Heel jog

C SET

(Two minutes at each station; allow extra time to move to next station.)

Station 1 Noodles:

Bicycle race: Sit on noodle as if riding a bicycle and pedal with arms and legs; race until time is up.

Bicycle ride: Partner A is the handlebars with the noodle around his or her waist, and partner B is the bicycle rider, straddling the noodle. Halfway through they change positions.

Station 2 Kickboards:

Canoe: Partners stand one behind the other as if in a canoe. Partner A paddles on the R, and partner B paddles on the L. They switch every 10 seconds.

Balance challenge: Partners face each other standing on one foot. They push and pull to create turbulence and switch feet halfway through.

Station 3 Dumbbells:

Bird: When one partner does a lat pull-down, the other does arm lift to sides.

See saw: Partners hold dumbbells down at sides. When one partner squats, the other stands.

Station 4 Aquatic Steps:

See saw 2: Partners stand on two steps facing each other. When one partner squats, the other stands.

Chase: One partner follows the leader forward, backward, or sideways over and around the step. They switch leader halfway through.

D SET

Knee-high jog

Skip rope

In-line skate

Kick forward

Kick forward, neutral position

Crossover kick, neutral position

Crossover kick and sweep out, neutral position

Jacks tuck

Tuck ski

Cross-country ski, suspended

Cross-country ski

E SET

(Repeat circuit with new partner, one minute at each station; allow extra time to move to next station.)

STRETCH

Knee-high jog

Lift heels one at a time

Squat

Arms sweep side to side

Bowstring pull to R side

Bowstring pull to L side

R leg kicks side and crosses front, kicks side and crosses back

L leg kicks side and crosses front, kicks side and crosses back

R leg kicks forward and back

R quad stretch

L leg kicks forward and back

L quad stretch

Inhale and exhale

CHAPTER 4

Shallow-Water Lesson Plans for Classes With Two Objectives

At times you may wish to combine two objectives in a single class, such as when your class meets only twice a week or during the recovery season. In that case, your class will start with a 5-minute warm-up and 30 minutes of cardiorespiratory fitness training. Then you can spend 20 minutes on your second objective. The second objective can be strength training, core strength training, or fun activities. The class will end with 5 minutes of stretching. The following lesson plans are divided into two sections.

Section 1. 30-Minute Cardiorespiratory Fitness. The 12 lesson plans of continuous cardio in chapter 3, Shallow-Water Lesson Plans for Classes With a Single Objective, have been shortened to 30 minutes.

Section 2. 20-Minute Aquatic Endings. The strength-training classes have been shortened to 20-minute sessions. Any of these 20 sessions can be used as an aquatic ending following one of the 30-minute cardio lesson plans.

Section 3. 20-Minute Fun Activities. This section includes four 20-minute sessions of fun activities and eight games. Use one of the fun activities or choose two or more games to play after your 30-minute cardio lesson plan during the recovery season or during any season to give your class a break when they have been working especially hard.

By mixing and matching the cardio in section 1 with the activities in sections 2 and 3, you can create an almost endless variety of lesson plans for your two-objective classes.

SECTION 1: 30-MINUTE CARDIORESPIRATORY FITNESS

▶ Shallow-Water 30-Minute Cardio Lesson Plan 1

MOVEMENT IN TWO PLANES

EQUIPMENT
None

WARM-UP
Knee-high jog

Run tires

Rocking horse to R side

Kick side to side

Rocking horse to L side

Jumping jacks

Inner-thigh lift

Hopscotch

Straddle jog

A SET
R quad kick, travel sideways R

Knee-high jog with paddlewheel

L quad kick, travel sideways L

Knee-high jog with paddlewheel

Knee-high jog, travel backward

Kick forward, travel forward

Knee-high jog, travel backward

Kick forward, neutral position, travel forward

Jump backward

Knee-high jog, travel forward

Knee lift, straighten and power press-down, travel forward

Knee-high jog with breaststroke and knee-high jog push forward, alternate

Knee-high jog, faster, and knee-high jog, alternate

B SET
Inner-thigh lift

Jumping jacks

Frog jump, neutral position

Jacks tuck

Hopscotch

C SET
Cross-country ski, travel sideways R

Knee-high jog with hand waves

Cross-country ski, travel sideways L

Knee-high jog with hand waves

Knee-high jog, travel backward

Cross-country ski, neutral position, travel forward

Knee-high jog, travel backward

Cross-country ski, suspended, travel forward

Cross-country ski, travel backward

Knee-high jog, travel forward

Lunge walk

Knee-high jog with standing row and knee-high jog with unison jog press, alternate

Knee-high jog, faster and knee-high jog, alternate

D SET
Inner-thigh lift

Jumping jacks

Frog jump, neutral position

Jacks tuck

Hopscotch

20 minutes aquatic endings or fun activities

Stretch: hip flexors, quadriceps, gastrocnemius, hamstrings, inner thigh, outer thigh

▶ Shallow Water 30-Minute Cardio Lesson Plan 2

TURNS AND CIRCLES

EQUIPMENT
None

WARM-UP
Instructor's choice

A SET
Knee-high jog, R shoulder sweep out 2× and L shoulder sweep out 2×

Knee-high jog with unison arm swing

Jumping jacks, doubles 1×, jacks cross 2×

Knee-high jog with reverse breaststroke, travel backward

Rocking horse R, travel forward

Knee-high jog with reverse breaststroke, travel backward

Rocking horse L, travel forward

Knee-high jog with standing row, travel backward

Skip rope, travel forward

Knee-high jog with standing row, travel backward

Skip rope, travel forward

Crossover kick

Crossover kick, doubles

Jacks cross 3-1/2× and half turn

Jacks cross, R leg in front, circle clockwise

Jacks cross, L leg in front, circle counterclockwise

Knee-high jog

B SET

Knee-high jog with double-arm press-down 2× and lat pull-down 2×

Jumping jacks with unison arm swing

Cross-country ski and mini ski, alternate

Jump backward

Jacks tuck with breaststroke, travel forward

Jump backward

Jacks tuck with breaststroke, travel forward

Knee-high jog with standing row, travel backward

Inner-thigh lift, travel forward

Knee-high jog with standing row, travel backward

Inner-thigh lift, travel forward

Crossover kick, doubles

Crossover kick, doubles, one low and one high

Cross-country ski 3-1/2× and half turn

Cross-country ski, suspended, circle clockwise and counterclockwise

Knee-high jog

C SET

Knee-high jog, punch down R, L and punch across R, L

Cross-country ski with unison arm swing

Jumping jacks and mini cross, alternate

Knee-high jog with reverse breaststroke, travel backward

Cross-country ski, travel forward

Knee-high jog with reverse breaststroke, travel backward

Cross-country ski, travel forward

Knee-high jog with standing row, travel backward

Leap forward

Knee-high jog with standing row, travel backward

Leap forward

Crossover kick, doubles, one low and one high

Crossover kick and sweep out

Jacks cross 3-1/2× and half turn

Jacks cross, R leg in front, circle clockwise

Jacks cross, L leg in front, circle counterclockwise

Knee-high jog

20 minutes aquatic endings or fun activities

Stretch: shoulders, pectorals, hip flexors, gastrocnemius, hamstrings, outer thigh

▶ Shallow-Water 30-Minute Cardio Lesson Plan 3

INCREASING COMPLEXITY

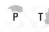

EQUIPMENT

None

WARM-UP

Instructor's choice

A SET

Jumping jacks

Jumping jacks with elbows bent

Inner-thigh lift

Straddle jog with shoulder blade squeeze

Rocking horse R, travel backward

Rocking horse L, travel forward

Jump backward

Knee-high jog, travel forward

Cross-country ski, travel sideways R and L

Cross-country ski with unison arm swing

Cross-country ski with rotation

Knee-high jog

B SET

Jumping jacks

Jumping jacks, arms cross in front and in back

Hopscotch

Straddle jog with shoulder blade squeeze

Rocking horse L, travel backward

Rocking horse R, travel forward

Jump backward

Leap forward

Cross-country ski, travel backward and forward

Cross-country ski, clap hands

Cross-country ski with rotation, hands together

Knee-high jog

C SET

Jumping jacks

Jumping jacks, palms touch in front and in back

Inner-thigh lift 1×, hopscotch 1×

Straddle jog with shoulder blade squeeze

Rocking horse R, travel backward and forward

Rocking horse L, travel backward and forward

Jump backward

Skate kick, travel forward

Cross-country ski with quarter turn

Cross-country ski with forearm press

Lunge walk

Walk on a tightrope

20 minutes aquatic endings or fun activities

Stretch: hamstrings, outer thigh, quadriceps, hip flexors, gastrocnemius, upper back

▶ Shallow-Water 30-Minute Cardio Lesson Plan 4

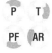

BLOCK CHOREOGRAPHY WITH FIVE MOVES

EQUIPMENT

None

WARM-UP

Instructor's choice

A SET

Knee-high jog

Kick forward

Jumping jacks

In-line skate

Cross-country ski

B SET

Knee-high jog, punch forward and side

Chorus-line kick

Jumping jacks with diagonal turn

Skate kick with pumping arms

Cross-country ski, two easy and one with power

C SET

Knee-high jog, push across and slice back

High kick

Jumping jacks, doubles

Knee lift and lunge R

Knee lift and lunge L

Cross-country ski, four easy and four with power

D SET

Knee-high jog with breaststroke

Kick forward with lat pull-down

Jumping jacks with arms out of the water

Skate kick with pumping arms

Cross-country ski, two easy and one with power

E SET

Knee-high jog, punch across

Crossover kick

Jumping jacks, syncopate

Kick and lunge R

Kick and lunge L

Cross-country ski, four easy and four with power

F SET

Knee-high jog

Kick forward, neutral position, travel backward

Jumping jacks, neutral position, travel forward

In-line skate

Skip rope

20 minutes aquatic endings or fun activities

Stretch: quadriceps, hip flexors, inner thigh, hamstrings, pectorals, upper back

▶ Shallow-Water 30-Minute Cardio Lesson Plan 5

DOUBLE LADDER

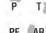

EQUIPMENT

None

TEACHING TIP

In a double ladder, two exercises, such as jumping jacks and side kick (karate), are paired. Perform each exercise for 10 seconds, then 20 seconds, and then 30 seconds, as if ascending a ladder. Next, descend the ladder, performing each exercise for 20 seconds and then 10 seconds. The third double ladder pairs rocking horse to the side with kick side to side. Perform the first rocking horse to the right side for 10 seconds, kick side to side for 10 seconds, then rocking horse to the left side for 20 seconds, and so on, alternating sides. Each double ladder takes 3 minutes.

WARM-UP

Instructor's choice

A SET

Kick forward

Crossover kick

Kick side to side

Heel jog

Skip rope

Cross-country ski

Double ladder: 10, 20, 30, 20, and 10 seconds

Jumping jacks

Side kick (karate)

B SET

Kick forward, doubles

Crossover kick, doubles, one low and one high

Jumping jacks

Hopscotch, doubles

Knee swing forward, back, forward, and down

Cross-country ski, doubles

Double ladder: 10, 20, 30, 20, and 10 seconds

Front kick (karate)

Cross-country ski

C SET

High kick

Skate kick, crossover kick, sweep out and center

Jacks cross

Hopscotch

Knee lift and lunge R

Knee lift and lunge L

Cross-country ski with rotation

Double ladder: 10, 20, 30, 20, and 10 seconds

Rocking horse to the side

Kick side to side

20 minutes aquatic endings or fun activities

Stretch: hamstrings, outer thigh, quadriceps, hip
flexors, gastrocnemius, ankles

▶ Shallow-Water 30-Minute Cardio Lesson Plan 6

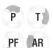
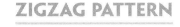
ZIGZAG PATTERN

EQUIPMENT

None

WARM-UP

Instructor's choice

A SET

In, in, out, out

Jumping jacks

Jumping jacks with diagonal turn

Crossover kick

Tuck and hold with reverse breaststroke, travel
backward

Knee-high jog, travel forward

Jump backward

Knee-high jog, travel in a zigzag

Skateboard R

Skateboard L

Kick forward

Kick forward, neutral position

Squat, R shoulder sweep out and in

Squat, L shoulder sweep out and in

Knee-high jog

Crab walk sideways

B SET

In, in, out, out

Jumping jacks

Jumping jacks with diagonal turn

Crossover kick, doubles, one low and one high

Tuck and hold with reverse breaststroke, travel
backward

Run 3× and hurdle 1×, travel forward

Jump backward

Cross-country ski, travel in a zigzag

Skate kick

Cross-country ski

Cross-country ski, neutral position

R leg sweeps out and in, neutral position,

L leg sweeps out and in, neutral position,

Knee-high jog

Rocking horse to R side, travel sideways R

Rocking horse to L side, travel sideways L

C SET

In, in, out, out

Jumping jacks

Jumping jacks with diagonal turn

Crossover kick and sweep out

Tuck and hold with reverse breaststroke, travel
forward

Leap forward

Jump backward

Bicycle, suspended, travel in a zigzag

Skateboard jump R

Skateboard jump L

Tuck ski

Cross-country ski, neutral position

Kick forward 3× and hold, one leg sweeps out and in 1×, neutral position

Knee-high jog

Run tires, travel sideways R and L

20 minutes aquatic endings or fun activities

Stretch: upper back, lower back, hamstrings, outer thighs, quadriceps, hip flexors

▶ Shallow-Water 30-Minute Cardio Lesson Plan 7

CARDIO WITH WALL EXERCISES

EQUIPMENT

None

WARM-UP

Instructor's choice

A SET

Straddle jog, clap hands

Jumping jacks, clap hands

Inner-thigh lift

Jacks cross

Run to one side of the pool and back to the wall

Climb wall, one foot on wall and one on floor

Cross-country ski, travel backward

Knee-high jog, travel forward

Kick forward, travel backward

Knee-high jog, travel forward

Crossover kick

B SET

Straddle jog, palms touch in back

Jumping jacks, palms touch in back

Hopscotch

Jacks cross

Run to one side of the pool and back to the wall

Climb wall, both feet on wall and down to floor

Cross-country ski, clap hands, travel backward

Knee-high jog, travel forward

Kick forward, clap hands, travel backward

Knee-high jog, travel forward

Chorus-line kick

C SET

Straddle jog, open and close doors

Jumping jacks, open and close doors

Inner-thigh lift and hopscotch, alternate

Jacks cross

Run to one side of the pool and back to the wall

Climb wall, one foot on wall and one on floor

Cross-country ski with unison arm swing, travel backward

Knee-high jog, travel forward

Kick forward with unison arm swing, travel backward

Knee-high jog, travel forward

Crossover kick, doubles, one low and one high

20 minutes aquatic endings or fun activities

Stretch: lower back, hamstrings, inner thigh, hip flexors, gastrocnemius, shoulders

▶ Shallow-Water 30-Minute Cardio Lesson Plan 8

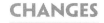

CHANGES

EQUIPMENT

None

WARM-UP

Instructor's choice

A SET

Knee-high jog with jog press

Run tires, reach side to side

Jumping jacks

Squat

Tuck and hold with reverse breaststroke, travel backward

Tuck and hold with breaststroke, travel forward

Cross-country ski with R arm swing, L hand on hip

Knee-high jog with jog press

Run tires, reach side to side

Jumping jacks

Squat

Tuck and hold with reverse breaststroke, travel backward

Tuck and hold with breaststroke, travel forward

Cross-country ski with L arm swing, R hand on hip

Cross-country ski 3× and hold

Cross-country ski 3× and bounce center

Cross-country ski, neutral position

Tuck ski

Jacks tuck

Knee-high jog

B SET

Knee-high jog, punch forward and side

Run tires with hand waves

Jumping jacks with diagonal turn

Kick and squat

Jump backward

Frog jump, travel forward

Cross-country ski, single, single, double

Knee-high jog, punch forward and side

Run tires with hand waves

Jumping jacks with diagonal turn

Kick and squat

Jump backward

Frog jump, travel forward

Cross-country ski, single, single, double

Cross-country ski with rotation

Tuck ski with rotation

Cross-country ski, tuck, diagonal turn and center

Jacks tuck

Knee-high jog

20 minutes aquatic endings or fun activities

Stretch: hamstrings, hip flexors, quadriceps, gastrocnemius, outer thigh, shoulders

▶ Shallow-Water 30-Minute Cardio Lesson Plan 9

BLOCK CHOREOGRAPHY WITH SIX MOVES

EQUIPMENT

None

WARM-UP

Instructor's choice

A SET

Knee-high jog

Run tires

Jumping jacks

Cross-country ski

Kick forward

Heel jog

B SET

Knee-high jog with pumping arms

Run tires with shoulder blade squeeze

Jumping jacks, clap hands

Cross-country ski with windshield wiper arms

Kick forward with triceps extension

Heel jog with forearm press

C SET

Leap forward

Leap sideways

Jumping jacks with arms out of the water

Cross-country ski, full ROM

High kick

Skate kick

D SET

Hip curl, suspended

Frog jump, neutral position

Jumping jacks, suspended

Tuck ski, neutral position

Kick forward, suspended, emphasize quadriceps

Kick forward, suspended, emphasize hamstrings

F SET

Crossover knees

Inner-thigh lift

Jacks cross

Cross-country ski with rotation

Crossover kick

Hopscotch

G SET

In, in, out, out

Cross-country ski 1×, jumping jacks 1×

R leg kicks forward and back

In, in, out, out

Cross-country ski 1×, jumping jacks 1×

L leg kicks forward and back

20 minutes aquatic endings or fun activities

Stretch: quadriceps, hip flexors, hamstrings, outer thigh, inner thigh, pectorals

▶ Shallow-Water 30-Minute Cardio Lesson Plan 10

LAYER TECHNIQUE

EQUIPMENT

None

WARM-UP

Jumping jacks squat

Jumping jacks

Inner-thigh lift

Hopscotch

Heel jog

Cross-country ski

Knee-high jog

Kick forward

A SET

Jumping jacks squat

Jumping jacks

Jumping jacks 1×, kick forward 1×

Inner-thigh lift

Inner-thigh lift R

Inner-thigh lift L

Hopscotch

Heel jog

Cross-country ski

Cross-country ski 3× and hold

Knee-high jog

Knee-high jog 3× and hold

Kick forward

Kick forward, neutral position

B SET

Jumping jacks squat

Jumping jacks 1×, kick forward 1×

Jumping jacks 1×, skate kick 1×

Inner-thigh lift R

Inner-thigh lift L

Inner-thigh lift, doubles

Hopscotch

Heel jog

Cross-country ski 3× and hold

Cross-country ski 2× and cross-country ski with power 1×

Knee-high jog 3× and hold

Knee-high jog 3× and hold with kayak row

Kick forward, neutral position

Hold R leg up, L leg kicks forward, suspended

Hold L leg up, R leg kicks forward, suspended

C SET

Jumping jacks squat

Jumping jacks 1×, skate kick 1×

Jumping jacks 2× and jumping jacks, doubles 1×

Inner-thigh lift, doubles

Inner-thigh lift R and hopscotch L, alternate

Inner-thigh lift L and hopscotch R, alternate

Hopscotch

Heel jog

Cross-country ski 2× and cross-country ski with power 1×

Cross-country ski with lat pull-down

Knee-high jog 3× and hold with kayak row

Tuck and down

Hold R leg up, L leg kicks forward, suspended

Hold L leg up, R leg kicks forward, suspended

Hold R leg up, L leg kicks forward 3× suspended and down

Hold L leg up, R leg kicks forward 3× suspended and down

20 minutes aquatic endings or fun activities

Stretch: latissimus dorsi, upper back, hip flexors, gastrocnemius, hamstrings, inner thigh

▶ Shallow-Water 30-Minute Cardio Lesson Plan 11

TABATA TIMING 1

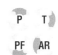

EQUIPMENT

None

WARM-UP

Instructor's choice

A SET

Knee-high jog, push forward, travel backward

Straddle jog, clap hands

Knee-high jog, hands cupped, travel forward

Straddle jog with shoulder blade squeeze

Knee-high jog, push forward, travel backward

Straddle jog, clap hands

Knee-high jog, hands cupped, travel forward

Straddle jog with shoulder blade squeeze

Tabata 8 sets (4 minutes):

Cross-country ski (20 seconds)

In-line skate (10 seconds)

B SET

Straddle jog with reverse breaststroke, travel backward

Rocking horse R with shoulder blade squeeze

Straddle jog with breaststroke, travel forward

Rocking horse L with arm curl

Straddle jog with reverse breaststroke, travel backward

Rocking horse L with shoulder blade squeeze

Straddle jog with breaststroke, travel forward

Rocking horse R with arm curl

Tabata 8 sets (4 minutes):

Kick forward (20 seconds)

Squat (10 seconds)

C SET

Heel jog with unison arm swing, travel backward

Jumping jacks with bowstring pull to R side

Heel jog with triceps kick back, travel forward

Jumping jacks with bowstring pull to L side

Heel jog with unison arm swing, travel backward

Jumping jacks with bowstring pull to R side

Heel jog with triceps kick back, travel forward

Jumping jacks with bowstring pull to L side

Tabata 8 sets (4 minutes):

Jacks tuck (20 seconds)

Run tires (10 seconds)

20 minutes aquatic endings or fun activities

Stretch: hip flexors, quadriceps, gastrocnemius, outer thigh, hamstrings, lower back

▶ Shallow-Water 30-Minute Cardio Lesson Plan 12

TABATA TIMING 2

EQUIPMENT

None

WARM-UP

Instructor's choice

A SET

Tabata repeat 4× (4 minutes):

Knee lift, doubles (20 seconds)

Knee-high jog (10 seconds)

Knee-high jog, syncopate (20 seconds)

Knee-high jog (10 seconds)

One-minute break:

Walk backward (30 seconds)

Walk forward (30 seconds)

B SET

Tabata repeat 4× (4 minutes):

R quad kick (20 seconds)

Kick forward (10 seconds)

L quad kick (20 seconds)

Kick forward (10 seconds)

One-minute break:

Walk backward, big steps (30 seconds)

Walk forward, big steps (30 seconds)

C SET

Tabata repeat 4× (4 minutes):

Kick side to side, doubles (20 seconds)

Straddle jog (10 seconds)

Kick side to side (20 seconds)

Straddle jog (10 seconds)

One-minute break:

Step sideways R (30 seconds)

Step sideways L (30 seconds)

D SET

Tabata repeat 4× (4 minutes):

Hopscotch (20 seconds)

Heel jog (10 seconds)

In-line skate (20 seconds)

Heel jog (10 seconds)

One-minute break:

Knee-high jog, travel backward (30 seconds)

Lunge walk (30 seconds)

E SET

Tabata repeat 4× (4 minutes):

Tuck ski, doubles (20 seconds)

Lunge R (10 seconds)

Tuck ski (20 seconds)

Lunge L (10 seconds)

One-minute break:

Knee-high jog, travel backward (30 seconds)

Crossover step, travel forward (30 seconds)

F SET

Tabata repeat 4× (4 minutes):

Jumping jacks (20 seconds)

Run tires (10 seconds)

Jumping jacks, syncopate (20 seconds)

Run tires (10 seconds)

One-minute break:

Step sideways R (30 seconds)

Step sideways L (30 seconds)

20 minutes aquatic endings or fun activities

Stretch: quadriceps, gastrocnemius, hamstrings, outer thigh, pectorals, upper back

SECTION 2: 20-MINUTE AQUATIC ENDINGS

▶ Shallow-Water 20-Minute Strength Training 1

HAND POSITIONS

EQUIPMENT

None

A SET

R shoulder sweep in, hand slicing, squat position

L shoulder sweep in, hand slicing, squat position

R shoulder sweep in, hand cupped, squat position

L shoulder sweep in, hand cupped, squat position

B SET

R shoulder sweep out, hand slicing, squat position

L shoulder sweep out, hand slicing, squat position

R shoulder sweep out, hand open, squat position

L shoulder sweep out, hand open, squat position

C SET

R bowstring pull, hand fisted, lunge position

L bowstring pull, hand fisted, lunge position

R bowstring pull, hand cupped, lunge position

L bowstring pull, hand cupped, lunge position

D SET

R arm curl, hand slicing, lunge position

L arm curl, hand slicing, lunge position

R arm curl, palm faces direction of motion, lunge position

L arm curl, palm faces direction of motion, lunge position

E SET 4 MINUTES

R forearm press, palm up, hand slicing, squat position

L forearm press, palm up, hand slicing, squat position

R forearm press, hand open, squat position

L forearm press, hand open, squat position

▶ Shallow-Water 20-Minute Strength Training 2

LEVER LENGTH

EQUIPMENT

None

A SET

Clamshells R

Clamshells L

R leg kicks side

L leg kicks side

B SET

Squat

Squat and jump

Squat travel sideways R and L

C SET

R quad kick

L quad kick

Kick and lunge R

Kick and lunge L

D SET

R hamstring curl

L hamstring curl

R leg kicks back

L leg kicks back

E SET

Up on toes and down

Jump and land toe-ball-heel

Walk on toes

Walk on heels

▶ Shallow-Water 20-Minute Strength Training 3

INERTIA AND FRONTAL RESISTANCE

EQUIPMENT

None

TEACHING TIP

In a pyramid, you perform one exercise 4× and then its pair 4×, then each exercise 2×, and finally you alternate one of each exercise.

A SET

Breaststroke, lunge position

Reverse breaststroke, lunge position

Kick forward

Skate kick

Breaststroke and reverse breaststroke, pyramid 4×, 2×, 1×, lunge position

Kick forward and skate kick, pyramid 4×, 2×, 1×

B SET

Double-arm press-down, lunge position

Lat pull-down, lunge position

Cross-country ski

Jumping jacks

Double-arm press-down and lat pull-down, pyramid 4×, 2×, 1×, lunge position

Cross-country ski and jumping jacks, pyramid 4×, 2×, 1×

C SET

Standing row, lunge position

Unison push forward, lunge position

Inner-thigh lift

Hopscotch

Standing row and unison push forward, pyramid 4×, 2×, 1×, lunge position

Inner-thigh lift and hopscotch, pyramid 4×, 2×, 1×

D SET

Triceps extension, lunge position

Arm curl, lunge position

R quad kick

L quad kick

Skateboard R

Skateboard L

Triceps extension and arm curl, pyramid 4×, 2×, 1×, lunge position

R quad kick and skateboard R, pyramid 4×, 2×, 1×

L quad kick and skateboard L, pyramid 4×, 2×, 1×

▶ Shallow-Water 20-Minute Strength Training 4

ACCELERATION 1

EQUIPMENT

None

A SET

Shoulder blade squeeze, lunge position

Standing row, lunge position

Breaststroke, lunge position

Arm lift to sides with elbows bent, lunge position

Unison arm swing, lunge position

Knee-high jog, one lap

B SET

R shoulder sweep out, squat position

L shoulder sweep out, squat position

R shoulder sweep in, squat position

L shoulder sweep in, squat position

Lat pull-down, lunge position

Palms touch in back, lunge position

Chest press, lunge position

Clap hands, lunge position

Knee-high jog, one lap

C SET

Forearm press, squat position

Forearm press side to side, squat position

Arm curl, squat position

Open and close doors, squat position

Unison jog press, squat position

Push forward, squat position

Knee-high jog, one lap

D SET

Wall push-ups

Knee-high jog, one lap

Climb the wall, one foot on the wall and one on the floor

Knee-high jog, one lap

▶ **Shallow-Water 20-Minute Strength Training 5**

ACCELERATION 2

EQUIPMENT

None

A SET

R leg kicks forward

L leg kicks forward

Knee lift and lunge R

Knee lift and lunge L

R leg kicks forward and back

L leg kicks forward and back

Cross-country ski

Knee-high jog, one lap

B SET

R leg kicks side

L leg kicks side

R side kick (karate)

L side kick (karate)

R leg kicks side, crosses front, kicks side, crosses back

L leg kicks side, crosses front, kicks side, crosses back

Jacks cross

Knee-high jog, one lap

C SET

R hamstring curl

L hamstring curl

Skateboard R

Skateboard L

R quad kick

L quad kick

Rocking horse R

Rocking horse L

Knee-high jog, one lap

D SET

Climb the wall, both feet on the wall and down to the floor

Knee-high jog, one lap

Push off the wall with both feet and run back

Knee-high jog, one lap

▶ **Shallow-Water 20-Minute Strength Training 6**

ACTION AND REACTION

EQUIPMENT

None

A SET

Knee-high jog with standing row, travel backward

Knee-high jog, travel forward

Knee-high jog with breaststroke, travel backward

Knee-high jog, travel forward

Knee-high jog with double-arm press-down, travel backward

Knee-high jog with double-arm lift, travel forward

B SET

Knee-high jog with shoulder sweep out, travel backward

Knee-high jog with shoulder sweep in, travel forward

Knee-high jog with forearm press, travel backward

Knee-high jog, travel forward

Knee-high jog with triceps kick back, travel backward

Knee-high jog, push forward, travel forward

C SET

Knee lift, straighten and power press-down, travel backward

High kick, travel forward

Jumping jacks, neutral position, travel backward and forward

Heel jog, travel backward

Kick forward, neutral position, travel forward

D SET

Walk on toes

Walk on heels

Lunge walk backward

Lunge walk forward

Squat, travel sideways R and L

▶ Shallow-Water 20-Minute Strength Training 7

T

PF

BUOYANT EQUIPMENT— NOODLES

A SET

(Noodle in hands)

Rocking horse R, plunge noodle in front

Rocking horse L, pull noodle toward chest

Jumping jacks with double-arm press-down

Cross-country ski, noodle in R hand

Cross-country ski, noodle in L hand

Jumping jacks, noodle in R hand

Jumping jacks, noodle in L hand

Jumping jacks, touch ends in front

Jumping jacks with forearm press, noodle in back

Cross-country ski, push ends forward

Run tires with triceps extension

Knee-high jog, plunge R

Knee-high jog, plunge L

B SET

(Foot on a noodle)

Hip extension R

Hip extension L

Standing leg press R

Standing leg press L

Standing leg press to R side

Standing leg press to L side

C SET

(Sit on noodle like a swing)

Seated jacks

Seated kick

Seated kick with L shoulder sweep out, circle clockwise

Seated kick with R shoulder sweep out, circle counterclockwise

Point and flex feet

Hip hike

▶ Shallow-Water 20-Minute Strength Training 8

BUOYANT EQUIPMENT— DUMBBELLS

T

PF

A SET

Clap hands, lunge position

Knee-high jog

(With dumbbells)

Chest fly at 45-degree angle, lunge position

Knee-high jog

B SET

Arm swing, lunge position

Knee-high jog

(With dumbbells)

Cross-country ski

Knee-high jog

C SET

Lat pull-down, lunge position

Knee-high jog

(With dumbbells)

Lat pull-down, lunge position

Knee-high jog

D SET

Triceps extension, lunge position

Knee-high jog

(With dumbbells)

Triceps extension, lunge position

Knee-high jog

E SET

Clamshells R

Clamshells L

Knee-high jog

Jumping jacks with power, suspended

Knee-high jog

F SET

R leg kicks side

L leg kicks side

Knee-high jog

Jacks cross

Knee-high jog

H SET

(With dumbbells)

Lunge walk, hold dumbbells down at sides
Walk, one lap

▶ Shallow-Water 20-Minute Strength Training 9

BUOYANT EQUIPMENT— DUMBBELLS (CONCENTRIC AND ECCENTRIC CONTRACTIONS)

A SET

(With dumbbells)

Chest fly at 45-degree angle, lunge position
Cross-country ski with dumbbells as stabilizers
Chest fly at 45-degree angle, faster, lunge position
Cross-country ski, faster, with dumbbells as stabilizers
Chest fly at 45-degree angle, fast concentric and slow eccentric, lunge position
Cross-country ski, suspended, no dumbbells

B SET

(With dumbbells)

Lat pull-down, lunge position
Jumping jacks, neutral position, with dumbbells as stabilizers
Lat pull-down, faster, lunge position
Jumping jacks, faster, neutral position, with dumbbells as stabilizers
Lat pull-down, fast concentric and slow eccentric, lunge position
Jumping jacks, suspended, no dumbbells

C SET

(With dumbbells)

Double-arm press-down, lunge position
Kick forward, neutral position, with dumbbells as stabilizers
Double-arm press-down, faster, lunge position
Kick forward, faster, neutral position, with dumbbells as stabilizers
Double-arm press-down, fast concentric and slow eccentric, lunge position
Mermaid, suspended, no dumbbells

D SET

(With dumbbells)

Triceps extension, lunge position

Jumping jacks with dumbbells as stabilizers
Triceps extension, faster, lunge position
Jumping jacks, faster, with dumbbells as stabilizers
Triceps extension, fast concentric and slow eccentric, lunge position
Frog, suspended, no dumbbells

▶ Shallow-Water 20-Minute Strength Training 10

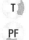

DRAG EQUIPMENT— WEBBED GLOVES OR PADDLES

A SET

R shoulder sweep out and slice in, lunge position
L shoulder sweep out and slice in, lunge position
Kick forward
R shoulder sweep in and slice out, lunge position
L shoulder sweep in and slice out, lunge position
Kick forward
Clap hands, faster, lunge position
Kick forward

B SET

R arm press-down and slice up, lunge position
L arm press-down and slice up, lunge position
Kick side to side
R arm lift and slice down, lunge position
L arm lift and slice down, lunge position
Kick side to side
Unison arm swing, faster, lunge position
Kick side to side

C SET

R lat pull-down and slice up, lunge position
L lat pull-down and slice up, lunge position
Heel jog
Arm lift to R side and slice down, lunge position
Arm lift to L side and slice down, lunge position
Heel jog
Lat pull-down and lift faster, lunge position
Heel jog

D SET

R triceps extension and slice up, lunge position
L triceps extension and slice up, lunge position

Rocking horse R

R arm curl and slice down, lunge position

L arm curl and slice down, lunge position

Rocking horse L

Arm curl, palms or paddles face direction of motion, faster, lunge position

Rocking horse R

Rocking horse L

▶ Shallow-Water 20-Minute Strength Training 11

DRAG EQUIPMENT—PADDLES

A SET

(With paddles held in hand brace position)

Breaststroke, lunge position

Cross-country ski, slice

Chest fly, lunge position

Cross-country ski, paddle face against water

Crossovers, lunge position

Jumping jacks, paddles cross in front slicing

Lat pull-down, lunge position

R shoulder sweep in and slice out, squat position

L shoulder sweep in and slice out, squat position

R shoulder sweep out and slice in, squat position

L shoulder sweep out and slice in, squat position

B SET

(With paddles held in freehold position)

Push forward R arm, squat position

Push forward L arm, squat position

Push forward R arm and L arm, alternate, squat position

Unison push forward, squat position

Pronate and supinate

C SET

(With paddles held in hand brace position)

Arms down at sides, bring R arm across to L shoulder, squat position

Arms down at sides, bring L arm across to R shoulder, squat position

Arms to sides 70 degrees, bring R arm down to L hip, squat position

Arms to sides 70 degrees, bring L arm down to R hip, squat position

Arm curl, lunge position

Rocking horse with triceps extension, hold paddles palms down

Forearm press, squat position

Arms sweep side to side, squat position

Arms sweep side to side, tandem stance (one foot in front of the other)

Lat pull-down, slice, stand on L foot

R lat pull-down, slice, stand on R foot

L lat pull-down, slice, stand on R foot

Upper-body twist, paddles extended to sides

▶ Shallow-Water 20-Minute Strength Training 12

RUBBERIZED EQUIPMENT— BANDS (CONCENTRIC AND ECCENTRIC CONTRACTIONS)

A SET

(With band)

R bowstring pull, lunge position

L bowstring pull, lunge position

R arm press-down, lunge position

L arm press-down, lunge position

Chest press, band behind back, lunge position

Arm lift to sides, band under knee

Arm curl, band under knee

R elbow sweep out

L elbow sweep out

Forearm press out, squat position

Knee-high jog

B SET

(With band, pause at the end range of motion, slow return)

R bowstring pull, lunge position

L bowstring pull, lunge position

R arm press-down, lunge position

L arm press-down, lunge position

Chest press, band behind back, lunge position

Arm lift to sides, band under knee

Arm curl, band under knee

R elbow sweep out

L elbow sweep out

Forearm press out, squat position

▶ Shallow-Water 20-Minute Strength Training 13

CIRCUIT CLASS 1

EQUIPMENT
Kickboards, paddles, dumbbells, noodles

A SET
Standing row with kickboard, lunge position
Knee-high jog
Lat pull-down with paddles in hand brace position, lunge position
Knee-high jog
Forearm press with paddles in freehold position, lunge position
Knee-high jog
Squat, dumbbells down at sides
Knee-high jog
Seated kick, sit on noodle like a swing
Knee-high jog
Standing leg press to R side, foot on a noodle
Standing leg press to L side, foot on a noodle
Knee-high jog
Up on toes and down, dumbbells down at sides
Knee-high jog
Fall forward, tuck, and stand, noodle in hands on surface of water
Knee-high jog
Upper-body twist, hold kickboard upright between palms
Knee-high jog

▶ Shallow-Water 20-Minute Strength Training 14

CIRCUIT CLASS 2

EQUIPMENT
Multiplane drag equipment, aquatic steps

A SET
(With multiplane drag equipment)
Standing row, lunge position
Double-arm press-down, lunge position
Arm swing, lunge position
Lat pull-down, lunge position
Chest fly, lunge position

R shoulder sweep out, squat position
L shoulder sweep out, squat position
R shoulder sweep in, squat position
L shoulder sweep in, squat position
Forearm press, squat position
Arm curl, squat position
Open and close doors, squat position
Triceps extension, squat position
Push forward, lunge position
Plunge down at sides, lunge position

B SET
(On aquatic step or floor)
Knee lift and lunge R, L foot on step
Knee lift and lunge L, R foot on step
Rocking horse R, R foot on step
Rocking horse L, L foot on step
Kick and lunge R, L foot on step
Kick and lunge L, R foot on step
Jumping jacks, land out on floor, land center on step
Cross-country ski, front foot on step
Cross-country ski, suspended over step
Squat on step
Skateboard R, L foot on step
Skateboard L, R foot on step
Step side to side, from floor to step to floor

▶ Shallow-Water 20-Minute Strength Training 15

FUNCTIONAL CORE STRENGTH 1

EQUIPMENT
None

A SET
Walk backward with hands on hips
Walk forward with hands on hips
Walk forward, R foot first, with L bowstring pull, R hand on hip
Walk forward, L foot first, with R bowstring pull, L hand on hip
Knee-high jog with toes in 3× and hold
Knee-high jog with toes out 3× and hold
Rocking horse R, 3× and hold
Rocking horse L, 3× and hold

Cross-country ski with R arm swing, L hand on hip

Cross-country ski with L arm swing, R hand on hip

Cross-country ski with feet wide, travel backward and forward

B SET

Jumping jacks squat

Jumping jacks

Jumping jacks with toes in

Jumping jacks with toes out

Crossover kick

Crossover kick and sweep out

Skate kick, crossover kick, sweep out and center

Hopscotch

Heel jog 3× and hold

Walk on toes

Lunge walk

Crossover step

Stand on R foot, arms sweep side to side

Stand on R foot, arms sweep side to side, eyes closed

Stand on L foot, turn head R and L

▶ Shallow-Water 20-Minute Strength Training 16

FUNCTIONAL CORE STRENGTH 2

EQUIPMENT

None

A SET

Walk backward with hands on hips

Walk forward with hands on hips

Step sideways with arms to sides 70 degrees

Knee-high jog with hands on hips, travel in a bowtie pattern

Kick and lunge R

Kick and lunge L

Brace core, arms down, turbulent hand movements

B SET

Cross-country ski, travel in a bowtie pattern

Cross-country ski

Cross-country ski, pause in center on toes, neutral position

Jumping jacks, heels out and toes in center, neutral position

Jumping jacks, neutral position

Jumping jacks

Jumping jacks, travel in a bowtie pattern

C SET

Kick forward with hands on hips

Crossover kick

Crossover kick and sweep out

Skate kick, crossover kick, sweep out and center

Kick and lunge R

Kick and lunge L

Inner-thigh lift

Kick side to side

Kick side to side with hands on hips

Hopscotch

Heel jog

Stand on L foot, turn head R and L

▶ Shallow-Water 20-Minute Strength Training 17

BALANCE 1

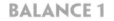
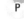

EQUIPMENT

None

A SET

Walk backward

Walk forward, R arm breaststroke and L arm crawl stroke

Walk backward

Walk forward, L arm breaststroke and R arm crawl stroke

Step sideways, R arm crosses in front, and L arm crosses in back

Step sideways, L arm crosses in front, and R arm crosses in back

Jumping jacks with arm swing

Cross-country ski with lat pull-down

Knee-high jog travel backward, forward, and sideways with quick change of direction

Step sideways R, look L

Step sideways L, look R

R leg kicks side and crosses midline

L leg kicks side and crosses midline

Clamshells R

Clamshells L

B SET

(Travel in a bowtie pattern)

Walk backward

Walk diagonally to front R corner, look L

Walk backward

Walk diagonally to front L corner, look R

Jumping jacks, travel backward

Cross-country ski, travel diagonally to front R corner

Jumping jacks, travel backward

Cross-country ski, travel diagonally to front L corner

Knee-high jog, travel diagonally to back R corner

Knee-high jog, travel forward

Knee-high jog, travel diagonally to back L corner

Knee-high jog, travel forward

▶ Shallow-Water 20-Minute Strength Training 18

BALANCE 2

EQUIPMENT

Paddles

A SET

Walk backward

Walk forward, circle both thumbs clockwise

Walk backward

Walk forward, circle both thumbs counterclockwise

Step sideways R 3× and squat

Step sideways L 3× and squat

Jumping jacks 1×, inner-thigh lift 1×

Cross-country ski and cross-country ski, neutral position, alternate

Knee-high jog, travel in a circle clockwise, look L

Knee-high jog, travel in a circle counterclockwise, look R

Stand on R foot, look R and L

Stand on L foot, look R and L

B SET

(With paddles)

Arms sweep side to side, hand brace, squat position

Double-arm press-down, hand brace, lunge position

Lat pull-down, hand brace, lunge position

Triceps extension, freehold, lunge position

Forearm press, freehold, lunge position

Arms sweep side to side, hand brace, tandem stance

Lat pull-down, hand brace, tandem stance

Triceps extension, freehold, tandem stance

Lat pull-down R, hand brace, stand on L foot

Lat pull-down L, hand brace, stand on R foot

Triceps extension R, freehold, stand on L foot

Triceps extension L, freehold, stand on R foot

▶ Shallow-Water 20-Minute Strength Training 19

PILATES FUSION 1

EQUIPMENT

Noodles

A SET

Tap R heel in front and toe in back

Tap L heel in front and toe in back

Knee lift and lunge R, pause on knee lift

Knee lift and lunge L, pause on knee lift

R leg kicks forward and back

L leg kicks forward and back

Kick and lunge R with double-arm press-down

Kick and lunge L with double-arm press-down

Kick and lunge R, arms sweep side to side

Kick and lunge L, arms sweep side to side

Knee-high jog, travel backward and forward

Straddle jog, travel sideways R and L

Heel jog, travel backward and forward

B SET

(Sit on noodle like a swing)

Seated kick, arms to sides 70 degrees

Seated jacks, arms to sides 70 degrees

Seated kick, R shoulder sweep out, circle counterclockwise

Seated kick, L shoulder sweep out, circle clockwise

Hip hike

C SET

(Noodle in posterior sling)
- Lower-body twist
- Pike and hold
- Pull R knee toward chest, lift and lower L leg
- Pull L knee toward chest, lift and lower R leg
- Pull R knee toward chest, hip roll
- Pull L knee toward chest, hip roll
- Flex R foot and lower, point R foot and lift
- Flex L foot and lower, point L foot and lift

▶ Shallow-Water 20-Minute Strength Training 20

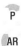

PILATES FUSION 2

EQUIPMENT
Dumbbells

A SET

- High kick and return
- High kick and return, travel backward and forward
- Skate kick and return
- Skate kick and return, travel backward and forward
- R leg kicks side and crosses midline
- L leg kicks side and crosses midline
- Jacks cross with power, grounded
- Inner-thigh lift
- Hopscotch
- Inner-thigh lift R and hopscotch R, alternate
- Inner-thigh lift L and hopscotch L, alternate
- Knee-high jog, travel backward and forward
- Straddle jog, travel sideways R and L
- Heel jog, travel backward and forward

B SET

(With dumbbells)
- Squat, slow, hold dumbbells down at sides
- R knee lift, extend knee, flex knee and lower, dumbbells on surface of water
- L knee lift, extend knee, flex knee and lower, dumbbells on surface of water
- Crossover kick toward opposite dumbbell
- Ankle circles to R side, dumbbells on surface of water
- Ankle circles to L side, dumbbells on surface of water
- Lat pull-down, slow return, squat position
- Alternating triceps extension, dumbbells upright, squat position
- Fall forward, tuck, and stand
- Fall forward and hold position, then pull back
- Stand on one foot and gently pulse dumbbells down
- Plank
- Plank scissors
- Side plank R
- Side plank pliers R
- Side plank L
- Side plank pliers L

SECTION 3: 20-MINUTE FUN ACTIVITIES

▶ Shallow-Water 20-Minute Fun Activities 1

CIRCUIT CLASS WITH PARTNERS   AR

EQUIPMENT
Noodles, dumbbells, kickboards, aquatic steps

TEACHING TIP
Two minutes at each station; allow extra time to move to next station. If you have an odd number of class participants, you will need to participate so that no one is left out.

Station 1 Noodles:
Bicycle race: Sit on noodle as if riding a bicycle and pedal with arms and legs; race until time is up.

Bicycle ride: Partner A is the handlebars with the noodle around his or her waist, and partner B is the bicycle rider, straddling the noodle. Halfway through they change positions.

Station 2 Kickboards:
Canoe: Partners stand one behind the other as if in a canoe. Partner A paddles on the R, and partner B paddles on the L. They switch every 10 seconds.

Balance challenge: Partners face each other standing on one foot. They push and pull to create turbulence and switch feet halfway through.

Station 3 Dumbbells:

Bird: When one partner does a lat pull-down, the other does arm lift to sides.

See saw 1: Partners hold dumbbells down at sides. When one partner squats, the other stands.

Station 4 Aquatic Steps:

See saw 2: Partners stand on two steps facing each other. When one partner squats, the other stands.

Chase: One partner follows the leader forward, backward, or sideways over and around the step. They switch leader halfway through.

▶ Shallow-Water 20-Minute Fun Activities 2

AR

SQUARE DANCE

EQUIPMENT

None

TEACHING TIP

Divide class into two lines facing each other. If you have an odd number of class participants, you will need to participate so that no one is left out.

A SET

Partners run forward, shake R hands, and return

Partners run forward, shake L hands, and return

Partners run forward, do sa do, and return

  (Pass on R and move around partner while facing same direction)

Partners run forward, high-five R, and return

Partners run forward, high-five L, and return

Partners run forward, high-ten, and return

Partners run forward, do sa do, and return

Partners run forward, hold R hands and kick, and return

Partners run forward, hold L hands and kick, and return

Partners run forward, face each other, hold hands and kick side to side, and return

Partners run forward, do sa do, and return

B SET

Partners run forward, swing their partner R, and return

Partners run forward, swing their partner L, and return

Partners run forward, swing their partner R and L, and return

Promenade

  (Partners at the head of the two lines run forward and then run through the lines to the end; the other partners follow.)

Weave the ring

  (Close the ends of the lines to form a circle and count off A, B, A, B, and so on. The A's circle clockwise, and the B's circle counterclockwise, weaving in and out of the ring.)

▶ Shallow-Water 20-Minute Fun Activities 3

YOU BE THE TEACHER

AR

EQUIPMENT

None

TEACHING TIP

The class is in a big circle.

Ask one participant to lead the class in his or her favorite cardio exercise. Then go around the circle until everyone has had a turn. Allow any participant who does not wish to lead an exercise to pass. The next time around the circle, ask for their favorite upper-body strength-training exercise, core strength exercise, lower-body strength-training exercise, balance exercise, stretch, and so on. Continue until 20 minutes are up.

▶ Shallow-Water 20-Minute Fun Activities 4

MODIFIED SYNCHRONIZED SWIMMING

AR

EQUIPMENT

Noodles

TEACHING TIP

Sit on a noodle as if riding a bicycle. The class is in a big circle. Count off A, B, A, B, and so on. If you have an odd number of class participants, you will need to participate so that no one is left out.

A SET

Bicycle, travel clockwise around the circle

A's stand up and raise arms

Bicycle, travel counterclockwise around the circle

B's stand up and raise arms

Seated kick, travel toward the center of the circle

Seated leg press with propeller scull, travel backward

Seated row, travel toward the center of the circle

Seated flutter kick with propeller scull, travel backward

B SET

Bicycle with L hand up, travel clockwise around the circle

Mermaid, circle clockwise

Bicycle with R hand up, travel counterclockwise around the circle

Mermaid, circle counterclockwise

Seated kick R, travel toward the center of the circle

Seated leg press with propeller scull, travel backward

Seated kick L, travel toward the center of the circle

Seated leg press with propeller scull, travel backward

C SET

A's bicycle toward the center of the circle; B's bicycle in place

A's bicycle and travel clockwise in the inner circle; B's bicycle and travel counterclockwise in the outer circle

A's seated flutter kick with propeller scull, travel backward; B's bicycle toward the center of the circle

B's bicycle and travel clockwise in the inner circle; A's bicycle and travel counterclockwise in the outer circle

B's seated flutter kick with propeller scull, travel backward; A's bicycle in place

D SET

Bicycle with R hand in the center of the circle, travel clockwise around the circle

Mermaid, circle clockwise

Bicycle with L hand in the center of the circle, travel clockwise around the circle

Mermaid, circle counterclockwise

Seated row, travel toward the center of the circle

Seated flutter kick with propeller scull, travel backward

A's link R arms with B to their R and circle clockwise

A's link L arms with B to their L and circle counterclockwise

A's stand up and raise arms

B's stand up and raise arms

Everyone stands up and raises arms

▶ Shallow-Water Fun Activities

GAMES AND RELAY RACES ⓐⓡ

TEACHING TIP

Choose one or more of these activities to play at the end of class.

1. Centipede (with noodles)

Everyone sits on a noodle as if riding a bicycle. They line up behind the instructor and hold the end of the noodle of the person in front of them with both hands. Everyone bicycles, and the instructor at the head of the line bicycles and does a breaststroke. Travel around the pool in straight lines, circles, spirals, or random patterns.

2. Bicycle race (with noodles)

Divide the group into two-person teams. One team member is the handlebars with the noodle around his or her waist, and the other team member is the bicycle rider, straddling the noodle. On signal, the person who is the handlebars in front runs and the bicycle rider bicycles to the end of the pool. Then they switch positions and return to the starting point. The first team to get to the starting point wins.

3. Rickshaw race (with noodles)

Divide the group into two-person teams. Each team has two noodles. The driver stands in front of the rider, holding the ends of both noodles under his or her arms. The rider holds the opposite ends of the two noodles under his or her arms. On signal, the drivers run to the end of the pool while the riders sit in a dining-room chair position, keeping their feet off the bottom of the pool and enjoying the ride. Then they switch positions and return to the starting point. The first team to get to the starting point wins.

4. Choo-choo train relay (with noodles)

Divide the group into two teams. Each person has a noodle around his or her waist. The team members line up behind the first person in line, the engine, holding the ends of the noodle belonging to the person in front of them. They run to the back of the pool and return. The engine then goes to the end of the line, and the second person in line becomes the new engine. This continues until the original engine is again at the front. The first team to finish wins.

5. Kayak race (with noodles)

Everyone in the class sits on a noodle as if riding a bicycle and crosses his or her ankles. Participants row with their arms to the end of the pool and back. The first one to get to the starting line wins.

6. Pass the ball (with two balls)

Form a circle with an even number of players. You must participate if necessary to have an even number. Count off A, B, A, B, and so on. Give one ball to a player on team A on one side of the circle and a second ball to a player on team B on the opposite side of the circle. On signal, one team member passes the ball to the next, both balls traveling clockwise around the circle. The team whose ball overtakes the other team's ball wins the game.

7. Eye–hand coordination (with balls)

Form a circle and have the group pass one ball around the circle. Add another ball so that now they are passing two balls around the circle. Keep adding balls.

8. Ball toss (with one ball for every set of partners)

Position the class in two lines of partners, facing each other. If you have an odd number of class participants, you have to participate so that everyone has a partner. Each set of partners has a ball, which they toss back and forth. After one minute, the partners each take a step backward so that the distance between them increases. They keep taking steps backward every minute until they run out of room.

9. Ball sweep relay (with two balls and two kickboards)

Divide the group into two teams. Give each team a ball and a kickboard. The first person on each team sweeps the ball with the kickboard to the back of the pool and returns to his or her team. The person hands off the ball and kickboard to the next team member. The team members repeat until each person has had a turn. The first team to get back with the ball and kickboard wins.

10. Obstacle course (with kickboards, noodles, balls, and so on)

Divide the class into two groups. Arrange one group in various locations in an obstacle course. They can jog in place pushing the water to create turbulence or create turbulence by holding the ends of kickboards and pushing them forward. Two participants can each hold one end of a noodle in a rainbow. One or more can have balls. The second group runs through the human obstacle course. They run through the turbulence, run under the noodle rainbow, and stop to catch a ball and throw it back. Use your imagination with whatever equipment you have. When the second group completes the obstacle course, they become the obstacles and the first group runs through the course.

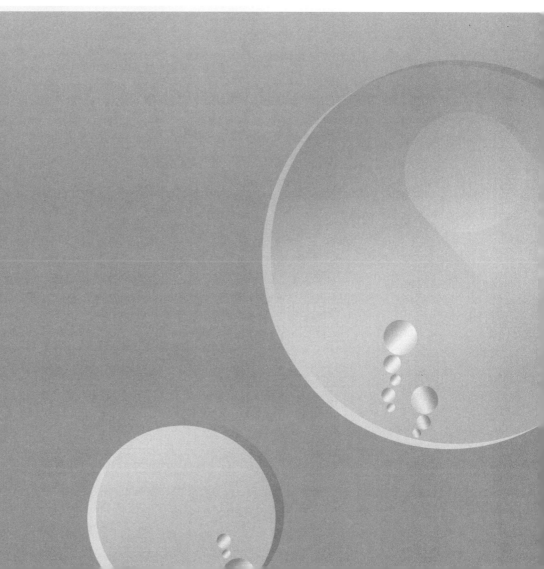

PART II

DEEP-WATER EXERCISE

CHAPTER 5

Deep-Water Periodization Stages

Deep-water exercise differs from shallow-water exercise in that participants are exercising in water that is over their heads. For safety's sake, they must wear a flotation device, such as a flotation belt, flotation vest, arm cuffs, or ankle cuffs. Sustaining neutral alignment in a vertical posture in deep water is difficult and tiring unless a flotation device is worn. Flotation belts, vests, and arm cuffs are comfortable for most participants. Ankle cuffs should be reserved for experienced participants because they are more challenging to use. Do not allow participants to use handheld equipment for flotation. The shoulder is not a weight-bearing joint. Hanging from handheld equipment puts pressure on the rotator cuff and shoulder stabilizers and may pinch the nerves, causing damage.

Maintaining good posture in deep water is important, just as it is in shallow water, but it is more difficult to achieve. Exercisers must aggressively engage the stabilizing muscles of the core to remain upright. They are used to having their center of gravity in the pelvic area on land, but in deep water they have to work with their center of buoyancy in the lungs. A common alignment error is leaning forward at the waist to bring the center of gravity and the center of buoyancy closer together. This stance might make the exercises easier to perform, but it inhibits the working muscles from doing their jobs and puts stress on the spine. Exercises are performed correctly when the spine in neutral, when the cervical, thoracic, and lumbar sections of the spine are aligned in their natural curves. After the spine is in neutral, the next step is to brace the core; only then are you ready to begin your workout. When the body is correctly aligned you can maximize the use of the water's resistance. Repeatedly performing an exercise incorrectly can cause microtrauma that eventually leads to an injury.

PRESEASON

The preseason establishes a baseline from which the following seasons progress. Your classes will include sessions of continuous cardiorespiratory fitness training, interval training to work on improving cardiorespiratory fitness, and strength training to work on improving muscular strength and endurance. You will want to emphasize good posture and performing the exercises correctly before you begin to increase resistance and add intensity in the following seasons.

Teaching your class to perform exercises correctly requires you to be familiar with the muscles of the body and with movement terminology. This information is available in your water fitness instructor certification manual. Table 5.1 provides the major movements and the muscles most involved. Joint motion involves prime movers, which are responsible for initiating the motion. Assistors are also involved, though to a lesser degree, as are stabilizers, which maintain joint integrity during the motion. The table includes only the prime

TABLE 5.1

Major Movements and Muscles Involved

Joint	Joint motion	Muscles most involved
Scapula	Abduction	Serratus anterior
	Adduction	Trapezius, rhomboids
Shoulder	Flexion	Anterior deltoid, pectoralis major, biceps
	Extension or hyperextension	Latissimus dorsi, triceps
	Abduction	Middle deltoid
	Adduction	Latissimus dorsi, pectoralis major
	Horizontal abduction	Posterior deltoid
	Horizontal adduction	Pectoralis major, anterior deltoid
	Lateral rotation	Rotator cuff
	Medial rotation	Latissimus dorsi, rotator cuff
Elbow	Flexion	Biceps
	Extension	Triceps
Trunk	Flexion	Rectus abdominis
	Extension	Erector spinae
	Lateral flexion	Obliques
	Rotation	Obliques
	Core stabilization	Transversus abdominis
Hip	Flexion	Iliopsoas
	Extension or hyperextension	Gluteus maximus, hamstrings
	Abduction	Gluteus medius
	Horizontal abduction	Tensor fasciae latae
	Adduction	Adductors
Knee	Flexion	Hamstrings
	Extension	Quadriceps
Ankle	Plantar flexion	Gastrocnemius, soleus
	Dorsiflexion	Tibialis anterior

Adapted, by permission, from Aquatic Exercise Association, 2018, *Aquatic fitness professional manual,* 7th ed. (Champaign, IL: Human Kinetics), 70.

movers. All movements begin with the spine in neutral alignment, the arms down at the sides, the palms facing forward, and the feet hip-distance apart.

Joint Range of Motion

Knowing the normal joint range of motion will help you know what you can expect of healthy participants. But you will want to limit the range of motion (ROM) of some movements for safety reasons. For example, normal shoulder flexion is 150 to 180 degrees. Flexing the shoulders to that angle takes the arms out of the water, which removes the buoyancy support of the arms. The weight of the arms then pushes the body down. Participants may find this feeling uncomfortable or even threatening. Most arm movement in deep water takes place under water because participants are submerged up to their necks. Participants are not as likely to move their arms in and out of the water as they might in a shallow-water class. But you need to be aware of other ROM concerns in deep water. When focusing on legs, participants may abduct their shoulders to the water's surface for balance. Shoulder impingement occurs between 80 and 120 degrees, and maintaining the shoulder within this area may provoke bursitis. In this case, bringing the hands below the water's surface to a shoulder abduction of 70 degrees is better (Ivens & Holder, 2011, p. 13). Shoulder adduction can continue beyond neutral 0 degrees if the hands are brought in front of the body. Participants, however, often round out their shoulders when they do this. Because you want to stress good posture, limit shoulder adduction to neutral 0 degrees or balance arm moves in front of the body with arm moves behind the body.

Bringing the arms to their full ROM in horizontal shoulder abduction during a chest stretch is acceptable. But forceful horizontal shoulder abduction exposes the head of the humerus to injury. Limit the ROM to 90 degrees by asking participants to keep their hands in their peripheral vision.

During hip flexion, as in a knee lift, the hip flexors tend to overpower the lower back when the ROM goes beyond 90 degrees. Cue to bring the upper leg parallel to the floor. Never touch a participant, especially to assist with his or her range of motion. A participant who has limitations in range of motion should be encouraged to see his or her doctor and get permission to participate in an exercise program. Table 5.2 lists joint range of motion with notations specific for use in deep water.

Now that you have reviewed the prime movers for the basic joint movements and the normal range of motion specific to deep-water exercise, we will take a look at how to perform the exercises used for cardiorespiratory fitness with good form.

Cardiorespiratory Fitness

Cardiorespiratory training is a constant through all four seasons. After all, the heart is the most important muscle in the body! During aerobic exercise, the muscles use oxygen to produce energy. The heart pumps blood to the lungs to collect the oxygen and then delivers it to the working muscles. Regular aerobic exercise both increases the ability of the lungs to hold air and strengthens the heart muscle so that it pumps a greater volume of blood with each stroke. As the cardiorespiratory system becomes more efficient, exercisers find that they are able to exercise longer. They experience many other health benefits as well, such as a reduced risk of coronary heart disease, adult onset diabetes, hypertension, and certain cancers (ACSM, 2017b). Therefore, one goal of the preseason is to be able to do continuous cardiorespiratory training at a moderate rate for 20 to 30 minutes without tiring. The American College of Sports Medicine (ACSM) recommends that adults get 150 minutes a week or more of moderate-intensity physical activity (ACSM, 2017b).

Basic Cardiorespiratory Exercises

The basic exercises used for cardiorespiratory training in a deep-water class are jog, bicycle, kick, cross-country ski, and jumping jacks. All other moves are variations of these five

Joint Movement Range of Motion

Joint	Joint motion	ROM
Shoulder	Flexion	150-180 degrees *In deep water, shoulder flexion should stop at 90 degrees.*
	Extension	To neutral 0 degrees
	Hyperextension	50-60 degrees
	Abduction	180 degrees *In deep water, stop at 90 degrees. Shoulder impingement occurs between 80 and 120 degrees; if arms are extended to the sides for any length of time, hold at 70 degrees.*
	Adduction	50 degrees *Participants often round out their shoulders when bringing palms together in front; stop at neutral 0 degrees.*
	Horizontal abduction	130 degrees *Stop at 90 degrees to avoid risk of shoulder injury when working against the water's resistance.*
Elbow	Flexion	140-150 degrees
	Extension	To neutral 0 degrees
Hip	Flexion	100-120 degrees *Stop at 90 degrees to avoid stress on the lower back.*
	Extension	To neutral 0 degrees
	Hyperextension	30 degrees
	Abduction	40-50 degrees
	Adduction	0-30 degrees
Knee	Flexion	130-150 degrees
	Extension	0-10 degrees
Ankle	Plantar flexion	40-50 degrees
	Dorsiflexion	20 degrees

exercises. Performing these exercises correctly means performing them with the spine in neutral. The following list describes the benefits as well as common mistakes to watch for.

JOG

Knee-high jog: *Benefit*: This exercise works multiple leg muscles, including the powerful iliopsoas, more commonly called the hip flexors. This exercise is good for burning calories. Beginners can do the move successfully. *Common mistakes*: (1) wobbling the shoulders from side to side, which takes the spine out of neutral, (2) flexing the elbows instead of pumping the arms from the shoulders, (3) bringing the knees too high, which may aggravate the sciatic nerve, and (4) leaning forward, which puts stress on the spine.

Crossover knees: *Benefit*: This exercise works the obliques. *Common mistake*: bringing opposite elbow to knee because twisting while flexing forward is hard on the back.

Straddle jog: *Benefit*: Jogging with the hips open works the gluteus medius. *Common mistake*: jogging with the feet too far apart, which makes this exercise the same as running tires.

Run tires: *Benefit*: The hips are open wider than with straddle jog on this exercise, increasing the range of motion. *Common mistake*: leaning the trunk from side to side, which puts stress on the lower back. Instead, the core muscles should be stabilized putting the focus on working the legs.

Ankle touch or inner-thigh lift: *Benefit*: This move improves hip flexibility by working on a diagonal. Hip flexibility is important for reducing the risk of falling. *Common mistakes*: (1) performing the exercise from a narrow instead of a wide stance, which makes it the same as a knee-high jog, and (2) leaning forward to reach the foot instead of bringing the foot up to the hand, which puts stress on the lower back. Calling the exercise an inner-thigh lift reduces this tendency.

Hopscotch: *Benefit*: This exercise works the hamstrings. *Common mistake*: leaning to the side to reach down to the foot instead of bringing the foot up toward the hand, which puts stress on the lower back.

Heel jog: *Benefit*: This exercise is another one for the hamstrings. *Common mistake*: bringing the knee up in front instead of lifting the heel up in back, which makes the exercise similar to a knee-high jog.

BICYCLE

Bicycle: *Benefit*: This exercise works multiple leg muscles. The bicycle is used in place of the rocking horse, which is used in only shallow water. The rocking horse requires a weight shift, which is not possible in deep water. If the exercise is attempted, the exerciser will end up arching the back. *Common mistakes*: (1) pedaling in a seated position instead of an upright position and (2) leaning forward, which puts stress on the spine.

KICK

Flutter kick: *Benefit*: The flutter kick works the hip flexors. Because it is a small move, it does not get the heart rate up as much as a larger move, even when you flutter kick fast. But the core muscles must tighten to stabilize the body and maintain the upright position. *Common mistake*: flutter kicking from the knees instead of the hips. Fast kicking from the knees is hard on the knee joints.

Kick forward: *Benefit*: The kick forward uses the quadriceps and hip flexors. *Common mistakes*: (1) performing the kick in a seated position instead of returning the hips to the fully extended position and (2) power popping the knees, that is, adding force at the end of the kick, which is hard on the knee joint.

High kick: *Benefit*: The high kick increases the range of motion, therefore increasing intensity. *Common mistakes*: (1) leaning backward to get the toes out of the water, which takes the spine out of neutral alignment, and (2) emphasizing the upward motion at the expense of the downward motion, which works the powerful hip flexors more than the weaker gluteus maximus.

Cossack kick: *Benefit*: The Cossack kick is used in place of the kick side to side, which is used only in shallow water. Kick side to side requires a weight shift, which is not possible in deep water. If the exercise is attempted, the lower back is stressed. The Cossack kick works the trapezius, quadriceps, and hamstrings. To perform the exercise, the core is stabilized, the shoulder blades are contracted, and the hips are open in a diamond position; the arms then reach to the sides at the same time as the legs kick to the sides.

Skate kick: *Benefit*: The kick backward works the gluteus maximus. *Common mistakes*: (1) bending the knee, which takes the work out of the gluteus maximus and puts it in the hamstrings, and (2) arching the back, which puts stress on the lower back. To avoid arching the back, lean forward slightly from the hips.

CROSS-COUNTRY SKI

Cross-country ski: *Benefit*: This exercise works the hip flexors and gluteus maximus, as well as the shoulders. It is a long-lever, high-intensity move, which burns calories. *Common mistakes*: (1) You want full hip flexion and hyperextension, but many people limit the range of motion to forward flexion, the same as a kick forward, especially when traveling backward. (2) The arm movement contributes to the intensity, but some people reduce it by pushing the hands forward instead of swinging the arms through their full range of motion.

JUMPING JACKS

Jumping jacks: *Benefit*: Jacks work the adductors and gluteus medius. The arms and legs work opposite in deep water to avoid bobbing and possibly submerging the head. *Common mistakes*: (1) trying to make the legs go too far apart, which is hard on the hip joints, (2) bending the knee when traveling sideways, which is the same as a Cossack kick, which works the quads and hamstrings instead of the hip adductors, and (3) pointing the toes out, which works the hip flexors instead of the gluteus medius.

You can create many variations of these exercises. Here are some examples:

- Try different arm movements, such as standing row, arm swing, lat pull-down, clap hands, arm curl, and forearm press. Use alternating arms or both arms in unison. If you use one arm or no arms, you will challenge your core muscles, because maintaining neutral posture will be harder.
- Vary the tempo. The speed at which exercises are performed in deep water is slower than in shallow water because the range of motion is greater. But you can still vary the tempo with pauses (3× and hold) or syncopate (slow, slow, quick, quick, quick).
- Change the working position. Exercises can be performed upright, at a diagonal angle, side lying, or seated.
- Add turns. You can do quarter turns, half turns, or full turns. Diagonal turns are quarter turns toward the right corner and then toward the left corner.
- Combine exercises. Putting two or more exercises together creates a new exercise.

Not every variation will work with every exercise, but using even a few variations will increase the number of exercises in your repertoire.

Exercisers are able to judge how hard they are working by using perceived exertion. One scale of perceived exertion (see table 5.3) uses numbers from 1 to 10. Each number corresponds to a percentage of maximum exertion.

The target heart rate for aerobic exercise is 50 to 80 percent of the maximum heart rate. Participants who are working somewhat easy (50 percent), with moderate effort (60 percent), somewhat hard (70 percent), and hard (80 percent) are working within their target heart rate. During the preseason, you will ask your participants to work at a minimum of 50 percent of their maximum exertion during the continuous cardiorespiratory training sessions.

Interval Training
Interval training is an effective way to improve cardiorespiratory fitness. During interval training the exerciser works in alternating periods of higher and lower intensity. The higher

TABLE 5.3

Scale of Perceived Exertion

Level 1	No effort
Level 2	Little effort
Level 3	Very easy
Level 4	Easy
Level 5	Somewhat easy
Level 6	Moderate
Level 7	Somewhat hard
Level 8	Hard
Level 9	Very hard
Level 10	Maximum effort

Adapted, by permission, from Aquatic Exercise Association, 2018, *Aquatic fitness professional manual,* 7th ed. (Champaign, IL: Human Kinetics), 12.

intensity is called work and the lower intensity is called recovery. One period of work plus one period of recovery is called a set. A group of sets is called a cycle. The length of the work compared with the length of the recovery is referred to as the work–recovery ratio. The recovery needs to be long enough that the class participant is able to recover sufficiently so that he or she can again increase intensity for the next work period. The recovery exercises can be a low-intensity version of the exercise used during the work, a functional movement such as a knee-high jog, or full range of motion movements to promote flexibility. Exercising at a level of exertion that the participant is able to sustain for only a short time improves the heart's muscular strength.

Interval training is appropriate for beginners and fit participants alike. Beginners will be able to increase their exertion for short periods because the exertion is followed by a period of active recovery. One way to cue for interval training in the preseason is to ask participants to increase their exertion from 50 percent (somewhat easy) to 60 percent of maximum levels (moderate). Remember that one person's moderate effort may not be the same as another's. For safety's sake, encourage your participants to modify the intensity to a level that is challenging for them rather than try to keep up with other participants.

When you ask participants to increase their intensity, most likely they will go faster, but speed is not the only way to increase intensity. So rather than just encouraging them to work harder, you can use cues that tell participants how to change an exercise to make it more intense. Begin with exercises that use large-muscle groups in the legs. Save small movements, complex moves, and core challenges for the warm-up, the cool-down, or the recovery period. You want to use exercises that will put a demand on the heart muscle and make it beat faster. Five intensity variables can be used for deep-water exercise:

1. **Range of motion**. Increasing the range of motion by changing an exercise from a short-lever move, with elbows and knees bent, to a long-lever move, with arms and legs fully extended (but not locked), is one way to increase intensity. Exercises can be performed with larger arm or leg movements, or with the feet farther apart, or you can cross the midline of the body. Perform the long-lever moves at the same speed as the short-lever moves for the highest intensity.

2. **Speed**. Any exercise becomes more intense when it is performed faster. The temptation, however, is to reduce the range of motion when increasing speed. Tiny moves are not an effective way to increase intensity. An exercise should not be performed so fast that the range of motion is lost or that good form is compromised.

3. **Elevation**. Elevation means performing an exercise in such a way that the shoulders are lifted out of the water. If you accelerate toward center in what is sometimes called a power pop, your shoulders will rise above the water and fall back down in a high-intensity move. This move can be done with a cross-country ski or a frog kick, for example. Exercisers can also use a scull to provide lift, such as with a jog or a bicycle.

4. **Acceleration**. Acceleration in deep water means pushing hard against the water's resistance in a power move.

5. **Travel**. Newton's law of inertia states that an object will remain at rest or in motion with constant velocity unless acted on by a net external force. Starting the body moving, stopping it once it is moving, or changing a movement requires more effort than continuing with the same movement. You can travel forward, backward, sideways, or on a diagonal. You can travel in patterns, such as a circle, square, bowtie pattern, zigzag, scatter pattern, or with quick changes of direction.

Let's look again at the basic exercises to see how these intensity variables can be used with each of them during interval training. The numbers following the name of the exercise represent the intensity variable being used. Not all variables can be used with every exercise.

JOG

Knee-high jog: (1) Run (focus on full extension of the hip). Steep climb (like climbing a ladder out of the pool). (2) Knee-high jog, faster. Sprint. Steep climb, faster. (3) Knee-high jog with elevation (scull to lift the shoulders). (4) Power run (pull the water forcefully with cupped hands). Steep climb with power. (5) Knee-high jog, travel. Run. Sprint. Power run.

Straddle jog: (3) Frog kick with elevation. (5) Straddle jog, travel.

Run tires: (2) Run tires, faster. (3) Run tires with elevation (scull to lift the shoulders). (5) Run tires, travel.

Inner-thigh lift: (1) Inner-thigh lift with full range of motion (ROM). (2) Inner-thigh lift, faster. (4) Inner-thigh lift with power. (5) Inner-thigh lift, travel.

Hopscotch: (1) Hopscotch with full range of motion (ROM). (2) Hopscotch, faster. (4) Hopscotch with power. (5) Hopscotch, travel.

Heel jog: (3) Breaststroke kick with elevation (lift the heels in back, abduct the hips, straighten the legs, and bring them forcefully to center). (5) Heel jog, travel.

BICYCLE

Bicycle: (1) Bicycle with full range of motion (ROM) (large circles). Bicycle tandem (in unison). (2) Bicycle, faster. (3) Bicycle with elevation (scull to lift the shoulders). (4) Bicycle with power. Bicycle tandem with power. (5) Bicycle, travel.

KICK

Flutter kick: (1) Star flutter kick (feet are apart). (2) Flutter kick, faster. Star flutter kick, faster. (3) Flutter kick with elevation (scull to lift the shoulders). (5) Flutter kick, travel.

Kick forward: (1) High kick. (2) Kick forward, faster. (4) Knee lift, straighten and power press-down. High kick, power down. High kick with power. (5) Kick forward, travel. High kick, travel.

Cossack kick: (5) Cossack kick, travel.

Skate kick: (1) Skate kick with full range of motion (ROM). (2) Skate kick, faster. (4) Skate kick with power. (5) Skate kick, travel.

CROSS-COUNTRY SKI

Cross-country ski: (1) Tuck ski with full extension. Cross-country ski with full range of motion (ROM). Cross-country ski with rotation. Helicopter ski (move arms and legs in semicircles instead of straight lines). (2) Mini ski, faster. Cross-country ski, faster. (3) Cross-country ski with elevation. Tuck ski together with elevation. (4) Cross-country ski with power. Helicopter ski with power. Cross-country ski, arms sweep side to side. (5) Cross-country ski, travel.

JUMPING JACKS

Jumping jacks: (1) Jacks cross. (2) Mini jacks, faster. Mini cross, faster. Jumping jacks, faster. (4) Jumping jacks, clap hands, with power. (5) Jumping jacks, travel.

Timing the Intervals   You can time intervals in many ways. During the preseason, you may wish to intersperse cycles of interval training among periods of continuous cardiorespiratory training. In effect, the cardio serves as a long period of recovery between the cycles of interval sets. The goal is to pull the interval sets together gradually and place them in the middle or at the end of your continuous cardio.

In general, your participants will aim for 60 percent of maximum effort (moderate) during the preseason. But occasionally introduce them to higher levels of intensity—70 percent (somewhat hard) in a rolling interval, a surge, or Tabata. Toward the end of the preseason, let them try working at 80 percent (hard) in a random interval set. An intensity of 80 percent of maximum effort is considered high-intensity interval training (HIIT). More information about Tabata is in the sidebar in chapter 1 on page 12.

The following are options for timing intervals in the preseason (Thielen, 2015):

INTERVAL 30

30 seconds of work to 90 seconds of recovery (1:3 ratio), 6 to 8 sets

INTERVAL 40

40 seconds of work to 80 seconds of recovery (1:2 ratio), 6 to 8 sets

INTERVAL 60

60 seconds of work to 2 minutes of recovery (1:2 ratio), 6 to 8 sets

REDUCED RECOVERY TIME

60 seconds of work to 30 seconds of recovery (2:1 ratio), 4 to 6 sets

ROLLING INTERVALS

1 minute at 50 percent, 1 minute at 60 percent, and 1 minute at 70 percent of maximum effort, 3 to 5 sets

SURGES

45 seconds at 60 percent, 15 seconds at 70 percent of maximum effort, and 1 minute of recovery (1:1 ratio), 4 to 8 sets

RANDOM INTERVALS

30 seconds of work to 30 seconds of recovery

45 seconds of work to 45 seconds of recovery

15 seconds at 50 percent of maximum effort, 15 seconds at 60 percent, 15 seconds at 70 percent, and 15 seconds at 80 percent to 1 minute of recovery (rolling interval)

45 seconds of work to 45 seconds of recovery

30 seconds of work to 30 seconds of recovery

1 cycle

PYRAMID

15 seconds of work to 45 seconds of recovery

20 seconds of work to 45 seconds of recovery

25 seconds of work to 45 seconds of recovery

30 seconds of work to 45 seconds of recovery

1 or more cycles

TABATA TIMING

20 seconds of work at 70 percent of maximum effort to 10 seconds of recovery

8 sets (2:1 ratio), 1 or more cycles

Muscular Strength and Endurance

Strength training is an important component of the periodization program. Some participants may wonder why they should strength train. Children's muscles grow larger and stronger as their bodies grow, and this muscle growth continues into adulthood until around age 30. After reaching a peak, muscle mass begins to decline with age. The prescription for preventing or reversing this loss of muscle mass is strength training. Maintaining or increasing muscular fitness can help prevent osteoporosis, decrease the risk of heart disease, reduce the risk of falling, and enhance the quality of life. The American College of Sports Medicine recommends that every adult perform activities that maintain or increase muscular strength and endurance for a minimum of two days a week. Adults over 65 should strength train two to three times a week (ACSM, 2017c). Strength training involves training both the muscles of the core and the muscles of the limbs to improve their muscular strength and endurance.

Neutral alignment is possible when the muscles that affect the spine, including the shoulder girdle, the trunk muscles, and the pelvic girdle, are balanced in strength. The core refers to the postural muscles of the trunk: transversus abdominis, rectus abdominis, internal and external obliques, erector spinae, latissimus dorsi, trapezius, rhomboids, serratus anterior, gluteus maximus, and hip abductors and adductors. The trapezius is involved in scapular stabilization. Strong hip abductors are important for maintaining balance. These muscles work together to maintain good posture and to support and move the shoulders, the back, and the hips.

In functional movement, the stabilizers activate before the prime movers. Specifically, the core muscles engage before the arms and legs move. The deep end of the pool is the perfect place to work on core strength. Exercisers must aggressively engage the stabilizing muscles of the core to remain upright. They will know immediately if they have not succeeded because they will feel off-balance and may randomly move around the pool. Sculling is an important skill to learn because it will assist in maintaining balance and alignment. In a scull, the exerciser holds the hands in front of his or her body almost flat. The participant sweeps in with the thumbs slightly up and sweeps out with the thumbs slightly down (see figure 5.1). With practice, most participants are able to achieve balance and control their movement through the water. But they may still have a tendency to streamline their bodies when they travel. They may bend forward at the hips, leading with the chest and allowing the water to slide down the rest of the body. This streamlining is an advantage for swimmers, but in deep-water exercise the goal is to present as much frontal resistance as possible. Deep-water participants need to move inefficiently if they are to use the maximum amount of physical effort. You will have to cue for vertical alignment often. Participants do not get the same feedback from gravity that they get on land, so more postural cues are necessary. The classic cue is "Ears over shoulders, over hips, over ankles."

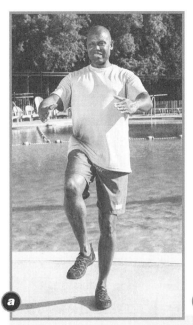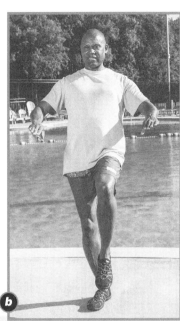

FIGURE 5.1 Scull: (*a*) sweep in and (*b*) sweep out.

You can also ask class participants to travel as if they have a book on their heads, to keep their chests up and their shoulders down, to relax their shoulders and brace the core, to maintain level shoulders and hips, to emphasize a lengthened spine, and to lengthen their bodies by pressing their heels down toward the floor. Have frequent posture checks and repeat your cues over and over. Any participant who is unable to achieve neutral posture, in spite of all your cues, may need to be referred to a doctor.

Some of the best exercises for training the core are functional exercises that mimic activities of daily living, such as running forward and backward, and running in multiple directions. Cross-country ski is another good core exercise that uses long levers with alternating arm and leg movement to create balance. You can challenge core muscles in a variety of ways, such as (1) using one arm only, keeping the other hand on the hip, (2) bracing the core and using one leg only, (3) performing off-axis moves such as leaning 45 degrees to the side, (4) holding a position and creating turbulence with the hands, and (5) performing exercises in a seated position. Avoid exercises that take the spine out of neutral alignment. Avoid leaning forward to touch the toes during a front kick. Forward flexion with rotation, such as a knee lift with opposite elbow to knee, puts a strain on the lower back. Prone flutter kicks at the pool wall result in hyperextension of the back. Pay careful attention to neutral alignment in your participants and demonstrate good posture at all times.

Although knowing movement terminology is important, you will not use those terms with class participants. Exercises have a wide variety of names, because terms are not standardized in the aquatics industry. For the purpose of this book, the following terms in table 5.4 will be used for strength-training exercises.

Muscle Pairs

If you refer to the table of table 5.1, you will notice that the body's muscles are organized in pairs of opposing muscle groups. Often one muscle in a pair is stronger than the opposing muscle. Although you will want to work both sets of opposing muscles (see table 5.5), you should cue your participants to place more force in the direction of the weaker muscle. You also want to be sure to stretch the stronger muscle.

Muscular Contractions

There are three types of muscle actions: isotonic, isometric and isokinetic. In isotonic contractions, the muscle shortens and lengthens and movement occurs at the joint. In

TABLE 5.4

Strength-Training Exercise Names

Exercise science terminology	Common terms
Scapula adduction	Standing row, crawl stroke, bowstring pull, shoulder blade squeeze
Shoulder flexion	Double-arm lift, arm swing forward
Shoulder extension or hyperextension	Double-arm press-down, arm swing back
Shoulder abduction	Arm lift to sides
Shoulder adduction	Lat pull-down
Shoulder horizontal abduction	Clap hands out, shoulder sweep out, breaststroke
Shoulder horizontal adduction	Clap hands in, shoulder sweep in, reverse breaststroke, chest fly, chest press
Shoulder lateral rotation	Forearm press out
Shoulder medial rotation	Forearm press in
Elbow flexion	Arm curl
Elbow extension	Triceps extension, push forward, triceps kick back
Elbow flexion with shoulder abducted 70 degrees	Close doors, side arm curl, elbow sweep in
Elbow extension with shoulder abducted 70 degrees	Open doors, elbow sweep out
Trunk flexion	Crunch
Trunk extension	Spine extension
Trunk lateral flexion	Side to side extension, hip hike
Trunk rotation	Upper-body twist, swirl
Hip flexion	Kick forward, knee swing forward
Hip extension or hyperextension	Kick back, hip extension, knee lift straighten and power press-down, knee swing back, standing leg press, seated leg press
Hip abduction	Kick side, leg lift side, dog hike
Hip adduction	Return kick side to center, standing leg press to the side
Hip horizontal abduction	Clamshells open, bent knee jacks out
Hip horizontal adduction	Clamshells close, bent knee jacks in
Knee flexion	Hamstring curl
Knee extension	Quad kick
Plantar flexion	Point feet
Dorsiflexion	Flex feet

Squats and lunges, which are used in shallow water, are not an option in deep water.

isometric contractions, muscle tension occurs but no movement occurs at the joint and muscle length does not change. Isokinetic muscle actions occur at a constant rate of speed regardless of the muscular force being used. Isokinetic muscle actions require specialized equipment and are not possible in water exercise. The type of muscle action that occurs

TABLE 5.5

Opposing Muscles

Muscle	Opposing muscle	Stronger muscle
Middle deltoid	Latissimus dorsi	Latissimus dorsi
Posterior deltoid	Pectoralis major	Pectoralis major
Biceps	Triceps	Biceps
Rectus abdominis	Erector spinae	Erector spinae
Gluteus medius	Adductors	Adductors
Hamstrings	Quadriceps	Quadriceps
Gastrocnemius	Tibialis anterior	Gastrocnemius

during strength training in water is an isotonic contraction. During an isotonic contraction, the muscle contracts, or shortens, and then lengthens causing movement at a joint. The shortening phase is called a concentric contraction, and the lengthening phase is called an eccentric action. Eccentric actions are not called contractions because the muscle is lengthening rather than contracting. In water the muscles are working against resistance in every direction. Both muscles in a muscle pair work concentrically. Eccentric actions will not occur unless certain types of equipment are used. Gains in strength are possible with concentric contractions alone. Eccentric actions are associated with delayed onset muscle soreness, which almost never happens in water exercise. This consideration may be important for participants who are new to strength training or who have a history of poor compliance to a fitness routine because they don't like the muscle soreness afterward.

Properties of Water

To produce gains in strength, greater-than-normal stress must be placed on the working muscles. Participants can move gently through the water in ways that do not put any stress on the limbs. Therefore, a person who is serious about improving his or her muscular strength must be intentional about overloading the muscles. Remember that the spine must be in neutral alignment before overloading the muscles in any strength-training exercise. In the preseason, muscles are overloaded by taking advantage of the properties of water.

Buoyancy   Archimedes principle states that a body will float if it displaces water weighing more than its own weight. Buoyancy is the upward force exerted on lighter-than-water objects submerged in water, including many participants and their limbs. Buoyancy helps objects float toward the surface of the water. Buoyancy also resists movement of buoyant objects toward the bottom of the pool.

What this means in practice is that movements toward the surface of the water (shoulder flexion, shoulder abduction, elbow flexion, hip flexion, hip abduction, knee flexion, and plantar flexion) are buoyancy assisted for most people. Movements toward the pool floor (shoulder extension, shoulder adduction, elbow extension, hip extension, hip adduction, knee extension and dorsiflexion) are buoyancy resisted.

Movement that is parallel to the water's surface (scapula abduction and adduction, shoulder horizontal abduction and adduction, shoulder rotation, and hip horizontal abduction and adduction) is buoyancy neutral. The effects of buoyancy can be counteracted in some cases by a change of position. Elbow flexion and extension can be done with the shoulders abducted at 70 degrees, making the movement buoyancy neutral. Knee flexion can be done in a seated position, making it buoyancy resisted.

Newton's Law of Inertia   Newton's law of inertia states that an object will remain at rest or in motion with constant velocity unless acted on by a net external force. Starting the body moving, stopping it once it is moving, or changing a movement requires more effort than continuing with the same movement. This effect is more pronounced in the water than on land because the water's resistance tends to slow movement quickly. This resistance is called drag resistance. The law of inertia can be used to create overload by changing movements or changing direction frequently.

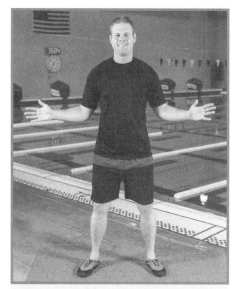

FIGURE 5.2 Resistor arms

Frontal Resistance Frontal resistance creates overload by increasing drag resistance. The larger the frontal surface area presented to the resistance of the water, the greater the energy required to move through the water. A larger surface area can be created by traveling forward with resistor arms (see figure 5.2) or by traveling forward with the legs farther apart. Traveling sideways presents less frontal resistance, except for very obese participants. You can increase frontal resistance while traveling sideways by performing exercises in the sagittal plane, such as a cross-country ski with both arms sweeping to the side.

Hand Positions A hand sliced sideways through the water encounters minimal resistance. A closed fist encounters more resistance. But an open hand or a cupped hand position with the fingers relaxed and slightly apart will pull water more effectively and encounter the most resistance.

Lever Length Lever length is another factor in creating overload for strength training. The longer the lever, the greater the drag resistance and the more force the muscle must use to move the limb. Although shoulder movement can be performed with the elbow bent, greater resistance is encountered when the elbow is extended (but not locked) and the wrist is in the neutral position. Although hip movement can be performed with the knee bent, greater resistance is encountered when the knee is extended (but not locked) and the ankle is plantar flexed.

Newton's Law of Acceleration Newton's law of acceleration states that the rate at which a body changes speed is directly related to the force applied. The law of acceleration can be used to create overload by pushing harder, or applying more force, against the water's resistance with the arms or legs. The harder you push the water, the harder the water pushes back. Double speed produces quadruple the force. But you are not simply trying to move faster; the goal is to move the limb through a greater range of motion at the same tempo or faster. The law of acceleration can be used to overcome the effects of buoyancy because force can be applied in any direction, including upward. In deep water, however, you will need to perform a compensating leg movement to prevent the head from going underwater. For example, you can move the arms and legs in opposition when doing jumping jacks. The law of acceleration is the primary means for overloading the muscles during strength training in water. It should be used consistently and intentionally, even when other means of increasing intensity are added. You want to accelerate through most of your range of motion, but you must also decelerate near the end of the movement to prevent the joint from going beyond its normal range of motion. A brief pause before moving the limb in the opposite direction will allow the acceleration to be more powerful and the overload more effective.

Newton's Law of Action and Reaction Newton's law of action and reaction states that every action causes an equal and opposite reaction. Newton discovered that forces occur in pairs, which he named action and reaction. These forces are obvious in water. For example, when you perform the action of sweeping the arms to the right, the reaction is that the body moves to the left. Swimmers use this law with their swim strokes. You cannot use impeding arm and leg movements in deep water as you can in shallow water. You can, however, use powerful arm movements to propel the body forward, backward, or sideways either with or without leg movements. If you are not moving the legs, the body can be upright or in a seated position. In any case, be sure to brace the core before beginning travel.

In the preseason, inertia, frontal resistance, hand positions, lever length, acceleration, and action and reaction are used to overload the muscles. Participants should be competent using the properties of water before resistance equipment is added in the transition season. Perform 8 to 10 exercises for the major muscle groups in a strength-training session. Aim for at least one set of 8 to15 repetitions of each exercise.

The tempo of music used in a deep-water class is not the same as that used in a shallow-water class. In deep-water exercise, the water surrounds 90 percent of the body and it therefore feels heavier. As a result, participants move slower and react slower. In addition, being fully suspended allows full range of movement. Not having a floor to push off from makes gaining speed difficult. The 134 beats per minute tempo used in a shallow-water strength-training session will be too fast for a deep-water class. A good choice is something around 126 beats per minute.

Flexibility

Stretch at the end of each class to increase range of motion. Choose either dynamic stretches, in which a joint slowly moves through its full range of motion, or static stretches, in which the stretch is held for 10 to 20 seconds. Spend at least 5 minutes on stretching.

DYNAMIC STRETCHES

Middle trapezius (upper back) and pectoralis major (pectorals): Round out the back and stretch the chest; sweep one arm across the chest and bowstring pull back.

Pectoralis major (pectorals): Stretch one arm to the side and bicycle in a circle away from the arm.

Deltoids (shoulders): One arm swings forward and back.

Iliopsoas (hip flexors) and gluteus maximus: Cross-country ski, slow and big (hip flexion and hyperextension).

Gluteus medius (outer thigh): Crossover step.

Hip adductors (inner thigh) and gluteus medius (outer thigh): Jacks cross, slow and big (hip abduction and adduction).

Quadriceps: Cross-country ski and hold with back knee bent.

Ankles: Circle the ankles.

STATIC STRETCHES

Upper trapezius (neck): Bring your ear toward your shoulder; look over your shoulder.

Middle trapezius (upper back): Hug yourself; round out your back as if hugging a barrel.

Pectoralis major (pectorals): Clasp hands behind your back.

Latissimus dorsi: Using the pool wall for support, raise one arm straight up.

Erector spinae (lower back): Using the pool wall for support, round out the back and rest the shins on the wall in a yoga child's pose.

Triceps: Using the pool wall for support, raise one arm up and bend the elbow.

Iliopsoas (hip flexors): Using the pool wall for support, perform a posterior pelvic tilt and extend one leg back.

Gluteus maximus: Using the pool wall for support, lift one knee and support it with the hand under the knee.

ARM MOVEMENT ASSISTING TRAVEL

The following upper-body moves can be used for travel forward, backward, and sideways.

Forward Assisted Arm Movement:
Propeller scull (hands down)
Standing row
Crawl stroke
Unison arm swing back
Double-arm press-down
Breaststroke
Breaststroke pull
Shoulder sweep out
Bicycle arms
Forearm press out
Triceps kick back

Backward Assisted Arm Movement:
Propeller scull (hands in front)
Push forward
Unison arm swing forward
Double-arm lift
Reverse breaststroke
Shoulder sweep in
Forearm press in
Arm curl

Sideways Assisted Arm Movement:
Sidestroke
Unison sidestroke
Shoulder sweep in (one arm)
Shoulder sweep out (one arm)
Lat pull-down (one arm)
Side arm curl

Hamstrings: Using the pool wall for support, walk up the wall and when the feet get close to the hands, straighten the legs.

Gluteus medius (outer thigh): Put one ankle on the opposite knee and sit down.

Hip adductors (inner thigh): Using the pool wall for support, perform a yoga tree pose; using the pool wall for support, walk up the wall, walk the feet wide apart, and then lean to one side, being careful that the knee does not extend beyond the toes

Quadriceps: Using the pool wall for support, lift one foot up behind the body with the knee pointed down and add a posterior pelvic tilt; the foot may be supported by the hand if the range of motion allows.

Gastrocnemius: Using the pool wall for support, brace the toes on the wall and press the heels down.

Preseason Lesson Plans

In the periodization program you devote some time to each of the requirements for cardio-respiratory fitness, strength, and flexibility, but unless your class meets five days a week, you will not be able to meet all the requirements in class. Encourage your participants to get additional exercise on the days that the class does not meet. A schedule might look like the following:

TWO ONE-HOUR CLASSES A WEEK

1. 5 minutes warm-up, 30 minutes cardiorespiratory training and 20 minutes strength training or core strength training, *or* 50 minutes strength training, 5 minutes stretching
2. 5 minutes warm-up, 50 minutes cardiorespiratory training with intervals, 5 minutes stretching

THREE ONE-HOUR CLASSES A WEEK

1. 5 minutes warm-up, 50 minutes cardiorespiratory training, 5 minutes stretching
2. 5 minutes warm-up, 50 minutes strength training or core strength training, 5 minutes stretching
3. 5 minutes warm-up, 50 minutes cardiorespiratory training with intervals, 5 minutes stretching

FIVE ONE-HOUR CLASSES A WEEK

1. 5 minutes warm-up, 50 minutes cardiorespiratory training, 5 minutes stretching
2. 5 minutes warm-up, 50 minutes strength training, 5 minutes stretching
3. 5 minutes warm-up, 50 minutes cardiorespiratory training with intervals, 5 minutes stretching
4. 5 minutes warm-up, 50 minutes strength training or core strength training, 5 minutes stretching
5. 5 minutes warm-up, 50 minutes cardiorespiratory training *or* cardiorespiratory training with intervals, 5 minutes stretching

TRANSITION SEASON

The transition season progresses from the baseline established in the preseason. Continue to emphasize good posture and correct performance of the exercises, although by now you should see improvements in your participants' form. Neutral spine and bracing the core has become second nature to them.

The focus of this season is improving the quality of their exercise by paying attention to how the arms and legs move the water. You want them to become more aware of how they use their hand positions to push and pull the water and how the water moves in reaction to their leg exercises. As their awareness grows, they will be able to maintain good body alignment in any working position. Being able to manipulate the water intentionally improves stability, prevents drifting in deep water, controls travel, and allows participants to use acceleration at will to increase intensity for intervals and strength training. During the transition season, cardiorespiratory training continues, interval training continues at a higher intensity including occasional HIIT sessions, and equipment is introduced in the sessions that focus on muscular strength.

Cardiorespiratory Fitness

Your participants should now be able to do continuous cardiorespiratory training at 50 percent of maximum effort for 30 minutes without tiring. Compliment them for their improvement in endurance. Begin to draw their attention to the quality of their movement. Relaxed fluid moves should now become more intentional. Remind them that the resistance of water is much greater than the resistance of air and encourage them to push it, pull it, and move it around with their arms and legs. Have them drag the water with them when they travel. You will be asking them to increase their exertion from 50 percent to 60 percent of maximum. They should work with moderate effort during their sessions of continuous cardiorespiratory training. They need to establish a base fitness level, which means that they need to be able to work at 60 percent of maximum effort for 30 minutes without tiring to be able to add regular sessions of high-intensity interval training (HIIT) to their workout schedule.

To increase the intensity, you can use interval training. Interval-training intensities increase from 60 percent of maximum effort to 70 percent (somewhat hard). You may still occasionally intersperse cycles of interval training between periods of cardiorespiratory training, but more often you will put all your intervals together in the middle or at the end of the cardio. You will also begin to include HIIT once every two weeks or even once a week toward the end of the transition season.

HIIT involves working at 80 percent of maximum effort or greater. After you reach 90 percent of maximum effort, you cross the anaerobic threshold. Working at 90 percent of maximum effort improves both aerobic and anaerobic fitness. During aerobic exercise, the muscles use oxygen to produce energy. In anaerobic exercise your body's demand for oxygen exceeds the oxygen supply available. Anaerobic exercise, therefore, is not dependent on oxygen from breathing but instead relies on energy sources that are stored in the muscles. The recovery period in anaerobic exercise is important. If the recovery period is shorter than the high-intensity period, then the body is unable to achieve full anaerobic recovery. Therefore, in most cases the recovery needs to be longer than the work. Besides improving fitness, HIIT has been shown to improve blood pressure, cardiovascular health, insulin sensitivity, cholesterol profiles, and abdominal fat and body weight. HIIT burns more calories than continuous cardiorespiratory training, especially after the workout. This occurs because the heart and lungs work hard to supply oxygen to the working muscles and after the exercise ends, the body has excess oxygen to consume. About two hours are needed to use up the excess oxygen. This postexercise period adds around 15 percent more calories to the overall workout energy expenditure (ACSM, 2017a).

HIIT in the transition season includes rolling intervals and surges during which participants get up to 80 percent of maximum effort (hard). In random intervals you might ask your participants to work at 80 percent to 90 percent (very hard) for 15 to 30 seconds. Introduce your participants to a Tabata Type class performed at 80 percent of maximum effort. This format has a recovery period shorter than the work period. Do not cue an active recovery but instead let the participants float in place to catch their breath. Include a transition period of 1 to 2 minutes of moderate activity between Tabata cycles.

If your participants have been following the progression of gradually increasing intensity levels up to this point, then they should be ready for HIIT. Nevertheless, you want to encourage everyone to modify the intensity of the work intervals to their preferred challenging level. Safety is always a priority. Ask everyone to focus on their own optimal training intensities rather than try to keep up with other participants.

The following are options for interval training during the transition season (Thielen, 2015).

INTERVAL 30

30 seconds of work to 60 seconds of recovery (1:2 ratio), 8 to 10 sets

INTERVAL 40

40 seconds of work to 60 seconds of recovery (1:1.5 ratio), 8 to 10 sets

INTERVAL 60

60 seconds of work to 90 seconds of recovery (1:1.5 ratio), 8 to 10 sets

REDUCED RECOVERY TIME

2 minutes of work to 1 minute of recovery (2:1 ratio), 3 to 4 sets

ROLLING INTERVALS

1 minute at 60 percent, 1 minute at 70 percent, and 1 minute at 80 percent of maximum effort, 3 to 5 sets

SURGES

45 seconds at 70 percent, 15 seconds at 80 percent of maximum effort, and 1 minute of recovery (1:1 ratio), 4 to 8 sets

RANDOM INTERVALS

15 seconds at 60 percent of maximum effort, 15 seconds at 70 percent, 15 seconds at 80 percent, and 15 seconds at 90 percent to 1 minute of recovery (rolling interval)

30 seconds of work to 30 seconds of recovery, 3 sets

15 seconds of work to 15 seconds of recovery, 4 sets

30 seconds at 60 percent of maximum effort, 30 seconds at 70 percent, 30 seconds at 80 percent, and 30 seconds at 90 percent to 1 minute of recovery (rolling interval)

1 cycle

PYRAMID

15 seconds of work to 30 seconds of recovery

20 seconds of work to 30 seconds of recovery

25 seconds of work to 30 seconds of recovery

30 seconds of work to 30 seconds of recovery

1 or more cycles

TABATA TYPE

20 seconds of work at 80 percent of maximum effort to 10 seconds of recovery

8 sets (2:1 ratio), 1 or more cycles

Muscular Strength and Endurance

In the transition season equipment is added to the program. Strength training in the water can be accomplished using only the properties of water. The muscular contractions are always concentric. As mentioned previously, gains in strength are possible with concentric contractions alone as long as greater-than-normal stress is placed on the muscle being trained. It is a misconception that eccentric muscle actions are better than concentric contractions at building muscle strength (AEA, 2017, p. 79). Eccentric muscle actions, however, can be added by using certain types of equipment. Equipment also increases the resistance beyond what is possible using only the properties of water.

Equipment Types

Three types of equipment are commonly available for use in deep water: buoyant, drag, and rubberized equipment. Before adding any equipment, remind your participants that they need to maintain neutral posture at all times to avoid injury.

Buoyant Equipment Buoyant equipment uses the buoyancy of the water for resistance. The equipment can either be held in the hands or attached to a limb. The most popular forms of handheld buoyant equipment are foam dumbbells and noodles. Buoyant ankle cuffs are attached to the ankles. Buoyant equipment floats, so the resistance occurs when the equipment is plunged toward the pool floor. The muscular contraction is concentric. When the buoyant equipment is raised, the same muscle lengthens against the resistance in an eccentric action. For example, in elbow extension the triceps shortens in a concentric contraction to press the equipment toward the pool floor. Then, to prevent the equipment from popping out of the water, the triceps maintains its tension as it lengthens in a controlled manner. The opposing muscle, the biceps, is not involved. This action is the opposite of using weighted equipment on land. In the same example, during elbow flexion the biceps shortens in a concentric contraction to lift the weight against gravity. Then, to avoid dropping the weight, the biceps maintains its tension as it lengthens in a controlled manner. The opposing muscle, the triceps, is not involved.

What this means is that only one muscle in a muscle pair is worked with buoyant equipment. When using weighted equipment on land, changing positions to work the other muscle of the pair is possible, but in deep water many of those positions are not possible. When buoyant equipment is moved parallel to the floor, such as when targeting the pectoralis major, the drag forces of the water come into play. But the main muscular contraction is an isometric contraction of the latissimus dorsi and lower trapezius to hold the buoyant equipment under water (AEA, 2018, p. 54). In the case of targeting the pectoralis major, movements parallel to the floor can be avoided by leaning forward 45 degrees and flutter kicking, if necessary, to maintain the spine in neutral alignment. The shoulders can now be horizontally adducted in a chest fly. The equipment can also be plunged diagonally downward to work the pectoralis major and triceps in a chest press. You must carefully observe your participants to make sure that they are able to maintain a neutral spine in this position. If they cannot, avoid these exercises. Ankle cuffs provide resistance for the legs during movements toward the pool floor, such as hip or knee extension. Buoyant equipment cannot be manipulated to provide resistance for trunk exercises in deep water. Handheld buoyant equipment, however, can be used for stabilization when performing crunches or side-to-side extensions. For more information about foam dumbbells, see the sidebar Exercise Safety With Foam Dumbbells in chapter 1.

Table 5.6 shows which muscles are worked with buoyant equipment.

EXERCISE SAFETY WITH HANDHELD DRAG EQUIPMENT

With hand held drag equipment, participants need to keep the wrist neutral rather than flex and extend it. Cue straight wrists and a loose grip. Good postural alignment must be maintained. A participant who has to throw his or her body weight into the exercise, elevates the shoulders, or loses range of motion when trying to increase the speed of the exercise is not ready to use drag equipment. The movement should be performed smoothly, with equal force in both directions, at the participant's full range of motion. After every set allow 30 to 60 seconds to rest and encourage participants to relax their shoulders and stretch their fingers.

TABLE 5.6

Muscle Actions With Buoyant Equipment in Deep Water

Motion	Muscle action	Note
Chest press (push)	Concentric pectoralis major, serratus anterior, anterior deltoid, and triceps	Lean forward 45 degrees
Chest press (pull)	Eccentric pectoralis major, serratus anterior, anterior deltoid, and triceps	Lean forward 45 degrees
Standing row	Isometric latissimus dorsi and lower trapezius, concentric middle trapezius, and rhomboids	Drag forces used
Shoulder flexion	Eccentric latissimus dorsi and triceps	
Shoulder extension or hyperextension	Concentric latissimus dorsi and triceps	
Shoulder abduction	Eccentric latissimus dorsi and pectoralis major	
Shoulder adduction	Concentric latissimus dorsi and pectoralis major	
Shoulder horizontal abduction	Eccentric pectoralis major and anterior deltoid	Lean forward 45 degrees
Shoulder horizontal adduction	Concentric pectoralis major and anterior deltoid	Lean forward 45 degrees
Shoulder lateral rotation	Isometric latissimus dorsi and lower trapezius, concentric rotator cuff	Drag forces used
Shoulder medial rotation	Isometric latissimus dorsi and lower trapezius, concentric rotator cuff	Drag forces used
Elbow flexion	Eccentric triceps	
Elbow extension	Concentric triceps	
Hip flexion	Eccentric gluteus maximus and hamstrings	Foot on a noodle or use ankle cuffs
Hip extension	Concentric gluteus maximus and hamstrings	Foot on a noodle or use ankle cuffs
Standing leg press (down)	Concentric gluteus maximus, hamstrings, and quadriceps	Foot on a noodle or use ankle cuffs
Standing leg press (return)	Eccentric gluteus maximus, hamstrings, and quadriceps	Foot on a noodle or use ankle cuffs
Hip abduction or standing leg press to side	Eccentric adductors	Foot on a noodle or use ankle cuffs
Hip adduction or standing leg press to side	Concentric adductors	Foot on a noodle or use ankle cuffs
Knee flexion	Eccentric quadriceps	Ankle cuffs
Knee extension	Concentric quadriceps	Ankle cuffs

Adapted from Aquatic Exercise Association, 2018, *Aquatic fitness professional manual,* 7th ed. (Champaign, IL: Human Kinetics), 86-87.

Drag Equipment Drag equipment increases the drag forces of the water by increasing surface area and creating turbulence. Drag equipment must either float or be attached to the hands for it to be practical to use in deep water. The most popular piece of drag equipment in deep water is webbed gloves. The smaller handheld equipment with multiple planes can also be used. Paddles and kickboards require the exerciser to be able to stabilize in a wide stance or a lunge position, so they are impractical in deep water. Large handheld drag equipment with multiple planes may cause an exerciser to sink when lifting it toward the water's surface, making it unsafe for deep water. The movement of the arms and legs with webbed gloves and handheld equipment with multiple planes (appropriate for deep water) feels natural, and for that reason, some participants prefer drag equipment to buoyant equipment. The muscular contraction with drag equipment is concentric in all directions, working both muscles in a muscle pair. But eccentric action of the opposing muscle also occurs at the end of the range of motion, slowing the movement down as the limb prepares to change direction (AEA, 2010, p. 121). For example, in elbow flexion the biceps shortens in a concentric contraction, but near the end of the range of motion, the triceps fires eccentrically to slow the motion so that the arm can stop and change direction. Then, the triceps contracts concentrically to extend the elbow.

Movement parallel to the floor using drag equipment does not involve any isometric contractions of the latissimus dorsi or lower trapezius, as when using buoyant equipment. Therefore, no special body positions are required to target any muscle group, making drag equipment ideal for those who are unable to maintain neutral alignment while leaning forward 45 degrees. Drag equipment cannot be manipulated to provide resistance for trunk exercises in deep water.

Table 5.7 shows the muscle contractions with drag equipment.

Rubberized Equipment Rubberized equipment works the same in water as on land. The resistance comes from the equipment itself rather than from buoyancy or the drag

TABLE 5.7

Muscle Actions With Drag Equipment in Deep Water

Motion	Muscle action
Chest press	Concentric pectoralis major, serratus anterior, anterior deltoids, and triceps
Standing row	Concentric trapezius and rhomboids
Shoulder flexion	Concentric anterior deltoid, pectoralis major, and biceps
Shoulder extension or hyperextension	Concentric latissimus dorsi and triceps
Shoulder abduction	Concentric middle deltoid
Shoulder adduction	Concentric latissimus dorsi and pectoralis major
Shoulder horizontal abduction	Concentric posterior deltoid
Shoulder horizontal adduction	Concentric pectoralis major and anterior deltoid
Shoulder lateral rotation	Concentric rotator cuff
Shoulder medial rotation	Concentric latissimus dorsi and rotator cuff
Elbow flexion	Concentric biceps
Elbow extension	Concentric triceps

Adapted from Aquatic Exercise Association, 2018, *Aquatic fitness professional manual*, 7th ed. (Champaign, IL: Human Kinetics), 86-87.

forces of the water. Rubberized equipment is available as straight bands, loops, and tubes. Pool chemicals and sunlight tend to break down rubberized equipment fairly quickly, so it must be inspected frequently. Chlorine-resistant rubberized equipment is now available. Both regular rubberized equipment and chlorine-resistant rubberized equipment will last longer if it is rinsed in fresh water after each use.

Not all the positions used with bands in shallow water will work in deep water. Attaching the band to a pool ladder or having a partner serve as an anchor is not practical because neither the exerciser nor the partner can stabilize against the floor. Instead, the band needs to be anchored to the nonworking arm or the nonworking leg or foot. To maintain the spine in neutral when doing exercises for the upper body, the participant may need to perform a stabilizing leg movement, such as a jog, cross-country ski, or jumping jack. Placing a band under the foot or positioning a loop around the legs in deep water is difficult for some participants. You must consider the participants' abilities when designing a class with rubberized equipment. The muscle being worked depends on the location of the anchor. The muscular contraction is concentric away from the anchor point and eccentric toward the anchor point. Table 5.8 shows the muscle contractions with rubberized equipment.

Strength Reps and Sets

Perform 8 to 10 exercises for the major muscle groups in a strength-training session. Aim for two or three sets of 8 to 15 repetitions of each exercise. Cue to relax the shoulders and the grip after each set with equipment.

Flexibility

Be sure to end all of your transition season classes with at least five minutes of stretching, focusing on the major muscles used during the class.

Transition Season Lesson Plans

Three sessions per week of 20 to 60 minutes of vigorous-intensity exercise meets the American College of Sports Medicine guidelines for cardiorespiratory exercise (ACSM, 2017b). By increasing the intensity of the interval sessions in the periodization program, your class comes closer to meeting these guidelines, but unless your class meets five days a week, you will not be able to meet all the requirements for cardiorespiratory fitness, strength and flexibility in class.

Encourage your participants to get additional exercise on the days that the class does not meet. A schedule might look like the following:

TWO ONE-HOUR CLASSES A WEEK

1. 5 minutes warm-up, 30 minutes cardiorespiratory training and 20 minutes strength training, *or* 50 minutes of strength training, 5 minutes stretching

2. 5 minutes warm-up, 50 minutes cardiorespiratory training with intervals (HIIT every other week), 5 minutes stretching

THREE ONE-HOUR CLASSES A WEEK

1. 5 minutes warm-up, 50 minutes cardiorespiratory training, 5 minutes stretching

2. 5 minutes warm-up, 50 minutes strength training, 5 minutes stretching

3. 5 minutes warm-up, 50 minutes cardiorespiratory training with intervals (HIIT every other week), 5 minutes stretching

TABLE 5.8

Muscle Actions With Rubberized Equipment in Deep Water

Motion	Muscle action	Notes
Chest press (push)	Concentric pectoralis major, serratus anterior, anterior deltoids, and triceps	Band wrapped around back
Chest press (return)	Eccentric pectoralis major, serratus anterior, anterior deltoids, and triceps	
Standing row (pull)	Concentric trapezius and rhomboids	Anchor in front
Standing row (return)	Eccentric trapezius and rhomboids	
Shoulder flexion	Eccentric latissimus dorsi and triceps	Anchor in front
Shoulder extension	Concentric latissimus dorsi and triceps	
Shoulder abduction	Concentric middle deltoid	Low anchor
Shoulder adduction	Eccentric middle deltoid	
Shoulder horizontal abduction	Concentric posterior deltoid	Anchor in front
Shoulder horizontal adduction	Eccentric posterior deltoid	
Shoulder lateral rotation	Concentric rotator cuff	Pull band apart, elbows anchored at waist
Shoulder medial rotation	Eccentric rotator cuff	
Elbow flexion	Eccentric triceps	High anchor
Elbow extension	Concentric triceps	
Elbow flexion	Concentric biceps	Low anchor
Elbow extension	Eccentric biceps	
Hip flexion	Concentric iliopsoas	Anchor in back
Hip extension	Eccentric iliopsoas	
Hip flexion	Eccentric gluteus maximus and hamstrings	Anchor in front
Hip extension	Concentric gluteus maximus and hamstrings	
Hip abduction	Concentric gluteus medius	Medial anchor
Hip adduction	Eccentric gluteus medius	
Horizontal hip abduction	Concentric tensor fasciae latae	Loop around thighs
Horizontal hip adduction	Eccentric tensor fasciae latae	
Knee flexion	Eccentric quadriceps	Seated, loop around feet anchor in back
Knee extension	Concentric quadriceps	
Knee flexion	Concentric hamstrings	Seated, loop around feet anchor in front
Knee extension	Eccentric hamstrings	
Plantar flexion	Concentric gastrocnemius and soleus	Foot on band
Dorsiflexion	Eccentric gastrocnemius and soleus	

Adapted from Aquatic Exercise Association, 2018, *Aquatic fitness professional manual,* 7th ed. (Champaign, IL: Human Kinetics), 87.

FIVE ONE-HOUR CLASSES A WEEK

1. 5 minutes warm-up, 50 minutes cardiorespiratory training with intervals, 5 minutes stretching
2. 5 minutes warm-up, 50 minutes strength training, 5 minutes stretching
3. 5 minutes warm-up, 50 minutes cardiorespiratory training, 5 minutes stretching
4. 5 minutes warm-up, 50 minutes strength training, 5 minutes stretching
5. 5 minutes warm-up, 50 minutes cardiorespiratory training with intervals (HIIT every other week), 5 minutes stretching

PEAK FITNESS SEASON

At last you have arrived at the season for peak fitness. The preseason and the transition season have prepared your participants for the highest level of fitness that they will achieve this year. Peak fitness can be maintained for a few months, but it cannot be sustained indefinitely before the body will need to rest. Peak fitness will be different for everyone. But your participants should notice that the exercises seem easier even though they are performing more repetitions. Compliment them on their good posture and ability to perform the exercises correctly. Draw their attention to the improvement in the quality of their moves, because they are now better able to push and pull and drag the water with them while maintaining a braced core. The focus of this season is to increase their power to go beyond the intensity levels they achieved in the previous season, including brief periods in their anaerobic zone. Your classes will consist of cardiorespiratory training, HIIT, and strength training with equipment using both concentric and eccentric muscle actions but focusing on the eccentric actions.

Cardiorespiratory Fitness

Your participants should now be able to do continuous cardiorespiratory training at 60 percent of maximum effort for 30 minutes without tiring. They may have noticed that as long as they maintain neutral posture, they can safely increase the intensity of their arm and leg movements. They may have to work a little harder to achieve a moderate level of effort. Now is the time for them to focus on using powerful arm and leg movements that assist travel to increase their speed of travel. Remind them not to streamline their bodies by bending forward at the hips. Ask them to increase their exertion from 60 percent to 70 percent of maximum. They should be working somewhat hard during their sessions of continuous cardiorespiratory training

Now that a base fitness level has been established, interval-training intensities can increase from 70 percent of maximum effort to 80 percent (hard). Your participants may also be ready to cross the anaerobic threshold regularly, so you will include more frequent cycles in which they work at 90 percent of maximum effort (very hard). To work at this level, you will need to employ additional strategies for increasing intensity. Instead of using one intensity variable, use two, such as full range of motion with power, elevation with power, or power with travel.

Another strategy is to work in two planes at the same time. You can do this by alternating one move in the frontal plane, such as a frog kick, with another move in the sagittal plane, such as tuck ski together. A second way to work in two planes is to combine a leg move in one plane with an arm move in a different plane. Examples include jumping jacks (frontal plane) with clap hands (transverse plane), cross-country ski (sagittal plane) with arms sweeping side to side (transverse plane), and high kick (sagittal plane) clap over (transverse plane) and under (frontal plane). You will no longer intersperse cycles of interval training between periods of cardiorespiratory training. You will instead perform all your interval cycles together.

All of your intervals during peak fitness are HIIT, but not all HIIT intervals are anaerobic. Rolling intervals, surges, random intervals, and Tabata Type intervals include sets in which you ask your participants to work at 90 percent of maximum effort for periods of 15-seconds up to 1 minute. Remember that 90 percent of maximum effort is different for everyone and that some may not be able to achieve that level of effort for 1 minute or even 15 seconds. Encourage all participants to modify the intensity of the work intervals to their preferred challenging level and focus on their own optimal training.

The following are options for interval training during peak fitness (Thielen, 2015):

INTERVAL 30

30 seconds of work to 30 seconds of recovery (1:1 ratio), 10 to 12 sets

INTERVAL 40

40 seconds of work to 40 seconds of recovery (1:1 ratio), 10 to 12 sets

INTERVAL 60

60 seconds of work to 60 seconds of recovery (1:1 ratio), 10 to 12 sets

REDUCED RECOVERY TIME

3 minutes of work to 90 seconds of recovery (2:1 ratio), 2 to 3 sets

ROLLING INTERVALS

1 minute at 70 percent of maximum effort, 1 minute at 80 percent, and 1 minute at 90 percent, 3 to 5 sets

SURGES

45 seconds at 80 percent of maximum effort, 15 seconds at 90 percent, and 1 minute of recovery (1:1 ratio), 4 to 8 sets

RANDOM INTERVALS

30 seconds at 60 percent of maximum effort, 30 seconds at 70 percent, 30 seconds at 80 percent, and 30 seconds at 90 percent to 1 minute of recovery (rolling interval)

15 seconds at 60 percent of maximum effort, 15 seconds at 70 percent, 15 seconds at 80 percent, and 15 seconds at 90 percent to 1 minute of recovery (rolling interval)

30 seconds of work to 30 seconds of recovery, 4 sets

20 seconds of work to 10 seconds of recovery, 8 sets (Tabata)

1 cycle

PYRAMID

15 seconds of work to 15 seconds of recovery

20 seconds of work to 15 seconds of recovery

25 seconds of work to 15 seconds of recovery

30 seconds of work to 15 seconds of recovery

1 or more cycles

TABATA TYPE

20 seconds of work at 90 percent of maximum effort to 10 seconds of recovery (2:1 ratio)

8 sets, 1 or more cycles

Muscular Strength and Endurance

In the transition season, equipment was added to the program. Strength training without equipment involves only concentric contractions. Drag equipment involves a minor amount of eccentric action. Buoyant and rubberized equipment involve both concentric and eccentric muscle actions. Gains in strength are possible with concentric contractions alone. Eccentric actions can also be used to improve strength, and they add variety to a strength-training program. Eccentric actions may also improve muscle coordination and balance (ACSM, 2017c).

During peak fitness, you will continue to use equipment when your participants are strength training. Now, however, you will emphasize the eccentric action. For this you will choose either buoyant or rubberized equipment. When they are using buoyant equipment, ask them to dynamically press the equipment down under the water and then pause for two seconds. Participants should control the upward movement so that it takes about four seconds to return to the starting position. Watch for elevated shoulders when using buoyant equipment. This action is an indication that the participants selected equipment that is too large for them.

When they are using rubberized equipment, ask participants to pull the equipment away from the anchor point as fully as range of motion allows and then pause for two seconds. They should control the release so that it takes about four seconds to return to the anchor point. Remember to cue to relax the shoulders and the grip after each set with equipment. Be aware that delayed onset muscle soreness is common 24 to 48 hours after eccentric exercise, so begin slowly. Start with eight repetitions of each exercise and gradually increase the number of repetitions over time.

During the transition season, you aimed for two or three sets of 8 to 15 repetitions of each exercise. During peak fitness you will aim for three sets. You have several options for performing the three sets and incorporating eccentric actions.

1. Perform the first set without equipment. Perform the second set with buoyant or rubberized equipment without emphasizing the eccentric actions. Perform the third set with the pause and slow return.

2. Perform one set without equipment. Perform the second set with drag equipment. Perform the third set with buoyant or rubberized equipment using the pause and slow return.

3. Perform two sets with buoyant or rubberized equipment without emphasizing the eccentric action. Perform the third set with the pause and slow return.

4. Perform one set without equipment. Then perform two sets with buoyant or rubberized equipment using the pause and slow return.

5. Perform one set with buoyant or rubberized equipment without emphasizing the eccentric action. Then perform two sets using the pause and slow return.

Flexibility

Be sure to end all of your peak fitness classes with at least five minutes of stretching, focusing on the major muscles used during the class.

Peak Fitness Lesson Plans

Three sessions per week of 20 to 60 minutes of vigorous-intensity exercise meets the American College of Sports Medicine guidelines for cardiorespiratory exercise (ACSM, 2017b). By including HIIT, your class comes closer to meeting these guidelines, but unless your class meets five days a week, you will not be able to meet all the requirements for cardiorespiratory fitness, strength, and flexibility in class. Encourage your participants to get additional exercise on the days that the class does not meet. A schedule might look like the following:

TWO ONE-HOUR CLASSES A WEEK

1. 5 minutes warm-up, 30 minutes cardiorespiratory training and 20 minutes strength training, *or* 50 minutes strength training, 5 minutes stretching
2. 5 minutes warm-up, 50 minutes cardiorespiratory training with HIIT, 5 minutes stretching

THREE ONE-HOUR CLASSES A WEEK

1. 5 minutes warm-up, 50 minutes cardiorespiratory training with HIIT, 5 minutes stretching
2. 5 minutes warm-up, 50 minutes strength training, 5 minutes stretching
3. 5 minutes warm-up, 50 minutes cardiorespiratory training with HIIT, 5 minutes stretching

FIVE ONE-HOUR CLASSES A WEEK

1. 5 minutes warm-up, 50 minutes cardiorespiratory training with HIIT, 5 minutes stretching
2. 5 minutes warm-up, 50 minutes strength training, 5 minutes stretching
3. 5 minutes warm-up, 50 minutes cardiorespiratory training with HIIT, 5 minutes stretching
4. 5 minutes warm-up, 50 minutes strength training, 5 minutes stretching
5. 5 minutes warm-up, 50 minutes cardiorespiratory training with HIIT, 5 minutes stretching

ACTIVE RECOVERY SEASON

Your participants have worked hard for most of the year. Now it is time to rest. Their muscles may have suffered from microtrauma caused by the months of continuous training. Their bodies need time to repair so that the microtrauma does not lead to a cumulative injury. They also need to rest to restore their energy reserves. But you do not have to cancel class. Fitness will continue as long as some training continues, so this period is called the active recovery season. Classes consist of low-intensity continuous cardiorespiratory training, core strength training, including balance exercises and Pilates, and fun activities such as partner classes, dance moves, modified synchronized swimming, games, and relay races. Be sure to stretch at the end of every class.

Active Recovery Lesson Plans

A schedule might look like the following:

TWO ONE-HOUR CLASSES A WEEK

1. 5 minutes warm-up, 30 minutes light cardiorespiratory training, 20 minutes core strength training, 5 minutes stretching
2. 5 minutes warm-up, 30 minutes light cardiorespiratory training, 20 minutes fun activities, 5 minutes stretching

THREE ONE-HOUR CLASSES A WEEK

1. 5 minutes warm-up, 30 minutes light cardiorespiratory training, 20 minutes core strength training, 5 minutes stretching
2. 5 minutes warm-up, 50 minutes core strength training, 5 minutes stretching
3. 5 minutes warm-up, 30 minutes light cardiorespiratory training, 20 minutes fun activities, 5 minutes stretching

FIVE ONE-HOUR CLASSES A WEEK

1. 5 minutes warm-up, 30 minutes light cardiorespiratory training, 20 minutes fun activities, 5 minutes stretching
2. 5 minutes warm-up, 50 minutes core strength training, 5 minutes stretching
3. 5 minutes warm-up, 50 minutes light cardiorespiratory training, 5 minutes stretching
4. 5 minutes warm-up, 30 minutes light cardiorespiratory training, 20 minutes fun activities, 5 minutes stretching
5. 5 minutes warm-up, 50 minutes core strength training, 5 minutes stretching

References

ACSM. (2017a). *High intensity interval training*. Retrieved from www.acsm.org/docs/brochures/high-intensity-interval-training.pdf

ACSM. (2017b). Quantity and quality of exercise for developing and maintaining cardiorespiratory, musculoskeletal, and neuromotor fitness in apparently healthy adults: Guidance for prescribing exercise. *Medicine & Science in Sports & Exercise 43*(7). Retrieved from http://journals.lww.com/acsm-msse/Fulltext/2011/07000/Quantity_and_Quality_of_Exercise_for_Developing.26.aspx

ACSM. (2017c). *Resistance training for health and fitness*. Retrieved from www.acsm.org/docs/brochures/resistance-training.pdf

AEA. (2010). *Aquatic fitness professional manual, sixth edition*. Champaign, IL; Human Kinetics.

AEA. (2018). *Aquatic fitness professional manual, seventh edition*. Champaign, IL; Human Kinetics.

Ivens, P., & Holder, C. (2011). *Do no harm*. Retrieved from www.aquaaerobics.com

Thielen, S. (March 21, 2015). *Intelligent intervals for the deep*. Presented at Metroplex Association of Aquatic Professionals Continuing Education Training, Plano, TX.

CHAPTER 6

Deep-Water Exercises and Cues

This chapter is a list of exercises used in the deep-water lesson plans. The list includes the basic cardiorespiratory exercises of jog, bicycle, kick, cross-country ski, and jumping jacks with multiple variations of each basic exercise. Wall exercises round out the cardio exercises. Following these are strength exercises for the upper body, abdominals, obliques, and lower body. Cues or descriptions of the exercise are included for those exercises that may need additional explanation. These exercises can be used to create new classes for cardiorespiratory fitness or strength training. Choose variations that use a full range of motion, speed, elevation, or acceleration and power when higher intensity is desired. Travel will also increase the intensity. Add equipment with the strength exercises to increase the resistance.

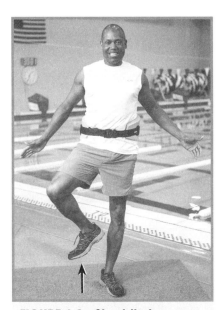

FIGURE 6.1 **Knee-high jog.**

FIGURE 6.2 **Straddle jog.**

CARDIORESPIRATORY EXERCISES

1. JOG

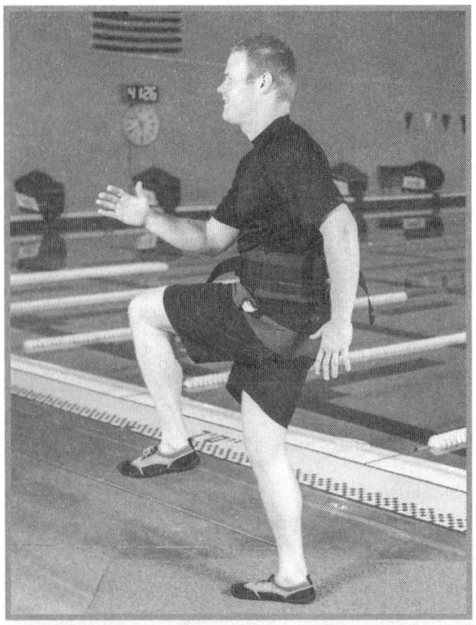

Knee-high jog—bring the knee up to hip level (see figure 6.1)

Knee-high jog, faster

Run—focus on full extension of the hip

Sprint—run at top speed

Power run—pull the water forcefully with cupped hands

Run 3× and hurdle

Steep climb—like climbing a ladder out of the pool

Steep climb, faster

Steep climb with power

Knee-high jog with elevation—scull to lift the shoulders

Knee lift, doubles—lift each knee 2×

Knee-high jog 3× and hold

Knee-high jog, syncopate—slow, slow, quick, quick, quick

Knee-high jog, diagonal—lean 45 degrees to the side with the spine in alignment; avoid turning to the side

Knee-high jog, side lying

Rock climb—lean forward 45 degrees; move arms and legs as if climbing a rock wall

Crossover knees—knees cross the midline

Crossover step—step across the midline

Crossover step 3× and half turn

Straddle jog—hips are open, but feet are close together (see figure 6.2)

Diamonds—pull the legs up in a diamond position and bring the arms down

Frog kick—lift the knees to the side, straighten the legs, and bring them to center

Frog kick with elevation—bring the legs forcefully to center

Run tires—hips are open and feet are wide apart, like running through tires at football practice

Run tires, faster

Run tires with elevation—scull to lift the shoulders

In, in, out, out—alternate feet in and out

Over the barrel travel sideways—like stepping over barrels one at a time

Inner-thigh lift or ankle touch—bring the inner thigh toward the opposite hand

Inner-thigh lift, full ROM

Inner-thigh lift, faster

Inner-thigh lift with power

Inner-thigh lift, one side

Inner-thigh lift, doubles—inner-thigh lift 2× on each side

Hopscotch—touch the heel in back with the opposite hand; if you can't reach the heel, just aim for it

Hopscotch, full ROM

Hopscotch, faster

Hopscotch with power

Hopscotch, one side

Hopscotch, doubles—touch heel 2× on each side

Heel jog—keep knees under hips and curl the hamstrings (see figure 6.3)

Breaststroke kick—lift the heels in back, abduct the hips, and straighten the legs to bring them to center

Breaststroke kick with elevation—bring the legs forcefully to center

Skateboard—stand with one foot as if on a skateboard and pedal with the other foot

Heel jog 3× and hold

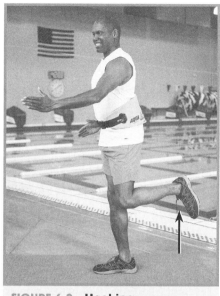

FIGURE 6.3 **Heel jog.**

2. BICYCLE

Bicycle—feet are under the body as if riding a unicycle (see figure 6.4)

Bicycle tandem—arms and legs pedal in unison

Bicycle, full ROM—large circles

Bicycle, faster

Bicycle with elevation—scull to lift the shoulders

Bicycle with power—pedal as if climbing a hill

Bicycle tandem with power

Bicycle one leg

Bicycle, doubles—pedal 2× with each foot

Bicycle 3× and hold

Bicycle, diagonal—lean 45 degrees to the side with the spine in alignment; avoid turning to the side

Bicycle, side lying

Bicycle, side lying, in a circle

Reverse bicycle—pedal backwards

Seated bicycle—as if on a recumbent bicycle

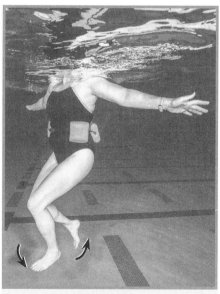

FIGURE 6.4 **Bicycle.**

3. KICK

Flutter kick—flutter kick from the hips, not the knees

Star flutter kick—feet are apart

Tuck and star flutter kick

Flutter kick, faster

Star flutter kick, faster

Flutter kick with elevation—scull to lift the shoulders

Flutter kick diagonal—lean 45 degrees to the side with the spine in alignment; avoid turning to the side

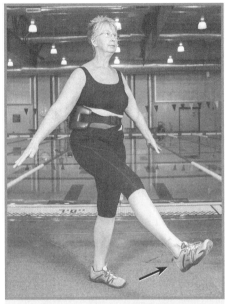

FIGURE 6.5 **Kick forward.**

Kick forward—keep knees soft; return the legs under the body after each kick (see figure 6.5)

Kick forward, faster

Knee lift, straighten, and power press-down

High kick

High kick and return—bring the foot to center before beginning the next kick

High kick, power down

High kick with power

High kick 7×, tuck, and turn—turn 180 degrees

High kick, clap over and under—clap the hands over the leg and then clap the hands under the leg

Kick forward, doubles—kick 2× with each leg

Kick forward, doubles, one low and one high

Chorus line kick—knee, down, kick, down

Seated kick

Mermaid—seated unison kick, like pumping a swing

Seated kick, faster

Seated kick, toes pointed or feet flexed

Seated kick 3× and hold

Seated kick, one leg

Crossover kick—kick across the midline

Crossover kick, doubles—kick across the midline 2× with each leg

Crossover kick, doubles, one low and one high

Crossover kick and sweep out—kick across the midline and then sweep the foot out to the side

Skate kick, crossover kick, sweep out, and center—kick back, kick across the midline, and then sweep the foot out to the side

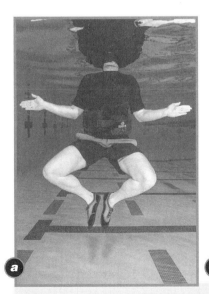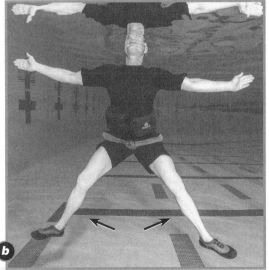

FIGURE 6.6 **Cossack kick: (a) start and (b) finish.**

Crossover kick and sweep out, doubles—kick across the midline and then sweep the foot out to the side 2× with each leg

Seated crossover kick

Seated crossover kick and sweep out

Seated kick 3×, crossover kick 1×

Seated kick 3× and hold; one leg sweeps out and in 1×

Cossack kick—legs are in a diamond position; then kick to the sides in unison (see figure 6.6)

Skate kick—kick backward with the leg straight; lean forward slightly to avoid arching the back (see figure 6.7)

Skate kick full ROM

Skate kick, faster

Skate kick and return—bring the foot to center before beginning the next kick

Skate kick with power

4. CROSS-COUNTRY SKI

Cross-country ski—work the arms and legs in opposition; swing the arms and legs forward and backward evenly (see figure 6.8)

Cross-country ski with knees bent 90 degrees—short-lever cross-country ski

Cross-country ski, full ROM

Cross-country ski with rotation—arm reaches across the midline

Helicopter ski—move arms and legs in semicircles instead of straight lines

Helicopter ski with power

Mini ski—short range of motion

Mini ski, faster

Cross-country ski, faster

Cross-country ski with elevation—pull the arms and legs together forcefully to lift the shoulders out of the water

Cross-country ski with power

Cross-country ski, arms sweep side to side

Cross-country ski, slow

Cross-country ski 3× and hold

Cross-country ski 3-1/2× and half turn—Ski R, L, R, L, R, L, R, and half turn

Cross-country ski 3× and tuck

Tuck ski—tuck the feet under the body

Tuck ski with full extension

Tuck ski with rotation—arm reaches across the midline

Tuck ski together—tuck, ski, and pull the legs together forcefully to lift the shoulders

Tuck ski, doubles—tuck ski 2× on each side

Tuck ski 3× and hold

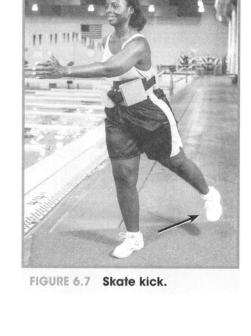

FIGURE 6.7 **Skate kick.**

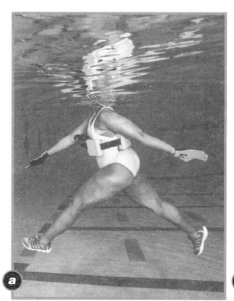 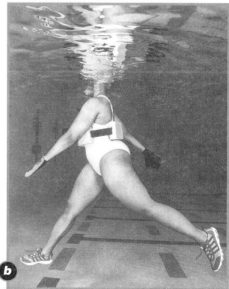

FIGURE 6.8 **Cross-country ski: (*a*) start and (*b*) finish.**

Cross-country ski, tuck, diagonal turn, and center—cross-country ski, tuck, hold the tuck and turn 45 degrees toward a corner, return to center

Cross-country ski, diagonal—lean 45 degrees to the side with the spine in alignment; avoid turning to the side

Cross-country ski, side lying

5. JUMPING JACKS

Jumping jacks—arms opposite legs to prevent bobbing (see figure 6.9)

Bent knee jacks—short-lever jumping jacks

Mini jacks—short range of motion

Mini jacks, faster

Jumping jacks, faster

Jumping jacks with power

Mini cross—using short range of motion, cross the ankles

Mini cross, faster

Jacks cross—begin with the feet apart and then cross the thighs

Jacks cross, faster

Jacks cross, R leg in front

Jacks cross, L leg in front

Jacks cross 3-1/2× and half turn—cross, out, cross, out, cross, out, cross, and half turn

Jumping jacks with diagonal turn—turn 45 degrees toward a corner when the feet come apart, feet come together in the center, turn 45 degrees to the opposite corner when the feet come apart again

Jumping jacks, pulse out or in

Jumping jacks, syncopate—slow, slow, quick, quick, quick

Jacks tuck—tuck the feet under the body

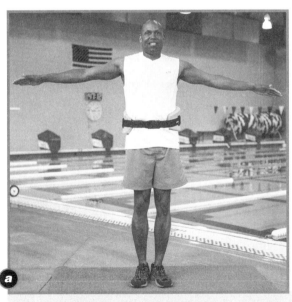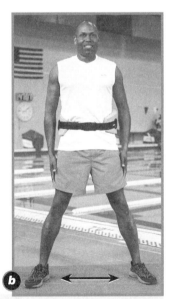

FIGURE 6.9 **Jumping jacks: (a) start and (b) finish.**

6. WALL EXERCISES

Breaststroke with feet on the wall

Reverse breaststroke in a kneeling position with back to the wall

Cross-country ski with back to the wall, heels tap the wall

Cross-country ski with both feet on the wall at twelve o'clock and six o'clock—tap the wall with the feet on an imaginary clock face

Cross-country ski with both feet on the wall at eleven o'clock and five o'clock

Cross-country ski with both feet on the wall at one o'clock and seven o'clock

Front kick (karate), heel taps wall, quarter turn, side kick (karate), heel taps wall—alternate taps to the front and taps to the side with the same foot

Push off the wall with both feet (see figure 6.10) and run back

Push off the wall with one foot (see figure 6.11), tuck, and breaststroke back

Push off the wall with both feet, side lying, tuck, and run back with sidestroke—run back to the wall sideways

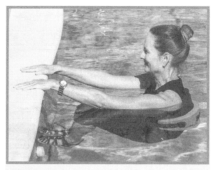

FIGURE 6.10 **Push off the wall with both feet.**

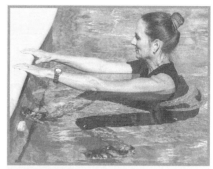

FIGURE 6.11 **Push off the wall with one foot.**

STRENGTH EXERCISES

7. UPPER BODY

Scapula adduction

Standing row (see figure 6.12)

Seated row

Kayak row—paddle with both hands; alternate right and left sides

Crawl stroke

Bowstring pull—hold the bow in front with one hand and pull the bowstring with the other hand

Bowstring pull to the side—hold the bow to the side with one hand and pull the bowstring with the other hand

Shoulder blade squeeze

Shoulder flexion and extension

Double-arm lift

Arm swing

Unison arm swing

Double-arm press-down (see figure 6.13)

Pumping arms

Shoulder abduction and abduction

Arm lift to sides

Arm lift to sides with elbows bent

Lat pull-down (see figure 6.14)

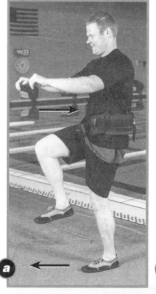
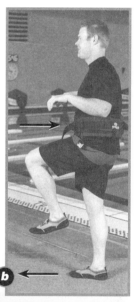

FIGURE 6.12 **Standing row: (*a*) start and (*b*) finish.**

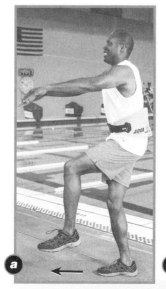
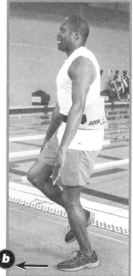

FIGURE 6.13 **Double-arm press-down: (*a*) start and (*b*) finish.**

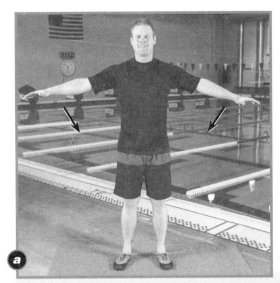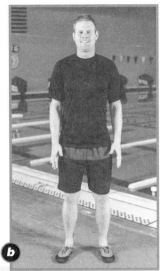

FIGURE 6.14 Lat pull-down: (*a*) start and (*b*) finish.

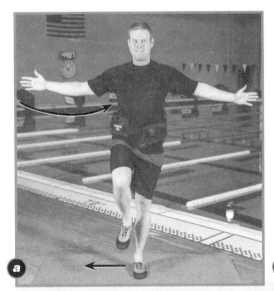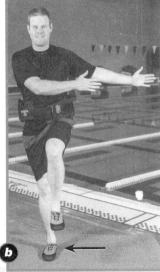

FIGURE 6.15 Shoulder sweep in: (*a*) start and (*b*) finish.

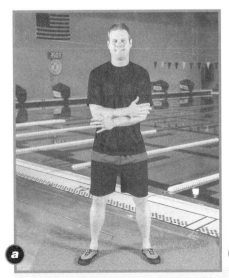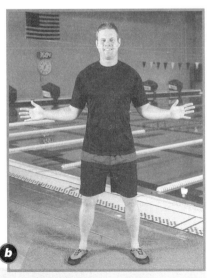

FIGURE 6.16 Forearm press: (*a*) start and (*b*) finish.

Arms cross in front and in back

Palms touch in front and in back

Palms touch in back

Windshield wiper arms—swing the arms side to side in front of the thighs

Shoulder horizontal abduction and adduction

Clap hands

Shoulder sweep, out or in (see figure 6.15)

Alternating sweep out

Alternating sweep in

Arms sweep side to side

Sidestroke

Unison sidestroke

Breaststroke—do the breaststroke with thumbs up to protect the shoulders

Reverse breaststroke

Breaststroke pull—small heart-shaped breaststroke with hands at navel level

Chest fly—with equipment

Chest press—push forward with the hands shoulder-distance apart

Shoulder lateral rotation

Forearm press (see figure 6.16)

Forearm press side to side

Resistor arms

Elbow flexion and extension

Arm curl

Triceps extension

Triceps kick back—elbows back, press back

Push forward—push forward with the hands in front of the chest

Unison push forward

Push across—push across the midline

Reach side to side—reach arms to side and then curl alternating arms toward the armpit

Open and close doors—arm curl with shoulders abducted

Side arm curl—one arm curls with shoulder abducted (see figure 6.17)

Elbow sweep—one arm triceps extension with shoulder abducted

Jog press—press alternating hands down at the sides

Unison jog press

Punch forward and side

Punch down

Punch across

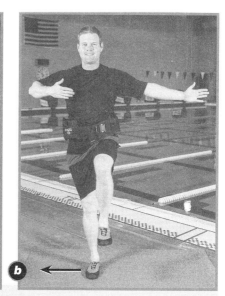

FIGURE 6.17 Side arm curl: (*a*) start and (*b*) finish.

Other arm and hand movements

Bring one arm across to opposite shoulder—start with arms down at sides (see figure 6.18)

Bring one arm down to opposite hip—start with arms to sides 70 degrees

Bicycle arms—pedal the hands in circles

Paddlewheel

Figure eight arms

Hand waves—hands are just above the surface of the water

Pronate and supinate—palms up, palms down

Wrist circles

Finger flicks—bend and straighten the fingers

Circle thumbs

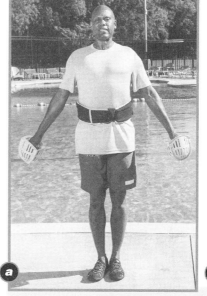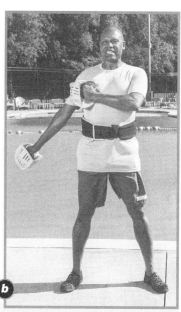

FIGURE 6.18 Bring arm across to opposite shoulder: (*a*) start and (*b*) finish.

Scull—sweep in with the thumbs slightly up and sweep out with the thumbs slightly down

Propeller scull—make figure eights with the hands in front of the body to travel backward or the hands down at the sides to travel forward

8. ABDOMINALS

Brace core, arms down, turbulent hand movements

Hold tuck, brace core, arms down, turbulent hand movements

T-hang—keep a slight bend in the elbows and shoulders relaxed

Tuck, mermaid, tuck, down and tuck, unison kick to the corners, tuck, down

Tuck and hold one leg extended, travel

Cross-country ski and hold, travel

Pike—extend legs in an L position; keep the knees together

Abdominal pike—tuck the feet under the body and pike, tuck and down to upright; keep the knees together

Abdominal pike and spine extension—tuck the feet under the body and pike, tuck and extend the legs back at a 45-degree angle; keep the knees together (see figure 6.19)

Log jump, forward and back—keep the knees together

Crunch, V position—bring chest toward the knees

Crunch—noodle under knees

Pull one knee toward chest; lift and lower other leg

Plank—hold noodle or dumbbells under the shoulders; the body is in a 45-degree angle with the spine in alignment

Plank scissors—one leg is hyperextended

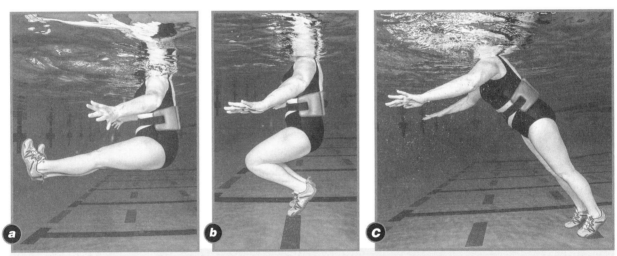

FIGURE 6.19 **Abdominal pike and spine extension: (a) pike, (b), tuck, and (c) spine extension.**

9. OBLIQUES

Brace core and sway legs side to side

Hip hike—lift one hip and then the other hip seated on a noodle

Log jump, side to side—keep the knees together

Log jump R, jacks tuck, log jump L, jacks tuck

Side extension, tuck and down—extend the legs to one side, tuck the feet under the body and down to upright; keep the knees together

Side extension, tuck and pike—extend the legs to one side, tuck the feet under the body and pike; keep the knees together

Side-to-side extension—extend the legs to one side, tuck the feet under the body, and then extend the legs to the other side; keep the knees together

Side-to-side extension with legs in a diamond position—maintain the diamond position throughout the move

Tuck and hold sidesaddle

Swirl—turn side to side with spine in alignment

Seated swirl

Seated swirl, pulse R 2× and L 2×

Swirl in a yoga tree pose—lift one knee to the side with that foot on the other leg anywhere between the knee and the ankle

Swirl with legs apart

Lower body twist—rotate the lower body side to side

Pelvic circles

Pull one knee toward chest, hip roll—legs extended in an L position

Side plank—hold noodle or dumbbell under one shoulder; the body is leaning in a 45-degree angle to the side with the spine in alignment (see figure 6.20)

Side plank pliers—top leg is abducted

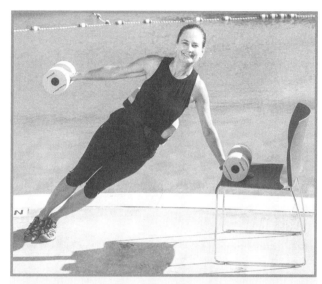

FIGURE 6.20 **Side plank.**

10. LOWER BODY

Knee lift—slow

Pull both knees up—slow

Quad kick—lift the knee and kick from the knee

Hold one leg up; other leg quad kick

Hold one leg up; other leg quad kick 3× and down

Hold one leg up; other leg quad kick and sweep out

Side quad kick—lift the knee to the side and kick from the knee

One knee swings forward and back

Leg lift—slow

One leg kicks forward

One leg kicks forward and back (see figure 6.21)

Leg lift side—slow

One leg kicks side

One leg kicks back

Knee lift, straighten, and power press-down

Hamstring curl—keep knees under hips and curl the hamstrings

Seated hamstring curl—seated kick with emphasis on hamstrings

Seated leg press—press the heels forward as if sitting in a leg press machine

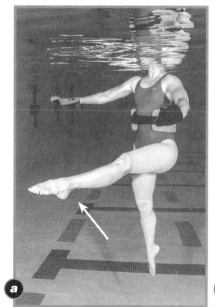 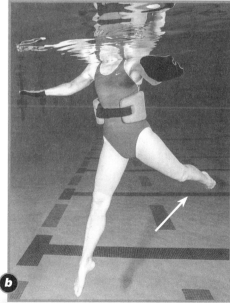

FIGURE 6.21 **One leg kicks forward and back: (a) start and (b) finish.**

Dog hike—hip abduction with knee flexed

Clamshells—horizontal hip abduction and adduction with knee flexed

Point and flex feet

Leg circles—circle from the hips

Ankle circles

Seated kick—on a noodle

Seated jacks—on a noodle

Point and flex feet—on a noodle

Hip extension—foot on a noodle

Standing leg press—foot on a noodle

Standing leg press to the side—foot on a noodle

CHAPTER 7

Deep-Water Lesson Plans for Classes With a Single Objective

The following lesson plans are divided into three sections:

Section 1. The objective for the 12 lesson plans in the first section is cardiorespiratory fitness. Each lesson plan has four versions:

1. Continuous cardio
2. Preseason intervals
3. Transition season intervals
4. Peak fitness intervals

Section 2. The objective for the 15 lesson plans in the second section is strength training. Four lesson plans use the properties of water for strength training, three lessons use buoyant equipment, two lessons use drag equipment, one lesson uses rubberized equipment, two circuit classes use a variety of equipment, and three lesson plans focus on core strength. The lesson plans that use the properties of water for strength training will mainly be used in the preseason. The lesson plans that focus on eccentric muscle actions will mainly be used in the peak fitness season. The remaining lesson plans can be used during the transition season or the peak fitness season. The core strength lesson plans are especially helpful during the preseason if you have participants that need to work on their posture. Core strength is also a focus during the recovery season.

Section 3. This single lesson plan of fun partner activities is designed for the recovery season. Additional fun activities can be found in chapter 8.

SECTION 1: CARDIORESPIRATORY FITNESS

▶ **Deep-Water Cardio Lesson Plan 1**

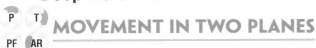

MOVEMENT IN TWO PLANES

EQUIPMENT
Deep-water belts

TEACHING TIP
This lesson plan alternates sets of exercises in the sagittal plane with sets of exercises in the frontal plane. The exercises in the frontal plane begin with ankle touch or inner-thigh lift (see figure 7.1). Perform the exercise with the spine in neutral, bringing the ankle up toward the hand. If your participants tend to lean forward to reach the ankle, call the exercise an inner-thigh lift instead.

WARM-UP
Knee-high jog
Run tires
Inner-thigh lift
Hopscotch
Jumping jacks
Jacks tuck
Tuck ski
Flutter kick

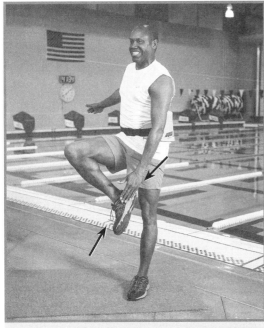

FIGURE 7.1 Ankle touch or inner-thigh lift.

A SET
Flutter kick, diagonal, travel sideways R
Knee-high jog with paddlewheel
Flutter kick, diagonal, travel sideways L
Knee-high jog with paddlewheel
Knee-high jog with reverse breaststroke, travel backward
Kick forward with breaststroke, travel forward
Knee-high jog with reverse breaststroke, travel backward
Seated kick, travel forward
Flutter kick with reverse breaststroke, travel backward
Knee-high jog with pumping arms, travel forward
Knee lift, straighten and power press-down, travel forward
Knee-high jog with breaststroke, travel forward and knee-high jog, alternate
Knee-high jog, faster and knee-high jog, alternate

B SET
Inner-thigh lift
Jumping jacks
Frog kick
Jacks tuck
Hopscotch

C SET
Cross-country ski, diagonal, travel sideways R
Knee-high jog with hand waves
Cross-country ski, diagonal, travel sideways L
Knee-high jog with hand waves
Knee-high jog, push forward, travel backward
Cross-country ski, travel forward
Knee-high jog, push forward, travel backward
Tuck ski, travel forward
Cross-country ski, travel backward
Knee-high jog with crawl stroke, travel forward
Rock climb, travel forward
Knee-high jog with standing row, travel forward and knee-high jog, alternate
Knee-high jog, faster and knee-high jog, alternate

D SET
Inner-thigh lift
Jumping jacks
Frog kick

Jacks tuck

Hopscotch

E SET

Bicycle, diagonal, travel sideways R

Knee-high jog with finger flicks

Bicycle, diagonal, travel sideways L

Knee-high jog with finger flicks

Knee-high jog with propeller scull, travel backward

Bicycle, no hands, travel forward

Knee-high jog with propeller scull, travel backward

Bicycle with bicycle arms, travel forward

Reverse bicycle, travel backward

Knee-high jog with pumping arms, travel forward

Skateboard R with breaststroke pull, travel forward

Skateboard L with breaststroke pull, travel forward

Knee-high jog with double-arm press-down, travel forward and knee-high jog, alternate

Knee-high jog, faster and knee-high jog, alternate

F SET

Inner-thigh lift

Jumping jacks

Frog kick

Jacks tuck

Hopscotch

COOL-DOWN

R leg kicks forward and back

L leg kicks forward and back

Clamshells R

Clamshells L

Tuck and hold with lat pull-down

Brace core, arms down, turbulent hand movements

Helicopter ski

Log jump, side to side

Bicycle, side lying R, circle clockwise

Bicycle, side lying L, circle counterclockwise

Side extension, tuck and pike, alternate R and L

Abdominal pike and spine extension

Log jump, forward and back

Seated swirl

Stretch: hip flexors, quadriceps, gastrocnemius, hamstrings, inner thigh, outer thigh

▶ Deep-Water Work Lesson Plan 1

INTERVAL 30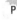

EQUIPMENT

Deep-water belts

TEACHING TIP

Deep-water cardio lesson plan 1 is modified to include interval training. Interval 30 in the preseason is 30 seconds of work to 90 seconds of recovery (1:3 ratio). The intensity level is 60 percent.

Level 6 (60 percent HR max)—Moderate

WARM-UP

Knee-high jog

Run tires

Inner-thigh lift

Hopscotch

Jumping jacks

Jacks tuck

Tuck ski

Flutter kick

A SET

Flutter kick, diagonal, travel sideways R

Knee-high jog with paddlewheel

Flutter kick, diagonal, travel sideways L

Knee-high jog with paddlewheel

Work: Knee lift, straighten and power press-down (30 seconds)

Recovery: Knee-high jog with propeller scull, travel backward (30 seconds)

Seated kick (30 seconds)

Knee-high jog with propeller scull, travel forward (30 seconds)

Work: Knee lift, straighten and power press-down (30 seconds)

Recovery: Knee-high jog with propeller scull, travel backward (30 seconds)

Seated kick (30 seconds)

Knee-high jog with propeller scull, travel forward (30 seconds)

Knee-high jog with breaststroke, travel forward and knee-high jog, alternate

Knee-high jog, faster and knee-high jog, alternate

B SET

Inner-thigh lift

Jumping jacks

Frog kick

Jacks tuck

Hopscotch

C SET

Cross-country ski, diagonal, travel sideways R

Knee-high jog with hand waves

Cross-country ski, diagonal, travel sideways L

Knee-high jog with hand waves

Work: Tuck ski with full extension (30 seconds)

Recovery: Knee-high jog with propeller scull, travel backward (30 seconds)

Cross-country ski with knees bent 90 degrees (30 seconds)

Knee-high jog with propeller scull, travel forward (30 seconds)

Work: Cross-country ski, full ROM (30 seconds)

Recovery: Knee-high jog with propeller scull, travel backward (30 seconds)

Cross-country ski with knees bent 90 degrees (30 seconds)

Knee-high jog with crawl stroke, travel forward (30 seconds)

Knee-high jog with standing row, travel forward and knee-high jog, alternate

Knee-high jog, faster and knee-high jog, alternate

D SET

Inner-thigh lift

Jumping jacks

Frog kick

Jacks tuck

Hopscotch

E SET

Bicycle, diagonal, travel sideways R

Knee-high jog with finger flicks

Bicycle, diagonal, travel sideways L

Knee-high jog with finger flicks

Work: Bicycle, full ROM (30 seconds)

Recovery: Knee-high jog with propeller scull, travel backward (30 seconds)

Skateboard R (30 seconds)

Knee-high jog with propeller scull, travel forward (30 seconds)

Work: Bicycle, full ROM (30 seconds)

Recovery: Knee-high jog with propeller scull, travel backward (30 seconds)

Skateboard L (30 seconds)

Knee-high jog with propeller scull, travel forward (30 seconds)

Knee-high jog with double-arm press-down, travel forward and knee-high jog, alternate

Knee-high jog, faster and knee-high jog, alternate

F SET

Inner-thigh lift

Jumping jacks

Frog kick

Jacks tuck

Hopscotch

COOL-DOWN

R leg kicks forward and back

L leg kicks forward and back

Clamshells R

Clamshells L

Tuck and hold with lat pull-down

Brace core, arms down, turbulent hand movements

Helicopter ski

Log jump, side to side

Bicycle, side lying R, circle clockwise

Bicycle, side lying L, circle counterclockwise

Side extension, tuck and pike, alternate R and L

Abdominal pike and spine extension

Log jump, forward and back

Seated swirl

Stretch: hip flexors, quadriceps, gastrocnemius, hamstrings, inner thigh, outer thigh

▶ Deep-Water Interval Lesson Plan 1

INTERVAL 30

EQUIPMENT

Deep-water belts

TEACHING TIP

Interval 30 in the transition season is 30 seconds of work to 60 seconds of recovery (1:2 ratio). The intensity level is 70 percent.

Level 7 (70 percent HR max)—Somewhat hard

WARM-UP

Knee-high jog

Run tires

Inner-thigh lift

Hopscotch

Jumping jacks

Jacks tuck

Tuck ski

Flutter kick

A SET

Flutter kick, diagonal, travel sideways R

Knee-high jog with paddlewheel

Flutter kick, diagonal, travel sideways L

Knee-high jog with paddlewheel

Work: Flutter kick, faster (30 seconds)

Recovery: Knee-high jog with jog press (30 seconds)

Kick forward (30 seconds)

Work: Kick forward, faster (30 seconds)

Recovery: Knee-high jog with propeller scull, travel backward (30 seconds)

Flutter kick with breaststroke, travel forward (30 seconds)

Work: High kick (30 seconds)

Recovery: Knee-high jog with propeller scull, travel backward (30 seconds)

Seated kick, travel forward (30 seconds)

Knee-high jog with breaststroke, travel forward and knee-high jog, alternate

Knee-high jog, faster and knee-high jog, alternate

B SET

Inner-thigh lift

Jumping jacks

Frog kick

Jacks tuck

Hopscotch

C SET

Cross-country ski, diagonal, travel sideways R

Knee-high jog with hand waves

Cross-country ski, diagonal, travel sideways L

Knee-high jog with hand waves

Work: Mini ski, faster (30 seconds)

Recovery: Knee-high jog with unison jog press (30 seconds)

Cross-country ski (30 seconds)

Work: Cross-country ski, faster (30 seconds)

Recovery: Knee-high jog with propeller scull, travel backward (30 seconds)

Tuck ski with breaststroke, travel forward (30 seconds)

Work: Cross-country ski, faster (30 seconds)

Recovery: Knee-high jog with propeller scull, travel backward (30 seconds)

Tuck ski with breaststroke, travel forward (30 seconds)

Knee-high jog with standing row, travel forward and knee-high jog, alternate

Knee-high jog, faster and knee-high jog, alternate

D SET

Inner-thigh lift

Jumping jacks

Frog kick

Jacks tuck

Hopscotch

E SET

Bicycle, diagonal, travel sideways R

Knee-high jog with finger flicks

Bicycle, diagonal, travel sideways L

Knee-high jog with finger flicks

Work: Flutter kick, faster (30 seconds)

Recovery: Knee-high jog with arm curl (30 seconds)

Bicycle (30 seconds)

Work: Bicycle, faster (30 seconds)

Recovery: Knee-high jog with propeller scull, travel backward (30 seconds)

Skateboard R with breaststroke pull, travel forward (30 seconds)

Work: Bicycle, faster (30 seconds)

Recovery: Knee-high jog with propeller scull, travel backward (30 seconds)

Skateboard L with breaststroke pull, travel forward (30 seconds)

Knee-high jog with double-arm press-down, travel forward and knee-high jog, alternate

Knee-high jog, faster and knee-high jog, alternate

F SET

Inner-thigh lift

Jumping jacks

Frog kick

Jacks tuck

Hopscotch

COOL-DOWN

R leg kicks forward and back

L leg kicks forward and back

Clamshells R

Clamshells L

Tuck and hold with lat pull-down

Brace core, arms down, turbulent hand movements

Helicopter ski

Log jump, side to side

Bicycle, side lying R, circle clockwise

Bicycle, side lying L, circle counterclockwise

Side extension, tuck and pike, alternate R and L

Abdominal pike and spine extension

Log jump, forward and back

Seated swirl

Stretch: hip flexors, quadriceps, gastrocnemius, hamstrings, inner thigh, outer thigh

▶ Deep-Water Interval Lesson Plan 1

INTERVAL 30

EQUIPMENT

Deep-water belts

TEACHING TIP

Interval 30 in the peak fitness season is 30 seconds of work to 30 seconds of recovery (1:1 ratio). The intensity level is 80 percent. Level 8 is high-intensity interval training (HIIT). For safety's sake, encourage your participants to modify the intensity to a level that is challenging for them rather than try to keep up with other participants.

Level 8 (80 percent HR max)—Hard

WARM-UP

Knee-high jog

Run tires

Inner-thigh lift

Hopscotch

Jumping jacks

Jacks tuck

Tuck ski

Flutter kick

A SET

Flutter kick, diagonal, travel sideways R

Knee-high jog with paddlewheel

Flutter kick, diagonal, travel sideways L

Knee-high jog with paddlewheel

Kick forward

Kick forward, doubles

Kick forward, doubles, one low and one high

Knee-high jog with breaststroke, travel forward and knee-high jog, alternate

Knee-high jog, faster and knee-high jog, alternate

B SET

Inner-thigh lift

Jumping jacks

Frog kick

Jacks tuck

Hopscotch

C SET

Cross-country ski, diagonal, travel sideways R

Knee-high jog with hand waves

Cross-country ski, diagonal, travel sideways L

Knee-high jog with hand waves

Cross-country ski with knees bent 90 degrees

Cross-country ski

Tuck ski together

Knee-high jog with standing row, travel forward and knee-high jog, alternate

Knee-high jog, faster and knee-high jog, alternate

D SET

Inner-thigh lift

Jumping jacks

Frog kick

Jacks tuck

Hopscotch

E SET

Bicycle, diagonal, travel sideways R

Knee-high jog with finger flicks

Bicycle, diagonal, travel sideways L

Knee-high jog with finger flicks

Skateboard R with breaststroke pull, travel forward

Skateboard L with breaststroke pull, travel forward

Bicycle

Knee-high jog with double-arm press-down, travel forward and knee-high jog, alternate

Knee-high jog, faster and knee-high jog, alternate

G SET INTERVALS

Work: High kick, power down (30 seconds)

Recovery: Knee-high jog (30 seconds)

Work: High kick with power (30 seconds)

Recovery: Kick forward (30 seconds)

Work: High kick with power (30 seconds)

Recovery: Seated kick (30 seconds)

Work: Cross-country ski with elevation (30 seconds)

Recovery: Knee-high jog (30 seconds)

Work: Cross-country ski with power (30 seconds)

Recovery: Cross-country ski (30 seconds)

Work: Cross-country ski with rotation (30 seconds)

Recovery: Tuck ski (30 seconds)

Work: Bicycle with elevation (30 seconds)

Recovery: Skateboard R (30 seconds)

Work: Bicycle with power (30 seconds)

Recovery: Skateboard L (30 seconds)

Work: Bicycle, tandem with power (30 seconds)

Recovery: Knee-high jog (30 seconds)

Work: Bicycle, tandem with power (30 seconds)

Recovery: Knee-high jog (30 seconds)

F SET

Inner-thigh lift

Jumping jacks

Frog kick

Jacks tuck

Hopscotch

COOL-DOWN

R leg kicks forward and back

L leg kicks forward and back

Clamshells R

Clamshells L

Tuck and hold with lat pull-down

Brace core, arms down, turbulent hand movements

Helicopter ski

Log jump, side to side

Bicycle, side lying R, circle clockwise

Bicycle, side lying L, circle counterclockwise

Side extension, tuck and pike, alternate R and L

Abdominal pike and spine extension

Log jump, forward and back

Seated swirl

Stretch: hip flexors, quadriceps, gastrocnemius, hamstrings, inner thigh, outer thigh

▶ Deep-Water Cardio Lesson Plan 2

TURNS AND CIRCLES

EQUIPMENT

Deep-water belts

TEACHING TIP

Add interest and fun to your lesson plan with turns and circles. Practicing the turns in slow motion during the warm-up may be helpful. For the jacks cross 3-1/2× and half turn (see figure 7.2), cue, "Cross, out, cross, out, cross, out, cross and turn." For the cross-country ski 3-1/2× and half turn (see figure 7.3), cue, "Ski R, L, R, L, R, L, R, and turn." The cool-down uses travel in a bowtie pattern, which includes traveling diagonally to a corner. Turning to the corner and jogging forward is not the same as traveling diagonally. Instead, continue to face forward while moving diagonally toward the corner.

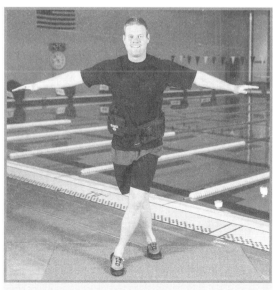

FIGURE 7.2 Jacks cross.

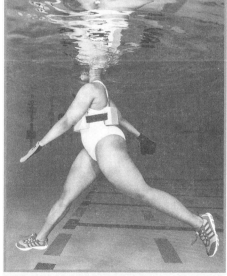

FIGURE 7.3 Cross-country ski.

WARM-UP

Instructor's choice

A SET

Knee-high jog, R shoulder sweep out 2× and L shoulder sweep out 2×

Knee-high jog with unison arm swing

Jumping jacks, pulse out and jacks cross, alternate

Knee-high jog with reverse breaststroke, travel backward

Skateboard R with breaststroke pull, travel forward

Knee-high jog with reverse breaststroke, travel backward

Skateboard L with breaststroke pull, travel forward

Knee-high jog, push forward, travel backward

Crossover step, travel forward

Knee-high jog, push forward, travel backward

Crossover step, travel forward

Crossover kick

Crossover kick, doubles

Jacks cross 3-1/2× and half turn

Jacks cross, R leg in front, circle clockwise

Jacks cross, L leg in front, circle counterclockwise

Knee-high jog

B SET

Knee-high jog with double-arm press-down 2× and lat pull-down 2×

Jumping jacks with unison arm swing

Cross-country ski and mini ski, alternate

Knee-high jog with reverse breaststroke, travel backward

Jacks tuck with breaststroke, travel forward

Knee-high jog with reverse breaststroke, travel backward

Jacks tuck with breaststroke, travel forward

Knee-high jog, push forward, travel backward

Jumping jacks with breaststroke, travel forward

Knee-high jog, push forward, travel backward

Jumping jacks with breaststroke, travel forward

Crossover kick, doubles

Crossover kick, doubles, one low and one high

Cross-country ski 3-1/2× and half turn

Helicopter ski

Knee-high jog

C SET

Knee-high jog, punch down R, L and punch across R, L

Cross-country ski with unison arm swing

Jumping jacks and mini cross, alternate

Knee-high jog with reverse breaststroke, travel backward

Cross-country ski, travel forward

Knee-high jog with reverse breaststroke, travel backward

Cross-country ski, travel forward

Knee-high jog, push forward, travel backward

Cross-country ski with alternating sweep out, travel forward

Knee-high jog, push forward, travel backward

Cross-country ski with alternating sweep out, travel forward

Crossover kick, doubles, one low and one high

Crossover kick and sweep out

Jacks cross 3-1/2× and half turn

Jacks cross, R leg in front, circle clockwise

Jacks cross, L leg in front, circle counterclockwise

Knee-high jog

D SET

Knee-high jog, open and close doors: open R, open L, close R, close L, and open close 2×

Bicycle with unison arm swing

Cross-country ski and tuck ski, alternate

Knee-high jog with reverse breaststroke, travel backward

Bicycle, tandem, travel forward

Knee-high jog with reverse breaststroke, travel backward

Bicycle, tandem, travel forward

Knee-high jog, push forward, travel backward

Bicycle R leg, travel forward

Knee-high jog, push forward, travel backward

Bicycle L, travel forward

Crossover kick and sweep out

Skate kick, crossover kick, sweep out and center

Cross-country ski 3-1/2× and half turn

Helicopter ski

Knee-high jog

COOL-DOWN

(Travel in a bowtie pattern)

Knee-high jog with propeller scull, travel backward

Knee-high jog with propeller scull, travel diagonally to front L corner

Knee-high jog with propeller scull, travel backward

Knee-high jog with propeller scull, travel diagonally to front R corner

Knee-high jog with propeller scull, travel diagonally backward to back L corner

Knee-high jog with propeller scull, travel forward

Knee-high jog with propeller scull, travel diagonally backward to back R corner

Knee-high jog with propeller scull, travel forward

Knee-high jog, travel in a circle clockwise, look L

Knee-high jog, travel in a circle counterclockwise, look R

Bicycle, diagonal R, circle clockwise

Bicycle, diagonal L, circle counterclockwise

Log jump, side to side

Bicycle, side lying R, circle clockwise

Bicycle, side lying L, circle counterclockwise

Side-to-side extension

Stretch: shoulders, pectorals, hip flexors, gastrocnemius, hamstrings, outer thigh

▶ Deep-Water Interval Lesson Plan 2

INTERVAL 40

EQUIPMENT

Deep-water belts

TEACHING TIP

Deep-water cardio lesson plan 2 is modified to include interval training. Interval 40 in the preseason is 40 seconds of work to 80 seconds of recovery (1:2 ratio). The intensity level is 60 percent.

Level 6 (60 percent HR max)—Moderate

WARM-UP

Instructor's choice

A SET

Knee-high jog, R shoulder sweep out 2× and L shoulder sweep out 2×

Knee-high jog with unison arm swing

Jumping jacks, pulse out and jacks cross, alternate

Knee-high jog with reverse breaststroke, travel backward

Skateboard R with breaststroke pull, travel forward

Knee-high jog with reverse breaststroke, travel backward

Skateboard L with breaststroke pull, travel forward

Work: Knee lift, straighten and power press-down (40 seconds)

Recovery: Crossover knees (20 seconds)

Knee-high jog (20 seconds)

Crossover knees (20 seconds)

Knee-high jog (20 seconds)

Work: Knee lift, straighten and power press-down (40 seconds)

Recovery: Crossover knees (20 seconds)

Knee-high jog (20 seconds)

Crossover knees (20 seconds)

Knee-high jog (20 seconds)

Jacks cross 3-1/2× and half turn

Jacks cross, R leg in front, circle clockwise

Jacks cross, L leg in front, circle counterclockwise

B SET

Knee-high jog with double-arm press-down 2× and lat pull-down 2×

Jumping jacks with unison arm swing

Cross-country ski and mini ski, alternate

Knee-high jog with reverse breaststroke, travel backward

Jacks tuck with breaststroke, travel forward

Knee-high jog with reverse breaststroke, travel backward

Jacks tuck with breaststroke, travel forward

Work: Jacks cross (40 seconds)

Recovery: Straddle jog (20 seconds)

Knee-high jog (20 seconds)

Straddle jog (20 seconds)

Knee-high jog (20 seconds)

Work: Jacks cross (40 seconds)

Recovery: Straddle jog (20 seconds)

Knee-high jog (20 seconds)

Straddle jog (20 seconds)

Knee-high jog (20 seconds)

Cross-country ski 3-1/2× and half turn

Helicopter ski

C SET

Knee-high jog, punch down R, L and punch across R, L

Cross-country ski with unison arm swing

Jumping jacks and mini cross, alternate

Knee-high jog with reverse breaststroke, travel backward

Cross-country ski, travel forward

Knee-high jog with reverse breaststroke, travel backward

Cross-country ski, travel forward

Work: Cross-country ski, full ROM (40 seconds)

Recovery: Heel jog (20 seconds)

Knee-high jog (20 seconds)

Heel jog (20 seconds)

Knee-high jog (20 seconds)

Work: Cross-country ski, full ROM (40 seconds)

Recovery: Heel jog (20 seconds)

Knee-high jog (20 seconds)

Heel jog (20 seconds)

Knee-high jog (20 seconds)

Jacks cross 3-1/2× and half turn

Jacks cross, R leg in front, circle clockwise

Jacks cross, L leg in front, circle counterclockwise

D SET

Knee-high jog, open and close doors: open R, open L, close R, close L, and open close 2×

Bicycle with unison arm swing

Cross-country ski and tuck ski, alternate

Knee-high jog with reverse breaststroke, travel backward

Bicycle, tandem, travel forward

Knee-high jog with reverse breaststroke, travel backward

Bicycle, tandem, travel forward

Work: Skate kick, full ROM (40 seconds)

Recovery: Bicycle R leg (20 seconds)

Knee-high jog (20 seconds)

Bicycle L leg (20 seconds)

Knee-high jog (20 seconds)

Work: Skate kick, full ROM (40 seconds)

Recovery: Bicycle R leg (20 seconds)

Knee-high jog (20 seconds)

Bicycle L leg (20 seconds)

Knee-high jog (20 seconds)

Cross-country ski 3-1/2× and half turn

Helicopter ski

COOL-DOWN

(Travel in a bowtie pattern)

Knee-high jog with propeller scull, travel backward

Knee-high jog with propeller scull, travel diagonally to front L corner

Knee-high jog with propeller scull, travel backward

Knee-high jog with propeller scull, travel diagonally to front R corner

Knee-high jog with propeller scull, travel diagonally backward to back L corner

Knee-high jog with propeller scull, travel forward

Knee-high jog with propeller scull, travel diagonally backward to back R corner

Knee-high jog with propeller scull, travel forward

Knee-high jog, travel in a circle clockwise, look L

Knee-high jog, travel in a circle counterclockwise, look R

Bicycle, diagonal R, circle clockwise

Bicycle, diagonal L, circle counterclockwise

Log jump, side to side

Bicycle, side lying R, circle clockwise

Bicycle, side lying L, circle counterclockwise

Side-to-side extension

Stretch: shoulders, pectorals, hip flexors, gastrocnemius, hamstrings, outer thigh

▶ Deep-Water Interval Lesson Plan 2

INTERVAL 40

EQUIPMENT

Deep-water belts

TEACHING TIP

Interval 40 in the transition season is 40 seconds of work to 60 seconds of recovery (1:1.5 ratio). The intensity level is 70 percent.

Level 7 (70 percent HR max)—Somewhat hard

WARM-UP

Instructor's choice

A SET

Knee-high jog, R shoulder sweep out 2× and L shoulder sweep out 2×

Knee-high jog with unison arm swing

Jumping jacks, pulse out and jacks cross, alternate

Knee-high jog with reverse breaststroke, travel backward

Skateboard R with breaststroke pull, travel forward

Knee-high jog with reverse breaststroke, travel backward

Skateboard L with breaststroke pull, travel forward

Knee-high jog with double-arm press-down 2× and lat pull-down 2×

Jumping jacks with unison arm swing

Cross-country ski and mini ski, alternate

Knee-high jog with reverse breaststroke, travel backward

Jacks tuck with breaststroke, travel forward

Knee-high jog with reverse breaststroke, travel backward

Jacks tuck with breaststroke, travel forward

Jacks cross 3-1/2× and half turn

Jacks cross, R leg in front, circle clockwise

Jacks cross, L leg in front, circle counterclockwise

Knee-high jog

B SET

Knee-high jog, punch down R, L and punch across R, L

Cross-country ski with unison arm swing

Jumping jacks and mini cross, alternate

Knee-high jog with reverse breaststroke, travel backward

Cross-country ski, travel forward

Knee-high jog with reverse breaststroke, travel backward

Cross-country ski, travel forward

Knee-high jog, open and close doors: open R, open L, close R, close L, and open close 2×

Bicycle with unison arm swing

Cross-country ski and tuck ski, alternate

Knee-high jog with reverse breaststroke, travel backward

Bicycle, tandem, travel forward

Knee-high jog with reverse breaststroke, travel backward

Bicycle, tandem, travel forward

Cross-country ski 3-1/2× and half turn

Helicopter ski

Knee-high jog

C SET INTERVALS

Work: Steep climb, faster (40 seconds)

Recovery: Crossover knees (30 seconds)

Knee-high jog (30 seconds)

Work: Knee-high jog, faster (40 seconds)

Recovery: Crossover knees (30 seconds)

Knee-high jog (30 seconds)

Work: Mini jacks, faster (40 seconds)

Recovery: Straddle jog (30 seconds)

Knee-high jog (30 seconds)

Work: Jumping jacks, faster (40 seconds)

Recovery: Straddle jog (30 seconds)

Knee-high jog (30 seconds)

Work: Mini ski, faster (40 seconds)

Recovery: Heel jog (30 seconds)

Knee-high jog (30 seconds)

Work: Cross-country ski, faster (40 seconds)

Recovery: Heel jog (30 seconds)

Knee-high jog (30 seconds)

Work: Mini ski, faster (40 seconds)

Recovery: Heel jog (30 seconds)

Knee-high jog (30 seconds)

Work: Bicycle, faster (40 seconds)

Recovery: Bicycle R leg (30 seconds)

Knee-high jog (30 seconds)

Work: Bicycle, faster (40 seconds)

Recovery: Bicycle L leg (30 seconds)

Knee-high jog (30 seconds)

COOL-DOWN

(Travel in a bowtie pattern)

Knee-high jog with propeller scull, travel backward

Knee-high jog with propeller scull, travel diagonally to front L corner

Knee-high jog with propeller scull, travel backward

Knee-high jog with propeller scull, travel diagonally to front R corner

Knee-high jog with propeller scull, travel diagonally backward to back L corner

Knee-high jog with propeller scull, travel forward

Knee-high jog with propeller scull, travel diagonally backward to back R corner

Knee-high jog with propeller scull, travel forward

Knee-high jog, travel in a circle clockwise, look L

Knee-high jog, travel in a circle counterclockwise, look R

Stretch: shoulders, pectorals, hip flexors, gastrocnemius, hamstrings, outer thigh

▶ Deep-Water Interval Lesson Plan 2

INTERVAL 40

PF

EQUIPMENT

Deep-water belts

TEACHING TIP

Interval 40 in the peak fitness season is 40 seconds of work to 40 seconds of recovery (1:1 ratio). The intensity level is 80 percent. Level 8 is high-intensity interval training (HIIT). For safety's sake, encourage your participants to modify the intensity to a level that is challenging for them rather than try to keep up with other participants.

Level 8 (80 percent HR max)—Hard

WARM-UP

Instructor's choice

A SET

Knee-high jog, R shoulder sweep out 2× and L shoulder sweep out 2×

Knee-high jog with unison arm swing

Jumping jacks, pulse out and jacks cross, alternate

Knee-high jog with reverse breaststroke, travel backward

Skateboard R with breaststroke pull, travel forward

Knee-high jog with reverse breaststroke, travel backward

Skateboard L with breaststroke pull, travel forward

Knee-high jog with double-arm press-down 2× and lat pull-down 2×

Jumping jacks with unison arm swing

Cross-country ski and mini ski, alternate

Knee-high jog with reverse breaststroke, travel backward

Jacks tuck with breaststroke, travel forward

Knee-high jog with reverse breaststroke, travel backward

Jacks tuck with breaststroke, travel forward

Jacks cross 3-1/2× and half turn

Knee-high jog

B SET

Knee-high jog, punch down R, L and punch across R, L

Cross-country ski with unison arm swing

Jumping jacks and mini cross, alternate

Knee-high jog with reverse breaststroke, travel backward

Cross-country ski, travel forward

Knee-high jog with reverse breaststroke, travel backward

Cross-country ski, travel forward

Knee-high jog, open and close doors: open R, open L, close R, close L, and open close 2×

Bicycle with unison arm swing

Cross-country ski and tuck ski, alternate

Knee-high jog with reverse breaststroke, travel backward

Bicycle, tandem, travel forward

Knee-high jog with reverse breaststroke, travel backward

Bicycle, tandem, travel forward

Cross-country ski 3-1/2× and half turn

Knee-high jog

C SET INTERVALS

Work: Steep climb with power (40 seconds)

Recovery: Crossover knees (20 seconds)
  Knee-high jog (20 seconds)

Work: Power run (40 seconds)

Recovery: Crossover knees (20 seconds)
  Knee-high jog (20 seconds)

Work: Power run (40 seconds)

Recovery: Crossover knees (20 seconds)
  Knee-high jog (20 seconds)

Work: Frog kick with elevation (40 seconds)

Recovery: Straddle jog (20 seconds)
  Knee-high jog (20 seconds)

Work: Frog kick with elevation (40 seconds)

Recovery: Straddle jog (20 seconds)
  Knee-high jog (20 seconds)

Work: Frog kick with elevation (40 seconds)

Recovery: Straddle jog (20 seconds)
  Knee-high jog (20 seconds)

Work: Cross-country ski with rotation (40 seconds)

Recovery: Heel jog (20 seconds)
  Knee-high jog (20 seconds)

Work: Cross-country ski with elevation (40 seconds)

Recovery: Heel jog (20 seconds)
  Knee-high jog (20 seconds)

Work: Tuck ski together (40 seconds)

Recovery: Heel jog (20 seconds)
  Knee-high jog (20 seconds)

Work: Bicycle with elevation (40 seconds)

Recovery: Bicycle, tandem (20 seconds)
  Knee-high jog (20 seconds)

Work: Bicycle with power (40 seconds)

Recovery: Bicycle R leg (20 seconds)
  Knee-high jog (20 seconds)

Work: Bicycle with power (40 seconds)

Recovery: Bicycle L leg (20 seconds)
  Knee-high jog (20 seconds)

COOL-DOWN

(Travel in a bowtie pattern)

Knee-high jog with propeller scull, travel backward

Knee-high jog with propeller scull, travel diagonally to front L corner

Knee-high jog with propeller scull, travel backward

Knee-high jog with propeller scull, travel diagonally to front R corner

Knee-high jog with propeller scull, travel diagonally backward to back L corner

Knee-high jog with propeller scull, travel forward

Knee-high jog with propeller scull, travel diagonally backward to back R corner

Knee-high jog with propeller scull, travel forward

Knee-high jog, travel in a circle clockwise, look L

Knee-high jog, travel in a circle counterclockwise, look R

Stretch: shoulders, pectorals, hip flexors, gastrocnemius, hamstrings, outer thigh

▶ Deep-Water Cardio Lesson Plan 3

INCREASING COMPLEXITY

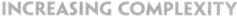

EQUIPMENT

Deep-water belts

TEACHING TIP

Another way to organize a lesson plan is to start with a set of basic exercises. Repeat those same exercises in the second set but insert additional exercises that may be new to your participants. For example, combine two moves to create a new move. This lesson plan combines jumping jacks (see figure 7.4) with kick forward (see figure 7.5) and with skate kick (see figure 7.6). Repeat the second set and insert even more exercises, so that each succeeding set is more complex than the preceding one.

WARM-UP

Instructor's choice

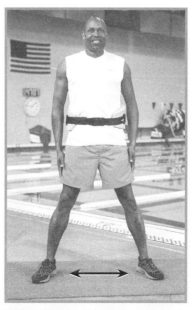

FIGURE 7.4　**Jumping jacks.**

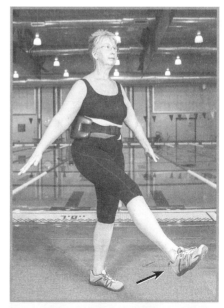

FIGURE 7.5　**Kick forward.**

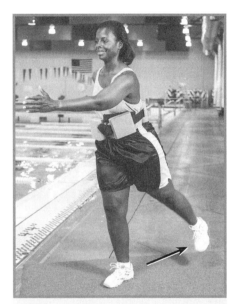

FIGURE 7.6 Skate kick.

A SET

Jumping jacks

Jumping jacks with elbows bent

Inner-thigh lift

Straddle jog with shoulder blade squeeze

Skateboard R with breaststroke pull, travel forward

Skateboard L with breaststroke pull, travel forward

Bicycle with breaststroke, one lap

Cross-country ski with unison sidestroke, travel sideways R and L

Cross-country ski with unison arm swing

Cross-country ski with rotation

Knee-high jog

B SET

Jumping jacks

Jumping jacks, arms cross in front and in back

Jumping jacks, pulse out

Jumping jacks 1×, kick forward 1×

Inner-thigh lift

Hopscotch

Straddle jog with shoulder blade squeeze

Skateboard L with breaststroke pull, travel forward

Skateboard R with breaststroke pull, travel forward

Bicycle with bicycle arms, one lap

Cross-country ski travel, backward and forward

Cross-country ski with unison arm swing

Cross-country ski, clap hands

Cross-country ski with rotation

Knee-high jog

C SET

Jumping jacks

Jumping jacks, palms touch in front and in back

Jumping jacks, pulse in

Jumping jacks 2×, jumping jacks, pulse out 4×

Jumping jacks 1×, kick forward 1×

Jumping jacks 1×, skate kick 1×

Inner-thigh lift 1×, hopscotch 1×

Straddle jog with shoulder blade squeeze

Skateboard R with breaststroke pull, one lap

Skateboard L with breaststroke pull, one lap

Bicycle, tandem, one lap

Cross-country ski, diagonal, travel sideways R and L

Cross-country ski with unison arm swing

Cross-country ski, clap hands

Cross-country ski with forearm press

Cross-country ski with rotation

Knee-high jog

COOL-DOWN

Jumping jacks

Jumping jacks 1×, kick forward 1×

Jumping jacks 1×, skate kick 1×

Skate kick

Kick forward

Seated kick

Seated kick 3× and hold

Tuck and hold R leg extended, reverse breaststroke, travel backward

Bicycle, no hands, travel forward

Seated kick 3× and hold

Tuck and hold L leg extended, reverse breaststroke, travel backward

Bicycle, tandem, travel forward

Mermaid

Stretch: hamstrings, outer thigh, quadriceps, hip flexors, gastrocnemius, upper back

▶ **Deep-Water Interval Lesson Plan 3**

INTERVAL 60

EQUIPMENT
Deep-water belts

TEACHING TIP
Deep-water cardio lesson plan 3 is modified to include interval training. Interval 60 in the preseason is 60 seconds of work to 2 minutes of recovery (1:2 ratio). The intensity level is 60 percent.

Level 6 (60 percent HR max)—Moderate

WARM-UP
Instructor's choice

A SET
Jumping jacks

Jumping jacks with elbows bent

Jumping jacks 2×, jumping jacks, pulse out 4×

Inner-thigh lift

Straddle jog with shoulder blade squeeze

Skateboard R with breaststroke pull, travel forward

Skateboard L with breaststroke pull, travel forward

Bicycle with breaststroke, one lap

Bicycle with bicycle arms, one lap

Knee-high jog

B SET
Jumping jacks

Jumping jacks, arms cross in front and in back

Jumping jacks 1×, kick forward 1×

Hopscotch

Straddle jog with shoulder blade squeeze

Skateboard L with breaststroke pull, travel forward

Skateboard R with breaststroke pull, travel forward

Bicycle with breaststroke, one lap

Bicycle, tandem, one lap

Knee-high jog

C SET INTERVALS
Work: Knee lift, straighten and power press-down (60 seconds)

Recovery: Flutter kick (30 seconds)

R leg kicks forward (30 seconds)

Flutter kick (30 seconds)

L kicks forward (30 seconds)

Work: Jacks cross (60 seconds)

Recovery: Run tires (30 seconds)

R leg kicks side (30 seconds)

Run tires (30 seconds)

L leg kicks side (30 seconds)

Work: Inner-thigh lift, full ROM (60 seconds)

Recovery: Cossack kick (30 seconds)

Straddle jog (30 seconds)

Cossack kick (30 seconds)

Straddle jog (30 seconds)

Work: Knee lift, straighten and power press-down (60 seconds)

Recovery: Flutter kick, toes pointed (30 seconds)

Crossover knees (30 seconds)

Flutter kick, feet flexed (30 seconds)

Crossover knees (30 seconds)

Work: Tuck ski with full extension (60 seconds)

Recovery: Heel jog (30 seconds)

R leg kicks back (30 seconds)

Heel jog (30 seconds)

L leg kicks back (30 seconds)

Work: Cross-country ski, full ROM (60 seconds)

Recovery: Knee-high jog (30 seconds)

Skateboard R (30 seconds)

Knee-high jog (30 seconds)

Skateboard L (30 seconds)

COOL-DOWN
Jumping jacks

Jumping jacks, palms touch in front and in back

Jumping jacks 1×, skate kick 1×

Inner-thigh lift 1×, hopscotch 1×

Straddle jog with shoulder blade squeeze

Skateboard R with breaststroke pull, one lap

Skateboard L with breaststroke pull, one lap

Bicycle with bicycle arms, one lap

Seated kick

Seated kick 3× and hold

Tuck and hold R leg extended, reverse breaststroke, travel backward

Bicycle, no hands, travel forward

Seated kick 3× and hold

Tuck and hold L leg extended, reverse breaststroke, travel backward

Bicycle, tandem, travel forward

Mermaid

Stretch: hamstrings, outer thigh, quadriceps, hip
flexors, gastrocnemius, upper back

▶ **Deep-Water Interval Lesson Plan 3**

INTERVAL 60

EQUIPMENT
Deep-water belts

TEACHING TIP
Interval 60 in the transition season is 60 seconds
of work to 90 seconds of recovery (1:1.5 ratio). The
intensity level is 70 percent.

Level 7 (70 percent HR max)—Somewhat hard

WARM-UP
Instructor's choice

A SET
Jumping jacks

Jumping jacks with elbows bent

Jumping jacks 2×, jumping jacks, pulse out 4×

Inner-thigh lift

Straddle jog with shoulder blade squeeze

Skateboard R with breaststroke pull, travel forward

Skateboard L with breaststroke pull, travel forward

Bicycle with breaststroke, one lap

Bicycle with bicycle arms, one lap

Knee-high jog

B SET
Jumping jacks

Jumping jacks, arms cross in front and in back

Jumping jacks 1×, kick forward 1×

Hopscotch

Straddle jog with shoulder blade squeeze

Skateboard L with breaststroke pull, travel forward

Skateboard R with breaststroke pull, travel forward

Bicycle with breaststroke, one lap

Bicycle, tandem, one lap

Knee-high jog

C SET INTERVALS
Work: Kick forward, faster (60 seconds)

Recovery: R leg kicks forward (30 seconds)

Kick forward (30 seconds)

L leg kicks forward (30 seconds)

Work: Jumping jacks, faster (60 seconds)

Recovery: R leg kicks side (30 seconds)

Run tires (30 seconds)

L leg kicks side (30 seconds)

Work: Inner-thigh lift, faster (60 seconds)

Recovery: Straddle jog (30 seconds)

Cossack kick (30 seconds)

Straddle jog (30 seconds)

Work: Skate kick, faster (60 seconds)

Recovery: Skateboard R (30 seconds)

Tuck ski (30 seconds)

Skateboard L (30 seconds)

Work: High kick (60 seconds)

Recovery: Flutter kick, toes pointed (30 seconds)

Crossover knees (30 seconds)

Flutter kick, feet flexed (30 seconds)

Work: Mini jacks, faster (60 seconds)

Recovery: Jumping jacks (30 seconds)

Jacks tuck (30 seconds)

Jumping jacks (30 seconds)

Work: Mini ski, faster (60 seconds)

Recovery: R leg kicks back (30 seconds)

Heel jog (30 seconds)

L leg kicks back (30 seconds)

Work: Cross-country ski, faster (60 seconds)

Recovery: Skateboard R (30 seconds)

Tuck ski (30 seconds)

Skateboard L (30 seconds)

COOL-DOWN
Jumping jacks

Jumping jacks, palms touch in front and in back

Jumping jacks 1×, skate kick 1×

Inner-thigh lift 1×, hopscotch 1×

Straddle jog with shoulder blade squeeze

Skateboard R 4×, skateboard L 4×, one lap

Bicycle with bicycle arms, one lap

Seated kick

Seated kick 3× and hold

Tuck and hold R leg extended, reverse breaststroke, travel backward

Bicycle, no hands, travel forward

Seated kick 3× and hold

Tuck and hold L leg extended, reverse breaststroke, travel backward

Bicycle, tandem, travel forward

Mermaid

Stretch: hamstrings, outer thigh, quadriceps, hip flexors, gastrocnemius, upper back

▶ **Deep-Water Interval Lesson Plan 3**

INTERVAL 60

EQUIPMENT

Deep-water belts

TEACHING TIP

Interval 60 in the peak fitness season is 60 seconds of work to 60 seconds of recovery (1:1 ratio). The intensity level is 80 percent. Level 8 is high-intensity interval training (HIIT). For safety's sake, encourage your participants to modify the intensity to a level that is challenging for them rather than try to keep up with other participants.

Level 8 (80 percent HR max)—Hard

WARM-UP

Instructor's choice

A SET

Jumping jacks

Jumping jacks with elbows bent

Jumping jacks 2×, jumping jacks, pulse out 4×

Inner-thigh lift

Straddle jog with shoulder blade squeeze

Skateboard R with breaststroke pull, travel forward

Skateboard L with breaststroke pull, travel forward

Bicycle with breaststroke, one lap

Bicycle with bicycle arms, one lap

Knee-high jog

B SET

Jumping jacks

Jumping jacks, arms cross in front and in back

Jumping jacks 1×, kick forward 1×

Hopscotch

Straddle jog with shoulder blade squeeze

Skateboard L with breaststroke pull, travel forward

Skateboard R with breaststroke pull, travel forward

Bicycle with breaststroke, one lap

Bicycle, tandem, one lap

Knee-high jog

C SET INTERVALS

Work: High kick, power down (60 seconds)

Recovery: R leg kicks forward (30 seconds)
  L leg kicks forward (30 seconds)

Work: Breaststroke kick with elevation (60 seconds)

Recovery: R leg kicks side (30 seconds)
  L leg kicks side (30 seconds)

Work: Inner-thigh lift with power (60 seconds)

Recovery: Straddle jog (30 seconds)
  Cossack kick (30 seconds)

Work: Cross-country ski with power (60 seconds)

Recovery: R leg kicks back (30 seconds)
  L leg kicks back (30 seconds)

Work: Cross-country ski with rotation (60 seconds)

Recovery: Tuck ski (30 seconds)
  Tuck ski with rotation (30 seconds)

Work: High kick 7×, tuck, and turn (60 seconds)

Recovery: Flutter kick, toes pointed (30 seconds)
  Flutter kick, feet flexed (30 seconds)

Work: Frog kick with elevation (60 seconds)

Recovery: Jumping jacks (30 seconds)
  Jacks tuck (30 seconds)

Work: Cross-country ski with power (60 seconds)

Recovery: R leg kicks forward and back (30 seconds)
  L leg kicks forward and back (30 seconds)

Work: Cross-country ski with rotation (60 seconds)

Recovery: Tuck ski (30 seconds)
  Tuck ski with rotation (30 seconds)

Work: Helicopter ski (60 seconds)

Recovery: Skateboard R (30 seconds)
  Skateboard L (30 seconds)

COOL-DOWN

Jumping jacks

Jumping jacks, palms touch in front and in back

Jumping jacks 1×, skate kick 1×

Inner-thigh lift 1×, hopscotch 1×

Straddle jog with shoulder blade squeeze

Skateboard R 4×, skateboard L 4×, one lap

Bicycle with bicycle arms, one lap

Seated kick

Seated kick 3× and hold

Tuck and hold R leg extended, reverse breast-stroke, travel backward

Bicycle, no hands, travel forward

Seated kick 3× and hold

Tuck and hold L leg extended, reverse breast-stroke, travel backward

Bicycle, tandem, travel forward

Mermaid

Stretch: hamstrings, outer thigh, quadriceps, hip flexors, gastrocnemius, upper back

▶ Deep-Water Cardio Lesson Plan 4

BLOCK CHOREOGRAPHY WITH FIVE MOVES

EQUIPMENT

Deep-water belts

TEACHING TIP

In block choreography you start with a set of basic moves, and in each succeeding set you change something about each move. This lesson plan uses just five moves—flutter kick (see figure 7.7), kick forward (see figure 7.8), jumping jacks (see figure 7.9), skate kick (see figure 7.10), and cross-country ski (see figure 7.11). It ends with an arm medley.

WARM-UP

Instructor's choice

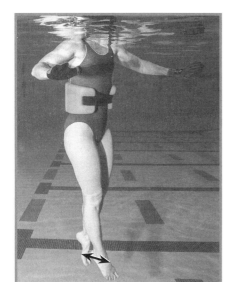

FIGURE 7.7 Flutter kick.

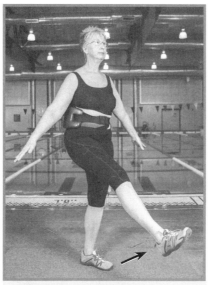

FIGURE 7.8 Kick forward.

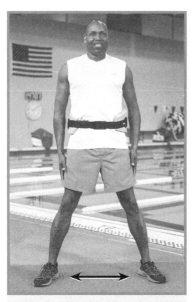

FIGURE 7.9 Jumping jacks.

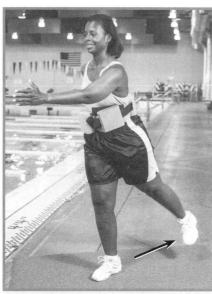

FIGURE 7.10 Skate kick.

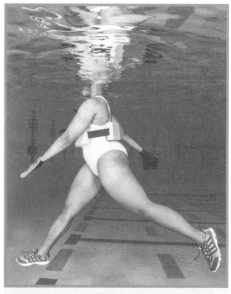

FIGURE 7.11 Cross-country ski.

A SET

Flutter kick

Kick forward

Jumping jacks

Heel jog

Cross-country ski

B SET

Flutter kick, punch forward and side

Chorus-line kick

Jumping jacks with diagonal turn

Skate kick with pumping arms

Cross-country ski, two easy and one with power

C SET

Flutter kick, push across and slice back

High kick

Jumping jacks, pulse out

R leg kicks forward and back

L leg kicks forward and back

Cross-country ski, four easy and four with power

D SET

Star flutter kick

Kick forward with lat pull-down

Jumping jacks, pulse in

Skate kick with pumping arms

Cross-country ski, two easy and one with power

E SET

Flutter kick, punch across

Crossover kick

Mini cross

R knee swings forward and back

L knee swings forward and back

Cross-country ski, four easy and four with power

F SET

Flutter kick with triceps extension

Crossover kick and sweep out

Jacks tuck

Skate kick with pumping arms

Cross-country ski, two easy and one with power

G SET

Flutter kick

Seated kick

Bent-knee jacks

Heel jog

Cross-country ski with knees bent 90 degrees

H SET

Straddle jog, clap hands

Straddle jog, shoulder sweep out R and L, alternate

Straddle jog, shoulder sweep in R and L, alternate

Straddle jog, clap hands with power

Knee-high jog with crawl stroke

Knee-high jog with R bowstring pull

Knee-high jog with L bowstring pull

Knee-high jog with standing row with power

Cross-country ski

Cross-country ski with R arm swing, L hand on hip

Cross-country ski with L arm swing, R hand on hip

Cross-country ski with unison arm swing with power

Straddle jog, open and close doors

Straddle jog, open and close R and L, alternate

Straddle jog, open R, open L, close R, close L with power

Straddle jog with forearm press

COOL-DOWN

Tuck, R shoulder sweep in, L hand on hip, circle clockwise

Tuck, L shoulder sweep in, R hand on hip, circle counterclockwise

Hold tuck, brace core, arms down, turbulent hand movements

Seated swirl

Tuck and hold sidesaddle R with reverse breaststroke, travel backward

Tuck and hold sidesaddle L with breaststroke, travel forward

Seated swirl

Stretch: quadriceps, hip flexors, inner thigh, hamstrings, pectorals, upper back

▶ Deep-Water Interval Lesson Plan 4

INTERVALS WITH REDUCED RECOVERY TIME 1

EQUIPMENT

Deep-water belts

TEACHING TIP

Deep-water cardio lesson plan 4 is modified to include interval training. Interval training with reduced recovery time in the preseason is 60 seconds of work to 30 seconds of recovery (2:1 ratio). The intensity level is 60 percent.

Level 6 (60 percent HR max)—Moderate

WARM-UP

Instructor's choice

A SET

Flutter kick

Kick forward

Jumping jacks

Heel jog

Cross-country ski

Work: Jacks cross (60 seconds)

Recovery: In, in, out, out (30 seconds)

Work: Jacks cross (60 seconds)

Recovery: Run tires (30 seconds)

B SET

Flutter kick, punch forward and side

Chorus-line kick

Jumping jacks with diagonal turn

Skate kick with pumping arms

Cross-country ski, two easy and one with power

C SET

Flutter kick, push across and slice back

High kick

Jumping jacks, pulse out

R leg kicks forward and back

L leg kicks forward and back

Cross-country ski, four easy and four with power

Work: Inner-thigh lift, full ROM (60 seconds)

Recovery: In, in, out, out (30 seconds)

Work: Hopscotch, full ROM (60 seconds)

Recovery: Run tires (30 seconds)

D SET

Star flutter kick

Kick forward with lat pull-down

Jumping jacks, pulse in

Skate kick with pumping arms

Cross-country ski, two easy and one with power

E SET

Flutter kick, punch across

Crossover kick

Mini cross

R knee swings forward and back

L knee swings forward and back

Cross-country ski, four easy and four with power

Work: Tuck ski with full extension (60 seconds)

Recovery: In, in, out, out (30 seconds)

Work: Cross-country ski, full ROM (60 seconds)

Recovery: Run tires (30 seconds)

F SET

Flutter kick

Seated kick

Bent-knee jacks

Heel jog

Cross-country ski with knees bent 90 degrees

COOL-DOWN

Straddle jog, clap hands

Straddle jog, shoulder sweep out R and L, alternate

Straddle jog, shoulder sweep in R and L, alternate

Straddle jog, clap hands with power

Knee-high jog with crawl stroke

Knee-high jog with R bowstring pull

Knee-high jog with L bowstring pull

Knee-high jog with standing row with power

Cross-country ski

Cross-country ski with R arm swing, L hand on hip

Cross-country ski with L arm swing, R hand on hip

Cross-country ski with unison arm swing with power

Straddle jog, open and close doors

Straddle jog, open and close R and L, alternate

Straddle jog, open R, open L, close R, close L with power

Straddle jog with forearm press

Yoga tree pose R, swirl

Yoga tree pose L, swirl

Stretch: quadriceps, hip flexors, inner thigh, hamstrings, pectorals, upper back

▶ Deep-Water Interval Lesson Plan 4

INTERVALS WITH REDUCED RECOVERY TIME 1

EQUIPMENT

Deep-water belts

TEACHING TIP

Interval training with reduced recovery time in the transition season is two minutes of work to one minute of recovery (2:1 ratio). The intensity level is 70 percent.

Level 7 (70 percent HR max)—Somewhat hard

WARM-UP

Instructor's choice

A SET

Flutter kick

Kick forward

Jumping jacks

Heel jog

Cross-country ski

Work: Mini jacks, faster (60 seconds)

Jumping jacks, faster (60 seconds)

Recovery: In, in, out, out (30 seconds)

Run tires (30 seconds)

B SET

Flutter kick, punch forward and side

Chorus-line kick

Jumping jacks with diagonal turn

Skate kick with pumping arms

Cross-country ski, two easy and one with power

C SET

Flutter kick, push across and slice back

High kick

Jumping jacks, pulse out

R leg kicks forward and back

L leg kicks forward and back

Cross-country ski, four easy and four with power

Work: Inner-thigh lift, faster (60 seconds)

Hopscotch, faster (60 seconds)

Recovery: In, in, out, out (30 seconds)

Run tires (30 seconds)

D SET

Star flutter kick

Kick forward with lat pull-down

Jumping jacks, pulse in

Skate kick with pumping arms

Cross-country ski, two easy and one with power

E SET

Flutter kick, punch across

Crossover kick

Jacks cross

R knee swings forward and back

L knee swings forward and back

Cross-country ski, four easy and four with power

Work: Mini ski, faster (60 seconds)

Skate kick, faster (60 seconds)

Recovery: In, in, out, out (30 seconds)

Run tires (30 seconds)

F SET

Flutter kick

Seated kick

Bent-knee jacks

Heel jog

Cross-country ski with knees bent 90 degrees

COOL-DOWN

Straddle jog, clap hands

Straddle jog, shoulder sweep out R and L, alternate

Straddle jog, shoulder sweep in R and L, alternate

Straddle jog, clap hands with power

Knee-high jog with crawl stroke

Knee-high jog with R bowstring pull

Knee-high jog with L bowstring pull

Knee-high jog with standing row with power

Cross-country ski

Cross-country ski with R arm swing, L hand on hip

Cross-country ski with L arm swing, R hand on hip

Cross-country ski with unison arm swing with power

Straddle jog, open and close doors

Straddle jog, open and close R and L, alternate

Straddle jog, open R, open L, close R, close L with power

Straddle jog with forearm press

Yoga tree pose R, swirl

Yoga tree pose L, swirl

Stretch: quadriceps, hip flexors, inner thigh, hamstrings, pectorals, upper back

▶ **Deep-Water Interval Lesson Plan 4**

INTERVALS WITH REDUCED RECOVERY TIME 1

PF

EQUIPMENT

Deep-water belts

TEACHING TIP

Interval training with reduced recovery time in the peak fitness season is 3 minutes of work to 90 seconds of recovery (2:1 ratio). The intensity level is 80 percent. Level 8 is high-intensity interval training (HIIT). For safety's sake, encourage your participants to modify the intensity to a level that is challenging for them rather than try to keep up with other participants.

Level 8 (80 percent HR max)—Hard

WARM-UP

Instructor's choice

A SET

Flutter kick

Kick forward

Jumping jacks

Heel jog

Cross-country ski

B SET

Flutter kick, punch forward and side

Chorus-line kick

Jumping jacks with diagonal turn

Skate kick with pumping arms

Cross-country ski, two easy and one with power

C SET

Flutter kick, push across and slice back

High kick

Jumping jacks, pulse out

R leg kicks forward and back

L leg kicks forward and back

Cross-country ski, four easy and four with power

D SET INTERVALS

Work: Inner-thigh lift with power (60 seconds)

Frog kick with elevation (60 seconds)

Breaststroke kick with elevation (60 seconds)

Recovery: In, in, out, out (30 seconds)

Run tires (30 seconds)

Knee-high jog (30 seconds)

Work: Hopscotch with power (60 seconds)

Frog kick with elevation (60 seconds)

Tuck ski together (60 seconds)

Recovery: In, in, out, out (30 seconds)

Run tires (30 seconds)

Knee-high jog (30 seconds)

E SET

Star flutter kick

Kick forward with lat pull-down

Jumping jacks, pulse in

Skate kick with pumping arms

Cross-country ski, two easy and one with power

F SET

Flutter kick, punch across

Crossover kick

Jacks cross

R knee swings forward and back

L knee swings forward and back

Cross-country ski, four easy and four with power

G SET

Flutter kick

Seated kick

Bent-knee jacks

Heel jog

Cross-country ski with knees bent 90 degrees

COOL-DOWN

Straddle jog, clap hands

Straddle jog, shoulder sweep out R and L, alternate

Straddle jog, shoulder sweep in R and L, alternate

Straddle jog, clap hands with power

Knee-high jog with crawl stroke

Knee-high jog with R bowstring pull

Knee-high jog with L bowstring pull

Knee-high jog with standing row with power

Cross-country ski

Cross-country ski with R arm swing, L hand on hip

Cross-country ski with L arm swing, R hand on hip

Cross-country ski with unison arm swing with power

Straddle jog, open and close doors

Straddle jog, open and close R and L, alternate

Straddle jog, open R, open L, close R, close L with power

Straddle jog with forearm press

Yoga tree pose R, swirl

Yoga tree pose L, swirl

Stretch: quadriceps, hip flexors, inner thigh, hamstrings, pectorals, upper back

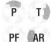

▶ Deep-Water Cardio Lesson Plan 5

DOUBLE LADDER

EQUIPMENT
Deep-water belts

TEACHING TIP
In a double ladder, two exercises, such as jumping jacks (see figure 7.12) and log jump, side to side (see figure 7.13) are paired. Perform each exercise for 10 seconds, then 20 seconds, and then 30 seconds, as if ascending a ladder. Next, descend the ladder, performing each exercise for 20 seconds and then 10 seconds. Each double ladder takes 3 minutes. This lesson plan concludes with some modified synchronized swimming just for fun.

WARM-UP
Instructor's choice

A SET
Kick forward
Crossover kick
Cossack kick
Heel jog
Bicycle
Cross-country ski
Double ladder: 10, 20, 30, 20, and 10 seconds
    Jumping jacks
    Log jump, side to side

B SET
Kick forward, doubles
Crossover kick, doubles, one low and one high
Jumping jacks
Hopscotch, doubles
Bicycle, doubles
Tuck ski together
Double ladder: 10, 20, 30, 20, and 10 seconds
    Flutter kick
    Cross-country ski

C SET
High kick
Skate kick, crossover kick, sweep out and center
Jacks cross
Hopscotch
Bicycle, tandem
Cross-country ski with rotation
Double ladder: 10, 20, 30, 20, and 10 seconds
    Bicycle
    Frog kick

D SET
Seated kick, R leg
Seated kick, L leg
Seated crossover kick and sweep out
Jacks tuck
Seated hamstring curl
Seated bicycle
Tuck ski
Knee-high jog, travel forward, hands on hips
Knee-high jog with resistor arms
Knee-high jog in multiple directions, hands on hips

COOL-DOWN: MODIFIED SYNCHRONIZED SWIMMING
(The class is in a big circle. Count off A, B, A, B, and so on. If you have an odd number of class participants, you will need to participate so that no one is left out.)
Bicycle travel clockwise around the circle
Flutter kick, A's do hand waves above the water
Bicycle travel counterclockwise around the circle
Flutter kick, B's do hand waves above the water
Seated kick, travel toward the center of the circle
Seated leg press with propeller scull, travel backward
Tuck and hold with seated row, travel toward the center of the circle

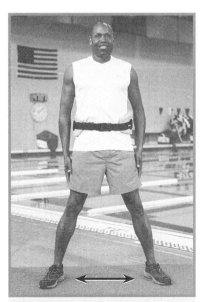

FIGURE 7.12 Jumping jacks.

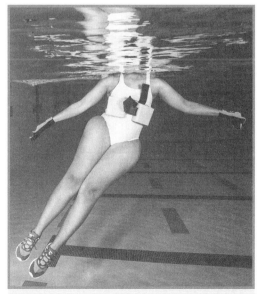

FIGURE 7.13 Log jump, side to side.

Seated flutter kick with propeller scull, travel backward

Bicycle with R hand in the center of the circle, travel clockwise around the circle

Mermaid, circle clockwise

Bicycle with L hand in the center of the circle, travel counterclockwise around the circle

Mermaid, circle counterclockwise

Stretch: hamstrings, outer thigh, quadriceps, hip flexors, gastrocnemius, ankles

▶ Deep-Water Interval Lesson Plan 5

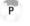

INTERVALS WITH REDUCED RECOVERY TIME 2

EQUIPMENT
Deep-water belts

TEACHING TIP
Deep-water cardio lesson plan 5 is modified to include interval training. The double ladder is dropped, and intervals using wall exercises are added. This is another lesson plan for intervals with reduced recovery time. In the preseason, this lesson plan involves 60 seconds of work to 30 seconds of recovery (2:1 ratio). Tapping the wall and pushing off the wall for 60 seconds effectively gets the heart rate into the target zone.

WARM-UP
Instructor's choice

A SET
Kick forward

Crossover kick

Cossack kick

Heel jog

Bicycle

Cross-country ski

Intervals (at the wall)

Work: R front kick (karate), heel taps wall, quarter turn, R side kick (karate), heel taps wall, with scull (60 seconds)

Recovery: Knee-high jog (30 seconds)

Work: L front kick (karate), heel taps wall, quarter turn, L side kick (karate), heel taps wall, with scull (60 seconds)

Recovery: Run tires (30 seconds)

B SET
Kick forward, doubles

Crossover kick, doubles, one low and one high

Jumping jacks

Hopscotch, doubles

Bicycle, doubles

Tuck ski together

Intervals (at the wall)

Work: Push off the wall with both feet (see figure 7.14) and run back (60 seconds)

Recovery: Knee-high jog (30 seconds)

Work: Push off the wall with one foot (see figure 7.15), tuck, and breaststroke back (60 seconds)

Recovery: Run tires (30 seconds)

C SET
High kick

Skate kick, crossover kick, sweep out and center

Jacks cross

Hopscotch

Bicycle, tandem

Cross-country ski with rotation

Intervals (at the wall)

Work: Push off the wall with both feet, side lying R, tuck, and run back with sidestroke (60 seconds)

Recovery: Knee-high jog (30 seconds)

Work: Push off the wall with both feet, side lying L, tuck, and run back with sidestroke (60 seconds)

Recovery: Run tires (30 seconds)

D SET
Seated kick R leg

Seated kick L leg

Seated crossover kick and sweep out

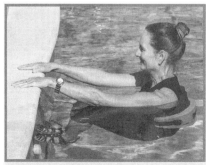

FIGURE 7.14 Push off the wall with both feet.

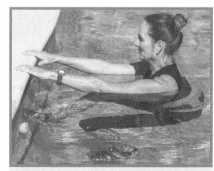

FIGURE 7.15 Push off the wall with one foot.

Jacks tuck

Seated hamstring curl

Seated bicycle

Tuck ski

Knee-high jog travel forward, hands on hips

Knee-high jog with resistor arms

Knee-high jog in multiple directions, hands on hips

COOL-DOWN: MODIFIED SYNCHRONIZED SWIMMING

(The class is in a big circle. Count off A, B, A, B, and so on. If you have an odd number of class participants, you will need to participate so that no one is left out.)

Bicycle travel clockwise around the circle

Flutter kick, A's do hand waves above the water

Bicycle travel counterclockwise around the circle

Flutter kick, B's do hand waves above the water

Seated kick, travel toward the center of the circle

Seated leg press with propeller scull, travel backward

Tuck and hold with seated row, travel toward the center of the circle

Seated flutter kick with propeller scull, travel backward

Bicycle with R hand in the center of the circle, travel clockwise around the circle

Mermaid, circle clockwise

Bicycle with L hand in the center of the circle, travel counterclockwise around the circle

Mermaid, circle counterclockwise

Stretch: hamstrings, outer thigh, quadriceps, hip flexors, gastrocnemius, ankles

▶ Deep-Water Interval Lesson Plan 5

INTERVALS WITH REDUCED RECOVERY TIME 2

EQUIPMENT

Deep-water belts

TEACHING TIP

The same wall exercises used in the preseason are used in the transition season in this lesson plan, but the duration of the interval doubles from one minute to two minutes. The recovery period is one minute long (2:1 ratio). Tapping the wall and pushing off the wall for two minutes effectively gets the heart rate into the target zone.

WARM-UP

Instructor's choice

A SET

Kick forward

Crossover kick

Cossack kick

Heel jog

Bicycle

Cross-country ski

B SET

Kick forward, doubles

Crossover kick, doubles, one low and one high

Jumping jacks

Hopscotch, doubles

Bicycle, doubles

Tuck ski together

C SET

High kick

Skate kick, crossover kick, sweep out and center

Jacks cross

Hopscotch

Bicycle, tandem

Cross-country ski with rotation

D SET INTERVALS

(At the wall)

Work: R front kick (karate), heel taps wall, quarter turn, R side kick (karate), heel taps wall, with scull (60 seconds)

L front kick (karate), heel taps wall, quarter turn, L side kick (karate), heel taps wall, with scull (60 seconds)

Recovery: Knee-high jog (30 seconds)

Run tires (30 seconds)

Work: Push off the wall with both feet and run back (60 seconds)

Push off the wall with one foot, tuck, and breaststroke back (60 seconds)

Recovery: Knee-high jog (30 seconds)

Run tires (30 seconds)

Work: Push off the wall with both feet, side lying R, tuck, and run back, with sidestroke (60 seconds)

Push off the wall with both feet, side lying L, tuck, and run back, with sidestroke (60 seconds)

Recovery: Knee-high jog (30 seconds)

Run tires (30 seconds)

E SET

Seated kick R leg

Seated kick L leg

Seated crossover kick and sweep out

Jacks tuck

Seated hamstring curl

Seated bicycle

Tuck ski

Knee-high, jog travel forward, hands on hips

Knee-high jog with resistor arms

Knee-high jog in multiple directions, hands on hips

COOL-DOWN: MODIFIED SYNCHRONIZED SWIMMING

(The class is in a big circle. Count off A, B, A, B, and so on. If you have an odd number of class participants, you will need to participate so that no one is left out.)

Bicycle travel clockwise around the circle

Flutter kick, A's do hand waves above the water

Bicycle travel counterclockwise around the circle

Flutter kick, B's do hand waves above the water

Seated kick, travel toward the center of the circle

Seated leg press with propeller scull, travel backward

Tuck and hold with seated row, travel toward the center of the circle

Seated flutter kick with propeller scull, travel backward

Bicycle with R hand in the center of the circle, travel clockwise around the circle

Mermaid, circle clockwise

Bicycle with L hand in the center of the circle, travel counterclockwise around the circle

Mermaid, circle counterclockwise

Stretch: hamstrings, outer thigh, quadriceps, hip flexors, gastrocnemius, ankles

▶ **Deep-Water Interval Lesson Plan 5**

INTERVALS WITH REDUCED RECOVERY TIME 2

EQUIPMENT

Deep-water belts

TEACHING TIP

The same wall exercises used in the preseason are used in the peak fitness season in this lesson plan, but the duration of the interval increases to 3 minutes. The recovery period is 90 seconds long (2:1 ratio). Tapping the wall and pushing off the wall for 3 minutes effectively gets the heart rate into the target zone.

WARM-UP

Instructor's choice

A SET

Kick forward

Crossover kick

Cossack kick

Heel jog

Bicycle

Cross-country ski

B SET

Kick forward, doubles

Crossover kick, doubles, one low and one high

Jumping jacks

Hopscotch, doubles

Bicycle, doubles

Tuck ski together

C SET

High kick

Skate kick, crossover kick, sweep out and center

Jacks cross

Hopscotch

Bicycle, tandem

Cross-country ski with rotation

D SET INTERVALS

(At the wall)

Work: R front kick (karate), heel taps wall, quarter turn, R side kick (karate), heel taps wall, with scull (60 seconds)

L front kick (karate), heel taps wall, quarter turn, L side kick (karate), heel taps wall, with scull (60 seconds)

Push off the wall with both feet and run back (60 seconds)

Recovery: Knee-high jog (30 seconds)

Run tires (30 seconds)

Heel jog (30 seconds)

Work: Push off the wall with one foot, tuck, and breaststroke back (60 seconds)

Push off the wall with both feet, side lying R, tuck, and run back with sidestroke (60 seconds)

Push off the wall with both feet, side lying L, tuck, and run back with sidestroke (60 seconds)

Recovery: Knee-high jog (30 seconds)

Run tires (30 seconds)

Heel jog (30 seconds)

E SET

Seated kick R leg

Seated kick L leg

Seated crossover kick and sweep out

Jacks tuck

Seated hamstring curl

Seated bicycle

Tuck ski

Knee-high jog, travel forward, hands on hips

Knee-high jog with resistor arms

Knee-high jog in multiple directions, hands on hips

COOL-DOWN: MODIFIED SYNCHRONIZED SWIMMING

(The class is in a big circle. Count off A, B, A, B, and so on. If you have an odd number of class participants, you will need to participate so that no one is left out.)

Bicycle, travel clockwise around the circle

Flutter kick, A's do hand waves above the water

Bicycle, travel counterclockwise around the circle

Flutter kick, B's do hand waves above the water

Seated kick, travel toward the center of the circle

Seated leg press with propeller scull, travel backward

Tuck and hold with seated row, travel toward the center of the circle

Seated flutter kick with propeller scull, travel backward

Bicycle with R hand in the center of the circle, travel clockwise around the circle

Mermaid, circle clockwise

Bicycle with L hand in the center of the circle, travel counterclockwise around the circle

Mermaid, circle counterclockwise

Stretch: hamstrings, outer thigh, quadriceps, hip flexors, gastrocnemius, ankles

▶ Deep-Water Cardio Lesson Plan 6

ZIGZAG PATTERN

EQUIPMENT

Deep-water belts

TEACHING TIP

When you travel in a zigzag pattern, you create a lot of turbulence, which adds to the intensity. This lesson plan travels in a zigzag pattern with knee-high jog (see figure 7.16), cross-country ski (see figure 7.17), bicycle (see figure 7.18), and jumping jacks (see figure 7.19). To travel in a zigzag with jumping jacks, travel sideways toward the left corner 4×, make a quarter turn, and travel sideways toward the right corner 4×.

WARM-UP

Instructor's choice

A SET

In, in, out, out

Jumping jacks

Jumping jacks with diagonal turn

Crossover kick

Seated kick and high kick, alternate, travel backward

Knee-high jog, travel forward

Tuck and hold with reverse breaststroke, travel backward

Knee-high jog, travel in a zigzag

Skateboard R with breaststroke pull, travel forward

Skateboard L with breaststroke pull, travel forward

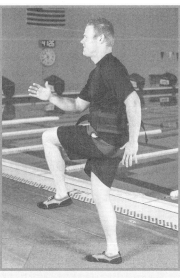

FIGURE 7.16 Knee-high jog.

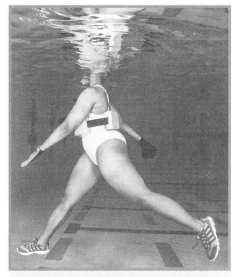

FIGURE 7.17 Cross-country ski.

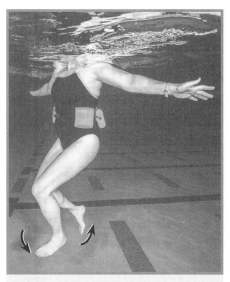

FIGURE 7.18 **Bicycle.**

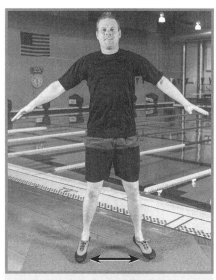

FIGURE 7.19 **Jumping jacks.**

Kick forward

Seated kick

Tuck and hold, R shoulder sweep out and in

Tuck and hold, L shoulder sweep out and in

Knee-high jog

Knee-high jog, diagonal, travel sideways R and L

B SET

In, in, out, out

Jumping jacks

Jumping jacks with diagonal turn

Crossover kick, doubles, one low and one high

Seated kick and high kick, alternate, travel backward

Run 3× and hurdle 1×, travel forward

Tuck and hold with reverse breaststroke, travel backward

Cross-country ski, travel in a zigzag

Skate kick

Cross-country ski

Tuck ski together

Tuck and hold, R leg sweeps out and in

Tuck and hold, L leg sweeps out and in

Knee-high jog

Cross-country ski, diagonal, travel sideways R and L

C SET

In, in, out, out

Jumping jacks

Jumping jacks with diagonal turn

Crossover kick and sweep out

Seated kick and high kick, alternate, travel backward

Bicycle, tandem, travel forward

Tuck and hold with reverse breaststroke, travel backward

Bicycle, travel in a zigzag

Bicycle R leg

Bicycle L leg

Bicycle

Tuck ski

Seated kick 3× and hold, one leg sweeps out and in 1×

Knee-high jog

Bicycle, diagonal, travel sideways R and L

D SET

In, in, out, out

Jumping jacks

Jumping jacks with diagonal turn

Skate kick, crossover kick, sweep out and center

Seated kick and high kick, alternate, travel backward

Jacks tuck with breaststroke, travel forward

Tuck and hold with reverse breaststroke, travel backward

Jumping jacks, travel in a zigzag

Frog kick

Jumping jacks

Jacks tuck

Seated kick 3×, crossover kick 1×

Knee-high jog

Bent-knee jacks, travel backward and forward

COOL-DOWN

Straddle jog with scull

Jumping jacks

Inner-thigh lift

Hopscotch

Jumping jacks

Jacks tuck

Jacks tuck with reverse breaststroke, travel backward

Tuck and hold with breaststroke, travel forward

Jacks tuck and pike

Log jump R, jacks tuck, log jump L, jacks tuck

Log jump, side to side

Mermaid

Stretch: upper back, lower back, hamstrings, outer thighs, quadriceps, hip flexors

▶ Deep-Water Interval Lesson Plan 6

ROLLING INTERVALS

EQUIPMENT

Deep-water belts

TEACHING TIP

Deep-water cardio lesson plan 6 is modified to include interval training. During rolling intervals an exercise is performed for one minute. It then rolls into a higher intensity level for one minute and finally rolls into an even higher intensity level for another minute. In the preseason, the intensity begins at level 5 and increases up to level 7.

Level 5 (50 percent HR max)—Somewhat easy

Level 6 (60 percent HR max)—Moderate

Level 7 (70 percent HR max)—Somewhat hard

WARM-UP

Instructor's choice

A SET

In, in, out, out

Jumping jacks

Jumping jacks with diagonal turn

Crossover kick

Seated kick and high kick, alternate, travel backward

Knee-high jog, travel forward

Tuck and hold with reverse breaststroke, travel backward

Knee-high jog, travel in a zigzag

Work: Knee-high jog 50 percent (1 minute)

Steep climb 60 percent (1 minute)

Steep climb, faster 70 percent (1 minute)

Recovery: Straddle jog (1 minute)

R side quad kick (30 seconds)

L side quad kick (30 seconds)

B SET

In, in, out, out

Jumping jacks

Jumping jacks with diagonal turn

Crossover kick, doubles, one low and one high

Seated kick and high kick, alternate, travel backward

Run 3× and hurdle 1×, travel forward

Tuck and hold with reverse breaststroke, travel backward

Cross-country ski, travel in a zigzag

Work: Cross-country ski with knees bent 90 degrees 50 percent (1 minute)

Tuck ski with full extension 60 percent (1 minute)

Cross-country ski, faster 70 percent (1 minute)

Recovery: Tuck ski (1 minute)

Bicycle R leg (30 seconds)

Bicycle L leg (30 seconds)

C SET

In, in, out, out

Jumping jacks

Jumping jacks with diagonal turn

Crossover kick and sweep out

Seated kick and high kick, alternate, travel backward

Bicycle, tandem, travel forward

Tuck and hold with reverse breaststroke, travel backward

Bicycle, travel in a zigzag

Work: Kick forward 50 percent (1 minute)

Knee lift, straighten and power press-down 60 percent (1 minute)

High kick 70 percent (1 minute)

Recovery: Knee-high jog (1 minute)

R quad kick (30 seconds)

L quad kick (30 seconds)

D SET

In, in, out, out

Jumping jacks

Jumping jacks with diagonal turn

Skate kick, crossover kick, sweep out and center

Seated kick and high kick, alternate, travel backward

Jacks tuck with breaststroke, travel forward

Tuck and hold with reverse breaststroke, travel backward

Jumping jacks, travel in a zigzag

Work: Jumping jacks 50 percent (1 minute)

Jacks cross 60 percent (1 minute)

Jumping jacks, faster 70 percent (1 minute)

Recovery: Jacks tuck (1 minute)

Log jump, side to side (1 minute)

COOL-DOWN

Straddle jog with scull

Jumping jacks

Inner-thigh lift

Hopscotch

Jumping jacks

Jacks tuck

Jacks tuck with reverse breaststroke, travel backward

Tuck and hold with breaststroke, travel forward

Jacks tuck and pike

Log jump R, jacks tuck, log jump L, jacks tuck

Log jump, side to side

Mermaid

Stretch: upper back, lower back, hamstrings, outer thighs, quadriceps, hip flexors

▶ Deep-Water Interval Lesson Plan 6

ROLLING INTERVALS

EQUIPMENT

Deep-water belts

TEACHING TIP

During rolling intervals an exercise is performed for one minute. It then rolls into a higher intensity level for one minute and finally rolls into an even higher intensity level for another minute. In the transition season, the intensity begins at level 6 and increases up to level 8. Level 8 is high-intensity interval training (HIIT). For safety's sake, encourage your participants to modify the intensity to a level that is challenging for them rather than try to keep up with other participants.

Level 6 (60 percent HR max)—Moderate

Level 7 (70 percent HR max)—Somewhat hard

Level 8 (80 percent HR max)—Hard

WARM-UP

Instructor's choice

A SET

In, in, out, out

Jumping jacks

Jumping jacks with diagonal turn

Crossover kick

Seated kick and high kick, alternate, travel backward

Knee-high jog, travel forward

Tuck and hold with reverse breaststroke, travel backward

Knee-high jog, travel in a zigzag

Work: Steep climb 60 percent (1 minute)

Knee-high jog, faster 70 percent (1 minute)

Steep climb with power 80 percent (1 minute)

Recovery: Straddle jog (1 minute)

R side quad kick (30 seconds)

L side quad kick (30 seconds)

B SET

In, in, out, out

Jumping jacks

Jumping jacks with diagonal turn

Crossover kick, doubles, one low and one high

Seated kick and high kick, alternate, travel backward

Run 3× and hurdle 1×, travel forward

Tuck and hold with reverse breaststroke, travel backward

Cross-country ski, travel in a zigzag

Work: Tuck ski with full extension 60 percent (1 minute)

Cross-country ski, faster 70 percent (1 minute)

Cross-country ski with elevation 80 percent (1 minute)

Recovery: Tuck ski (1 minute)

Bicycle R leg (30 seconds)

Bicycle L leg (30 seconds)

C SET

In, in, out, out

Jumping jacks

Jumping jacks with diagonal turn

Crossover kick and sweep out

Seated kick and high kick, alternate, travel backward

Bicycle, tandem, travel forward

Tuck and hold with reverse breaststroke, travel backward

Bicycle, travel in a zigzag

Work: Knee lift, straighten and power press-down 60 percent (1 minute)

High kick 70 percent (1 minute)

High kick, power down 80 percent (1 minute)

Recovery: Knee-high jog (1 minute)

> R quad kick (30 seconds)
>
> L quad kick (30 seconds)

D SET

In, in, out, out

Jumping jacks

Jumping jacks with diagonal turn

Skate kick, crossover kick, sweep out and center

Seated kick and high kick, alternate, travel backward

Jacks tuck with breaststroke, travel forward

Tuck and hold with reverse breaststroke, travel backward

Jumping jacks, travel in a zigzag

Work: Jacks cross 60 percent (1 minute)

> Jumping jacks, faster 70 percent (1 minute)
>
> Frog kick with elevation 80 percent (1 minute)

Recovery: Jacks tuck (1 minute)

> Log jump, side to side (1 minute)

COOL-DOWN

Straddle jog with scull

Jumping jacks

Inner-thigh lift

Hopscotch

Jumping jacks

Jacks tuck

Jacks tuck with reverse breaststroke, travel backward

Tuck and hold with breaststroke, travel forward

Jacks tuck and pike

Log jump R, jacks tuck, log jump L, jacks tuck

Log jump, side to side

Mermaid

Stretch: upper back, lower back, hamstrings, outer thighs, quadriceps, hip flexors

▶ Deep-Water Interval Lesson Plan 6

ROLLING INTERVALS

PF

EQUIPMENT

Deep-water belts

TEACHING TIP

During rolling intervals an exercise is performed for one minute. It then rolls into a higher intensity level

for one minute and finally rolls into an even higher intensity level for another minute. In the peak fitness season, the intensity begins at level 7 and increases up to level 9. Levels 8 and 9 are high-intensity interval training (HIIT). For safety's sake, encourage your participants to modify the intensity to a level that is challenging for them rather than try to keep up with other participants.

> Level 7 (70 percent HR max)—Somewhat hard
>
> Level 8 (80 percent HR max)—Hard
>
> Level 9 (90 percent HR max)—Very hard

WARM-UP

Instructor's choice

A SET

In, in, out, out

Jumping jacks

Jumping jacks with diagonal turn

Crossover kick

Seated kick and high kick, alternate, travel backward

Knee-high jog, travel forward

Tuck and hold with reverse breaststroke, travel backward

Knee-high jog, travel in a zigzag

B SET

In, in, out, out

Jumping jacks

Jumping jacks with diagonal turn

Crossover kick, doubles, one low and one high

Seated kick and high kick, alternate, travel backward

Run 3× and hurdle 1×, travel forward

Tuck and hold with reverse breaststroke, travel backward

Cross-country ski, travel in a zigzag

C SET INTERVALS

Work: Knee-high jog, faster 70 percent (1 minute)

> Steep climb with power 80 percent (1 minute)
>
> Steep climb with power, faster 90 percent (1 minute)

Recovery: Straddle jog (1 minute)

> R side quad kick (30 seconds)
>
> L side quad kick (30 seconds)

Work: Cross-country ski, faster 70 percent (1 minute)

> Cross-country ski with elevation 80 percent (1 minute)

Cross-country ski, arms sweep side to side 90 percent (1 minute)

Recovery: Tuck ski (1 minute)

Bicycle R leg (30 seconds)

Bicycle L leg (30 seconds)

Work: High kick 70 percent (1 minute)

High kick, power down 80 percent (1 minute)

High kick with lat pull-down 90 percent (1 minute)

Recovery: Knee-high jog (1 minute)

R quad kick (30 seconds)

L quad kick (30 seconds)

Work: Jumping jacks, faster 70 percent (1 minute)

Frog kick with elevation 80 percent (1 minute)

Frog kick with elevation and power 90 percent (1 minute)

Recovery: Jacks tuck (1 minute)

Log jump, side to side (1 minute)

D SET

In, in, out, out

Jumping jacks

Jumping jacks with diagonal turn

Crossover kick and sweep out

Seated kick and high kick, alternate, travel backward

Bicycle, tandem, travel forward

Tuck and hold with reverse breaststroke, travel forward

Bicycle, travel in a zigzag

E SET

In, in, out, out

Jumping jacks

Jumping jacks with diagonal turn

Skate kick, crossover kick, sweep out and center

Seated kick and high kick, alternate, travel backward

Jacks tuck with breaststroke, travel forward

Tuck and hold with reverse breaststroke, travel backward

Jumping jacks, travel in a zigzag

COOL-DOWN

Straddle jog with scull

Jumping jacks

Inner-thigh lift

Hopscotch

Jumping jacks

Jacks tuck

Jacks tuck with reverse breaststroke, travel backward

Tuck and hold with breaststroke, travel forward

Jacks tuck and pike

Log jump R, jacks tuck, log jump L, jacks tuck

Log jump, side to side

Mermaid

Stretch: upper back, lower back, hamstrings, outer thighs, quadriceps, hip flexors

▶ Deep-Water Cardio Lesson Plan 7

CARDIO WITH WALL EXERCISES

P T PF AR

EQUIPMENT

Deep-water belts

TEACHING TIP

Take advantage of the pool wall for some of your exercises. Here are two options:

1. Cross-country ski with both feet on the wall—pretend that a clock face is on the wall; tap twelve o'clock with one foot and six o'clock with the other, alternating feet (see figure 7.20).

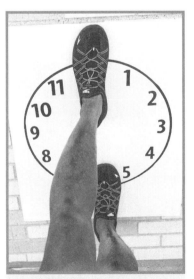

FIGURE 7.20 Twelve o'clock and six o'clock.

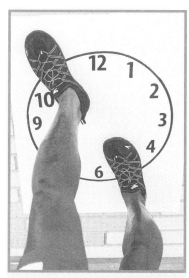

FIGURE 7.21 **Eleven o'clock and five o'clock.**

2. Cross-country ski with both feet on the wall at eleven o'clock and five o'clock—tilt your body slightly to the left on your imaginary clock face so that you tap eleven o'clock with one foot and five o'clock with the other, alternating feet (see figure 7.21).

WARM-UP

Instructor's choice

A SET

Straddle jog, clap hands

Jumping jacks, clap hands

Inner-thigh lift

Jacks cross

Run to one side of the pool and back to the wall

Breaststroke with feet on the wall

Cross-country ski, travel backward

Knee-high jog, travel forward

Kick forward with propeller scull, travel backward

Knee-high jog, travel forward

Crossover kick

B SET

Straddle jog, palms touch in back

Jumping jacks, palms touch in back

Hopscotch

Jacks cross

Run to one side of the pool and back to the wall

Cross-country ski with both feet on the wall at twelve o'clock and six o'clock

Cross-country ski with reverse breaststroke, travel backward

Knee-high jog, travel forward

Kick forward with reverse breaststroke, travel backward

Knee-high jog, travel forward

Chorus-line kick

C SET

Straddle jog, open and close doors

Jumping jacks, open and close doors

Inner-thigh lift R and hopscotch L, alternate

Jacks cross

Run to one side of the pool and back to the wall

Reverse breaststroke in a kneeling position with back to the wall

Cross-country ski with unison arm swing, travel backward

Knee-high jog, travel forward

Kick forward with unison arm swing, travel backward

Knee-high jog, travel forward

Crossover kick, doubles, one low and one high

D SET

Straddle jog with forearm press

Jumping jacks with forearm press

Inner-thigh lift L and hopscotch R, alternate

Jacks cross

Run to one side of the pool and back to the wall

Cross-country ski with both feet on the wall at eleven o'clock and five o'clock

Cross-country ski with both feet on the wall at one o'clock and seven o'clock

Cross-country ski, push forward, travel backward

Knee-high jog, travel forward

Kick forward, push forward, travel backward

Knee-high jog, travel forward

Crossover kick and sweep out

COOL-DOWN

Tuck ski

Tuck ski 3×, bent-knee jacks 1×

Bent-knee jacks 1×, seated kick 1×

Breaststroke kick 2×, abdominal pike 1×

Frog kick 2×, side extension 1×, alternate R and L

Side extension, tuck and down, alternate R and L

Side extension, tuck and down 2×, alternate R and L

Tuck and star flutter kick

Star flutter kick

Flutter kick, point and flex feet

Stretch: lower back, hamstrings, inner thigh, hip flexors, gastrocnemius, shoulders

▶ Deep-Water Interval Lesson Plan 7

SURGES 1

EQUIPMENT

Deep-water belts

TEACHING TIP

Deep-water cardio lesson plan 7 is modified to include interval training. In a surge in the preseason, an interval is performed at level 6 for 45 seconds and then bumped up to level 7 for 15 seconds.

Level 6 (60 percent HR max)—Moderate

Level 7 (70 percent HR max)—Somewhat hard

WARM-UP

Instructor's choice

A SET

Straddle jog, clap hands

Jumping jacks, clap hands

Inner-thigh lift

Jacks cross

Run to one side of the pool and back to the wall

Breaststroke with feet on the wall

Work: Cross-country ski full, ROM 60 percent (45 seconds)

Cross-country ski, faster 70 percent (15 seconds)

Recovery: Knee-high jog (1 minute)

Work: Knee lift, straighten and power press-down 60 percent (45 seconds)

High kick 70 percent (15 seconds)

Recovery: Knee-high jog (1 minute)

Crossover kick

B SET

Straddle jog, palms touch in back

Jumping jacks, palms touch in back

Hopscotch

Jacks cross

Run to one side of the pool and back to the wall

Cross-country ski with both feet on the wall at twelve o'clock and six o'clock

Work: Run 60 percent (45 seconds)

Sprint 70 percent (15 seconds)

Recovery: Knee-high jog (1 minute)

Work: Bicycle, full ROM 60 percent (45 seconds)

Bicycle, faster 70 percent (15 seconds)

Recovery: Knee-high jog (1 minute)

Chorus-line kick

C SET

Straddle jog, open and close doors

Jumping jacks, open and close doors

Inner-thigh lift R and hopscotch L, alternate

Jacks cross

Run to one side of the pool and back to the wall

Reverse breaststroke in a kneeling position with back to the wall

Work: Cross-country ski, full ROM 60 percent (45 seconds)

Cross-country ski, faster 70 percent (15 seconds)

Recovery: Knee-high jog (1 minute)

Work: Knee lift, straighten and power press-down 60 percent (45 seconds)

High kick 70 percent (15 seconds)

Recovery: Knee-high jog (1 minute)

Crossover kick, doubles, one low and one high

D SET

Straddle jog with forearm press

Jumping jacks with forearm press

Inner-thigh lift L and hopscotch R, alternate

Jacks cross

Run to one side of the pool and back to the wall

Cross-country ski with both feet on the wall at eleven o'clock and five o'clock

Cross-country ski with both feet on the wall at one o'clock and seven o'clock

Work: Run 60 percent (45 seconds)

Sprint 70 percent (15 seconds)

Recovery: Knee-high jog (1 minute)

Work: Bicycle, full ROM 60 percent (45 seconds)

Bicycle, faster 70 percent (15 seconds)

Recovery: Knee-high jog (1 minute)

Crossover kick and sweep out

COOL-DOWN

Tuck ski

Tuck ski 3×, bent-knee jacks 1×

Bent-knee jacks 1×, seated kick 1×

Breaststroke kick 2×, abdominal pike 1×

Frog kick 2×, side extension 1×, alternate R and L

Side extension, tuck and down, alternate R and L

Side extension, tuck and down 2×, alternate R and L

Tuck and star flutter kick

Star flutter kick

Flutter kick, point and flex feet

Stretch: lower back, hamstrings, inner thigh, hip flexors, gastrocnemius, shoulders

▶ Deep-Water Interval Lesson Plan 7

SURGES 1

EQUIPMENT

Deep-water belts

TEACHING TIP

In a surge in the transition season, an interval is performed at level 7 for 45 seconds and then bumped up to level 8 for 15 seconds. Level 8 is high-intensity interval training (HIIT). For safety's sake, encourage your participants to modify the intensity to a level that is challenging for them rather than try to keep up with other participants.

Level 7 (70 percent HR max)—Somewhat hard

Level 8 (80 percent HR max)—Hard

WARM-UP

Instructor's choice

A SET

Straddle jog, clap hands

Jumping jacks, clap hands

Inner-thigh lift

Jacks cross

Run to one side of the pool and back to the wall

Breaststroke with feet on the wall

Work: Cross-country ski, faster 70 percent (45 seconds)

Cross-country ski with rotation 80 percent (15 seconds)

Recovery: Knee-high jog (1 minute)

Work: High kick 70 percent (45 seconds)

High kick with power 80 percent (15 seconds)

Recovery: Knee-high jog (1 minute)

Crossover kick

B SET

Straddle jog, palms touch in back

Jumping jacks, palms touch in back

Hopscotch

Jacks cross

Run to one side of the pool and back to the wall

Cross-country ski with both feet on the wall at twelve o'clock and six o'clock

Work: Sprint 70 percent (45 seconds)

Power run 80 percent (15 seconds)

Recovery: Knee-high jog (1 minute)

Work: Bicycle, faster 70 percent (45 seconds)

Bicycle with power 80 percent (15 seconds)

Recovery: Knee-high jog (1 minute)

Chorus-line kick

C SET

Straddle jog, open and close doors

Jumping jacks, open and close doors

Inner-thigh lift R and hopscotch L, alternate

Jacks cross

Run to one side of the pool and back to the wall

Reverse breaststroke in a kneeling position with back to the wall

Work: Cross-country ski, faster 70 percent (45 seconds)

Cross-country ski with rotation 80 percent (15 seconds)

Recovery: Knee-high jog (1 minute)

Work: High kick 70 percent (45 seconds)

High kick with power 80 percent (15 seconds)

Recovery: Knee-high jog (1 minute)

Crossover kick, doubles, one low and one high

D SET

Straddle jog with forearm press

Jumping jacks with forearm press

Inner-thigh lift L and hopscotch R, alternate

Jacks cross

Run to one side of the pool and back to the wall

Cross-country ski with both feet on the wall at eleven o'clock and five o'clock

Cross-country ski with both feet on the wall at one o'clock and seven o'clock

Work: Sprint 70 percent (45 seconds)
  Power run 80 percent (15 seconds)
Recovery: Knee-high jog (1 minute)
Work: Bicycle, faster 70 percent (45 seconds)
  Bicycle with power 80 percent (15 seconds)
Recovery: Knee-high jog (1 minute)
Crossover kick and sweep out

COOL-DOWN
Tuck ski
Tuck ski 3×, bent-knee jacks 1×
Bent-knee jacks 1×, seated kick 1×
Breaststroke kick 2×, abdominal pike 1×
Frog kick 2×, side extension 1×, alternate R and L
Side extension, tuck and down, alternate R and L
Side extension, tuck and down 2×, alternate R and L
Tuck and star flutter kick
Star flutter kick
Flutter kick, point and flex feet
Stretch: lower back, hamstrings, inner thigh, hip flexors, gastrocnemius, shoulders

▶ Deep-Water Interval Lesson Plan 7

SURGES 1

EQUIPMENT
Deep-water belts

TEACHING TIP
In a surge in the peak fitness season, an interval is performed at level 8 for 45 seconds and then bumped up to level 9 for 15 seconds. Levels 8 and 9 are high-intensity interval training (HIIT). For safety's sake, encourage your participants to modify the intensity to a level that is challenging for them rather than try to keep up with other participants.
  Level 8 (80 percent HR max)—Hard
  Level 9 (90 percent HR max)—Very hard

WARM-UP
Instructor's choice

A SET
Straddle jog, clap hands
Jumping jacks, clap hands
Inner-thigh lift
Jacks cross
Run to one side of the pool and back to the wall

Breaststroke with feet on the wall
Crossover kick

B SET
Straddle jog, palms touch in back
Jumping jacks, palms touch in back
Hopscotch
Jacks cross
Run to one side of the pool and back to the wall
Cross-country ski with both feet on the wall at twelve o'clock and six o'clock
Chorus-line kick

C SET INTERVALS
Work: Cross-country ski with rotation 80 percent (45 seconds)
  Cross-country ski, arms sweep side to side 90 percent (15 seconds)
Recovery: Knee-high jog (1 minute)
Work: High kick with power 80 percent (45 seconds)
  High kick, clap over and under 90 percent (15 seconds)
Recovery: Knee-high jog (1 minute)
Work: Power run 80 percent (45 seconds)
  Skate kick with power, travel forward 90 percent (15 seconds)
Recovery: Knee-high jog (1 minute)
Work: Bicycle with power 80 percent (45 seconds)
  Bicycle with elevation and power 90 percent (15 seconds)
Recovery: Knee-high jog (1 minute)
Work: Cross-country ski with rotation 80 percent (45 seconds)
  Cross-country ski, arms sweep side to side 90 percent (15 seconds)
Recovery: Knee-high jog (1 minute)
Work: High kick with power 80 percent (45 seconds)
  High kick, clap over and under 90 percent (15 seconds)
Recovery: Knee-high jog (1 minute)
Work: Power run 80 percent (45 seconds)
  Skate kick with power, travel forward 90 percent (15 seconds)
Recovery: Knee-high jog (1 minute)
Work: Bicycle with power 80 percent (45 seconds)

Bicycle with elevation and power 90 percent (15 seconds)

Recovery: Knee-high jog (1 minute)

D SET

Straddle jog, open and close doors

Jumping jacks, open and close doors

Inner-thigh lift R and hopscotch L, alternate

Jacks cross

Run to one side of the pool and back to the wall

Reverse breaststroke in a kneeling position with back to the wall

Crossover kick, doubles, one low and one high

E SET

Straddle jog with forearm press

Jumping jacks with forearm press

Inner-thigh lift L and hopscotch R, alternate

Jacks cross

Run to one side of the pool and back to the wall

Cross-country ski with both feet on the wall at eleven o'clock and five o'clock

Cross-country ski with both feet on the wall at one o'clock and seven o'clock

Crossover kick and sweep out

COOL-DOWN

Tuck ski

Tuck ski 3×, bent-knee jacks 1×

Bent-knee jacks 1×, seated kick 1×,

Breaststroke kick 2×, abdominal pike 1×

Frog kick 2×, side extension 1×, alternate R and L

Side extension, tuck and down, alternate R and L

Side extension, tuck and down 2×, alternate R and L

Tuck and star flutter kick

Star flutter kick

Flutter kick, point and flex feet

Stretch: lower back, hamstrings, inner thigh, hip flexors, gastrocnemius, shoulders

▶ Deep-Water Cardio Lesson Plan 8

CHANGES

EQUIPMENT

Deep-water belts

TEACHING TIP

Changes in the flow of exercises challenge core strength. Try performing an exercise 3× and then pausing. Add tucks, diagonal turns, and rotation. Put one hand on the hip or bring the hands out of the water. Perform one exercise 3× and then another exercise 1×. Figure 7.22 shows cross-country ski, tuck, diagonal turn, and center from B set.

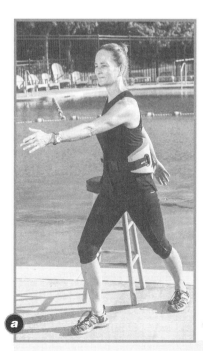 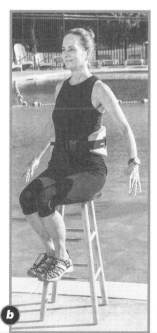 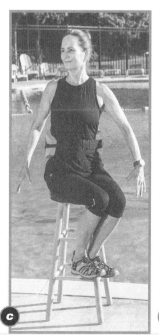 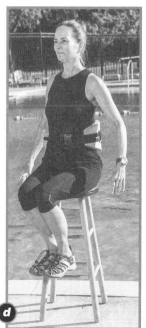

FIGURE 7.22 (*a*) cross-country ski, (*b*) tuck, (*c*) diagonal turn, (*d*) center.

WARM-UP

Instructor's choice

A SET

Knee-high jog with jog press

Run tires, reach side to side

Jumping jacks

Jacks tuck

Tuck and hold sidesaddle R with reverse breast-stroke, travel backward

Tuck and hold sidesaddle L with breaststroke, travel forward

Cross-country ski with R arm swing, L hand on hip

Knee-high jog with jog press

Run tires, reach side to side

Jumping jacks

Jacks tuck

Tuck and hold sidesaddle L with reverse breast-stroke, travel backward

Tuck and hold sidesaddle R with breaststroke, travel forward

Cross-country ski with L arm swing, R hand on hip

Cross-country ski 3× and hold

Cross-country ski 3× and tuck

Tuck ski

Jacks tuck

Knee-high jog

B SET

Knee-high jog, punch forward and side

Run tires with hand waves

Jumping jacks with diagonal turn

Jacks tuck 1×, seated kick 1×

Cross-country ski and hold R with reverse breaststroke, travel backward

Cross-country ski and hold L with breaststroke, travel forward

Helicopter ski

Knee-high jog, punch forward and side

Run tires with hand waves

Jumping jacks with diagonal turn

Jacks tuck 1×, seated kick 1×

Cross-country ski and hold L with reverse breast-stroke, travel backward

Cross-country ski and hold R with breaststroke, travel forward

Helicopter ski

Cross-country ski with rotation

Tuck ski with rotation

Cross-country ski, tuck, diagonal turn, and center

Jacks tuck

Knee-high jog

C SET

Knee-high jog with R bowstring pull

Run tires, clap hands

Jumping jacks with unison arm swing

Inner-thigh lift

Jacks tuck with reverse breaststroke, travel backward

Jacks tuck with breaststroke, travel forward

Knee-high jog with L bowstring pull

Run tires, clap hands

Jumping jacks with unison arm swing

Inner-thigh lift

Jacks tuck with reverse breaststroke, travel backward

Jacks tuck with breaststroke, travel forward

Cross-country ski, slow

Cross-country ski, slower

Cross-country ski, slowest, with power

Cross-country ski 3×, jumping jacks 1×

Tuck ski 3×, jacks tuck 1×

Jacks tuck

Knee-high jog

COOL-DOWN

Skateboard R with breaststroke pull, travel forward

Skateboard L with breaststroke pull, travel forward

Tuck, mermaid, tuck, down and tuck, unison kick to the corners, tuck, down

Bent-knee jacks

R side extension, tuck and down

L side extension, tuck and down

Abdominal pike and spine extension

Stretch: hamstrings, hip flexors, quadriceps, gas-trocnemius, outer thigh, shoulders

▶ **Deep-Water Lesson Plan 8**

SURGES 2

EQUIPMENT
Deep-water belts

TEACHING TIP
Deep-water cardio lesson plan 8 is modified to include interval training. This is another lesson plan for intervals with surges. In a surge in the preseason, an interval is performed at level 6 for 45 seconds and then bumped up to level 7 for 15 seconds.

Level 6 (60 percent HR max)—Moderate

Level 7 (70 percent HR max)—Somewhat hard

WARM-UP
Instructor's choice

A SET
Knee-high jog with jog press

Run tires, reach side to side

Jumping jacks

Jacks tuck

Tuck and hold sidesaddle R with reverse breast-stroke, travel backward

Tuck and hold sidesaddle L with breaststroke, travel forward

Cross-country ski with R arm swing, L hand on hip

Cross-country ski with L arm swing, R hand on hip

Cross-country ski 3× and hold

Cross-country ski 3× and tuck

Tuck ski

Jacks tuck

Knee-high jog

B SET INTERVALS
Work: Steep climb 60 percent (45 seconds)
  Steep climb, faster 70 percent (15 seconds)

Recovery: Straddle jog with shoulder blade squeeze (45 seconds)
  Jacks tuck (15 seconds)

Work: Cross-country ski, full ROM 60 percent (45 seconds)
  Cross-country ski, faster 70 percent (15 seconds)

Recovery: Straddle jog, clap hands (45 seconds)
  Jacks tuck (15 seconds)

Work: Jacks cross 60 percent (45 seconds)
  Mini cross, faster 70 percent (15 seconds)

Recovery: Jumping jacks (45 seconds)
  Jacks tuck (15 seconds)

Work: Steep climb 60 percent (45 seconds)
  Steep climb, faster 70 percent (15 seconds)

Recovery: Straddle jog with arm curl (45 seconds)
  Jacks tuck (15 seconds)

Work: Cross-country ski, full ROM 60 percent (45 seconds)
  Cross-country ski, faster 70 percent (15 seconds)

Recovery: Straddle jog with triceps extension (45 seconds)
  Jacks tuck (15 seconds)

Work: Jacks cross 60 percent (45 seconds)
  Mini cross, faster 70 percent (15 seconds)

Recovery: Straddle jog with forearm press (45 seconds)
  Jacks tuck (15 seconds)

C SET
Knee-high jog, punch forward and side

Run tires with hand waves

Jumping jacks with diagonal turn

Jacks tuck 1×, seated kick 1×

Cross-country ski and hold R with reverse breaststroke, travel backward

Cross-country ski and hold L with breaststroke, travel forward

Helicopter ski

Cross-country ski with rotation

Tuck ski with rotation

Cross-country ski, tuck, diagonal turn, and center

Jacks tuck

Knee-high jog

D SET
Knee-high jog with R bowstring pull

Knee-high jog with L bowstring pull

Run tires, clap hands

Jumping jacks with unison arm swing

Inner-thigh lift

Jacks tuck with reverse breaststroke, travel backward

Jacks tuck with breaststroke, travel forward

Cross-country ski, slow

Cross-country ski, slower

Cross-country ski, slowest, with power

Cross-country ski 3×, jumping jacks 1×

Tuck ski 3×, jacks tuck 1×

Jacks tuck

Knee-high jog

COOL-DOWN

Skateboard R with breaststroke pull, travel forward

Skateboard L with breaststroke pull, travel forward

Tuck, mermaid, tuck, down and tuck, unison kick to the corners, tuck, down

Bent-knee jacks

R side extension, tuck and down

L side extension, tuck and down

Abdominal pike and spine extension

Stretch: hamstrings, hip flexors, quadriceps, gastrocnemius, outer thigh, shoulders

▶ Deep-Water Interval Lesson Plan 8

SURGES 2

EQUIPMENT

Deep-water belts

TEACHING TIP

In a surge in the transition season, an interval is performed at level 7 for 45 seconds and then bumped up to level 8 for 15 seconds. Level 8 is high-intensity interval training (HIIT). For safety's sake, encourage your participants to modify the intensity to a level that is challenging for them rather than try to keep up with other participants.

Level 7 (70 percent HR max)—Somewhat hard

Level 8 (80 percent HR max)—Hard

WARM-UP

Instructor's choice

A SET

Knee-high jog with jog press

Run tires, reach side to side

Jumping jacks

Jacks tuck

Tuck and hold sidesaddle R with reverse breaststroke, travel backward

Tuck and hold sidesaddle L with breaststroke, travel forward

Cross-country ski with R arm swing, L hand on hip

Cross-country ski with L arm swing, R hand on hip

Cross-country ski 3× and hold

Cross-country ski 3× and tuck

Tuck ski

Jacks tuck

Knee-high jog

B SET INTERVALS

Work: Steep climb, faster 70 percent (45 seconds)

Steep climb with power 80 percent (15 seconds)

Recovery: Straddle jog with shoulder blade squeeze (45 seconds)

Jacks tuck (15 seconds)

Work: Cross-country ski, faster 70 percent (45 seconds)

Cross-country ski with rotation 80 percent (15 seconds)

Recovery: Straddle jog, clap hands (45 seconds)

Jacks tuck (15 seconds)

Work: Mini jacks, faster 70 percent (45 seconds)

Frog kick with elevation 80 percent (15 seconds)

Recovery: Jumping jacks (45 seconds)

Jacks tuck (15 seconds)

Work: Steep climb, faster 70 percent (45 seconds)

Steep climb with power 80 percent (15 seconds)

Recovery: Straddle jog with arm curl (45 seconds)

Jacks tuck (15 seconds)

Work: Cross-country ski, faster 70 percent (45 seconds)

Cross-country ski with rotation 80 percent (15 seconds)

Recovery: Straddle jog with triceps extension (45 seconds)

Jacks tuck (15 seconds)

Work: Mini jacks, faster 70 percent (45 seconds)

Frog kick with elevation 80 percent (15 seconds)

Recovery: Straddle jog with forearm press (45 seconds)

Jacks tuck (15 seconds)

C SET

Knee-high jog, punch forward and side

Run tires with hand waves

Jumping jacks with diagonal turn

Jacks tuck 1×, seated kick 1×

Cross-country ski and hold R with reverse breaststroke, travel backward

Cross-country ski and hold L with breaststroke, travel forward

Helicopter ski

Cross-country ski with rotation

Tuck ski with rotation

Cross-country ski, tuck, diagonal turn, and center

Jacks tuck

Knee-high jog

D SET

Knee-high jog with R bowstring pull

Knee-high jog with L bowstring pull

Run tires, clap hands

Jumping jacks with unison arm swing

Inner-thigh lift

Jacks tuck with reverse breaststroke, travel backward

Jacks tuck with breaststroke, travel forward

Cross-country ski, slow

Cross-country ski, slower

Cross-country ski, slowest, with power

Cross-country ski 3×, jumping jacks 1×

Tuck ski 3×, jacks tuck 1×

Jacks tuck

Knee-high jog

COOL-DOWN

Skateboard R with breaststroke pull, travel forward

Skateboard L with breaststroke pull, travel forward

Tuck, mermaid, tuck, down and tuck, unison kick to the corners, tuck, down

Bent-knee jacks

R side extension, tuck and down

L side extension, tuck and down

Abdominal pike and spine extension

Stretch: hamstrings, hip flexors, quadriceps, gastrocnemius, outer thigh, shoulders

▶ Deep-Water Interval Lesson Plan 8

SURGES 2

EQUIPMENT

Deep-water belts

TEACHING TIP

In a surge in the peak fitness season, an interval is performed at level 8 for 45 seconds and then bumped up to level 9 for 15 seconds. Levels 8 and 9 are high-intensity interval training (HIIT). For safety's sake, encourage your participants to modify the intensity to a level that is challenging for them rather than try to keep up with other participants.

Level 8 (80 percent HR max)—Hard

Level 9 (90 percent HR max)—Very hard

WARM-UP

Instructor's choice

A SET

Knee-high jog with jog press

Run tires, reach side to side

Jumping jacks

Jacks tuck

Tuck and hold sidesaddle R with reverse breaststroke, travel backward

Tuck and hold sidesaddle L with breaststroke, travel forward

Cross-country ski with R arm swing, L hand on hip

Cross-country ski with L arm swing, R hand on hip

Cross-country ski 3× and hold

Cross-country ski 3× and tuck

Tuck ski

Jacks tuck

Knee-high jog

B SET INTERVALS

Work: Steep climb with power 80 percent (45 seconds)

Steep climb with power, faster 90 percent (15 seconds)

Recovery: Straddle jog with shoulder blade squeeze (45 seconds)

Jacks tuck (15 seconds)

Work: Cross-country ski with rotation 80 percent (45 seconds)

Cross-country ski with rotation and power 90 percent (15 seconds)

Recovery: Straddle jog, clap hands (45 seconds)

Jacks tuck (15 seconds)

Work: Frog kick with elevation 80 percent (45 seconds)

Frog kick with elevation and power 90 percent (15 seconds)

Recovery: Jumping jacks (45 seconds)

Jacks tuck (15 seconds)

Work: Steep climb with power 80 percent (45 seconds)

Steep climb with power, faster 90 percent (15 seconds)

Recovery: Straddle jog with arm curl (45 seconds)

Jacks tuck (15 seconds)

Work: Cross-country ski with rotation 80 percent (45 seconds)

Cross-country ski with rotation and power 90 percent (15 seconds)

Recovery: Straddle jog with triceps extension (45 seconds)

Jacks tuck (15 seconds)

Work: Frog kick with elevation 80 percent (45 seconds)

Frog kick with elevation and power 90 percent (15 seconds)

Recovery: Straddle jog with forearm press (45 seconds)

Jacks tuck (15 seconds)

C SET

Knee-high jog, punch forward and side

Run tires with hand waves

Jumping jacks with diagonal turn

Jacks tuck 1×, seated kick 1×

Cross-country ski and hold R with reverse breaststroke, travel backward

Cross-country ski and hold L with breaststroke, travel forward

Helicopter ski

Cross-country ski with rotation

Tuck ski with rotation

Cross-country ski, tuck, diagonal turn, and center

Jacks tuck

Knee-high jog

D SET

Knee-high jog with R bowstring pull

Knee-high jog with L bowstring pull

Run tires, clap hands

Jumping jacks with unison arm swing

Inner-thigh lift

Jacks tuck with reverse breaststroke, travel backward

Jacks tuck with breaststroke, travel forward

Cross-country ski, slow

Cross-country ski, slower

Cross-country ski, slowest, with power

Cross-country ski 3×, jumping jacks 1×

Tuck ski 3×, jacks tuck 1×

Jacks tuck

Knee-high jog

COOL-DOWN

Skateboard R with breaststroke pull, travel forward

Skateboard L with breaststroke pull, travel forward

Tuck, mermaid, tuck, down and tuck, unison kick to the corners, tuck, down

Bent-knee jacks

R side extension, tuck and down

L side extension, tuck and down

Abdominal pike and spine extension

Stretch: hamstrings, hip flexors, quadriceps, gastrocnemius, outer thigh, shoulders

▶ Deep-Water Cardio Lesson Plan 9

BLOCK CHOREOGRAPHY WITH SIX MOVES

P T
PF AR

EQUIPMENT

Deep-water belts, dumbbells

TEACHING TIP

In block choreography you start with a set of basic moves and in each succeeding set you change something about each move. This lesson plan uses six basic moves—knee-high jog (see figure 7.23), run tires (see figure 7.24), jumping jacks (see figure 7.25), cross-country ski (see figure 7.26), kick forward (see figure 7.27), and heel jog (see figure 7.28). The moves are

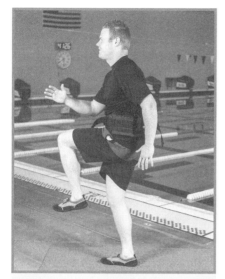

FIGURE 7.23 Knee-high jog.

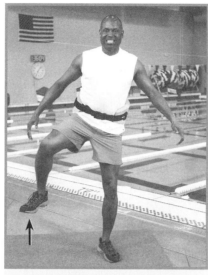

FIGURE 7.24 Run tires.

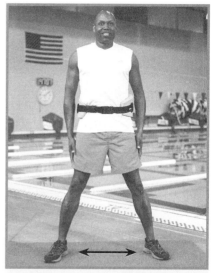

FIGURE 7.25 Jumping jacks.

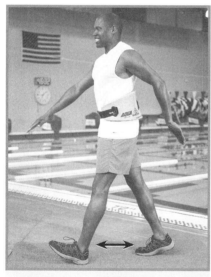

FIGURE 7.26 Cross-country ski.

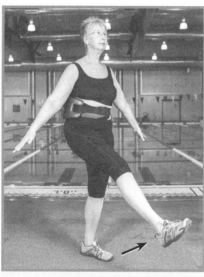

FIGURE 7.27 Kick forward.

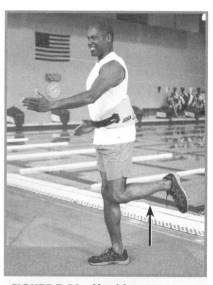

FIGURE 7.28 Heel jog.

modified by adding arm exercises, traveling, alternating intensity variables, adding elevation, increasing the range of motion, crossing the midline, and combining the moves.

WARM-UP

Instructor's choice

A SET

Knee-high jog

Run tires

Jumping jacks

Cross-country ski

Kick forward

Heel jog

B SET

Knee-high jog with pumping arms

Run tires with shoulder blade squeeze

Jumping jacks, clap hands

Cross-country ski with windshield wiper arms

Kick forward with triceps extension

Heel jog with forearm press

C SET

Knee-high jog with reverse breaststroke, travel backward

Run tires with breaststroke, travel forward

Jumping jacks, clap hands, travel backward

Cross-country ski, travel forward

Kick forward with unison arm swing, travel backward

Heel jog with unison arm swing, travel forward

D SET

Knee-high jog, faster and knee-high jog, alternate

Run tires, faster and run tires, alternate

Jumping jacks with power and jumping jacks, alternate

Cross-country ski with power and cross-country ski, alternate

High kick and kick forward, alternate

Skateboard R and heel jog, alternate

Skateboard L and heel jog, alternate

E SET

Knee-high jog

Frog kick with elevation

Jumping jacks

Tuck ski together

Kick forward

Breaststroke kick with elevation

F SET

Run

Over the barrel, travel sideways R and L

Jumping jacks with diagonal turn

Cross-country ski, full ROM

High kick

Skate kick

G SET

Crossover knees

Inner-thigh lift

Jacks cross

Tuck ski with rotation

Crossover kick

Hopscotch

H SET

In, in, out, out

Cross-country ski 1×, jumping jacks 1×

R leg kicks forward and back

In, in, out, out

Cross-country ski 1×, jumping jacks 1×

L leg kicks forward and back

COOL-DOWN

(With dumbbells)

Cross-country ski, upright, diagonal and side lying, alternate R and L

Side-to-side extension

Side-to-side extension with legs in a diamond position

Cross-country ski, side lying, tuck and pike, alternate R and L

Cross-country ski, side lying, tuck, pike, and crunch, alternate R and L

Stretch: quadriceps, hip flexors, hamstrings, outer thigh, inner thigh, pectorals

▶ Deep-Water Interval Lesson Plan 9

RANDOM INTERVALS

EQUIPMENT

Deep-water belts, dumbbells

TEACHING TIP

Deep-water cardio lesson plan 9 is modified to include interval training. In random intervals, the timing and duration varies so that the exercise session seems unpredictable to the participant. This example features two sets of 30-second intervals, two sets of 45-second intervals, and a set of rolling intervals in which the intensity increases every 15 seconds from level 5 to level 8. Level 8 is high-intensity interval training (HIIT). For safety's sake, encourage your participants to modify the intensity to a level that is challenging for them rather than try to keep up with other participants.

Level 5 (50 percent HR max)—Somewhat easy

Level 6 (60 percent HR max)—Moderate

Level 7 (70 percent HR max)—Somewhat hard

Level 8 (80 percent HR max)—Hard

WARM-UP

Instructor's choice

A SET

Knee-high jog

Run tires

Jumping jacks

Cross-country ski

Kick forward

Heel jog

B SET

Knee-high jog with pumping arms

Run tires with shoulder blade squeeze

Jumping jacks, clap hands

Cross-country ski with windshield wiper arms

Kick forward with triceps extension

Heel jog with forearm press

C SET

Knee-high jog with reverse breaststroke, travel backward

Run tires with breaststroke, travel forward

Jumping jacks, clap hands, travel backward

Cross-country ski, travel forward

Kick forward with unison arm swing, travel backward

Heel jog with unison arm swing, travel forward

D SET INTERVALS

Work: Run 60 percent (30 seconds)

Recovery: Knee-high jog (30 seconds)

Work: Knee lift, straighten and power press-down 60 percent (45 seconds)

Recovery: Kick forward (45 seconds)

Rolling interval:

Work: Cross-country ski 50 percent (15 seconds)

Cross-country ski, full ROM 60 percent (15 seconds)

Cross-country ski, faster 70 percent (15 seconds)

Cross-country ski with rotation 80 percent (15 seconds)

Recovery: Heel jog (1 minute)

Work: Knee lift, straighten and power press-down 60 percent (45 seconds)

Recovery: Kick forward (45 seconds)

Work: Run 60 percent (30 seconds)

Recovery: Knee-high jog (30 seconds)

E SET

Knee-high jog

Frog kick with elevation

Jumping jacks

Tuck ski together

Kick forward

Breaststroke kick with elevation

F SET

Run

Over the barrel, travel sideways R and L

Jumping jacks with diagonal turn

Tuck ski with full extension

High kick

Skate kick

G SET

Crossover knees

Inner-thigh lift

Jacks cross

Tuck ski with rotation

Crossover kick

Hopscotch

H SET

In, in, out, out

Cross-country ski 1×, jumping jacks 1×

R leg kicks forward and back

In, in, out, out

Cross-country ski 1×, jumping jacks 1×

L leg kicks forward and back

COOL-DOWN

(With dumbbells)

Cross-country ski, upright, diagonal and side lying, alternate R and L

Side-to-side extension

Side-to-side extension with legs in a diamond position

Cross-country ski, side lying, tuck and pike, tuck, alternate R and L

Cross-country ski, side lying, tuck, pike and crunch, alternate R and L

Stretch: quadriceps, hip flexors, hamstrings, outer thigh, inner thigh, pectorals

▶ Deep-Water Interval Lesson Plan 9

RANDOM INTERVALS

EQUIPMENT

Deep-water belts, dumbbells

TEACHING TIP

In random intervals, the timing and duration varies so that it seems unpredictable to the participant. This example features two sets of rolling intervals. In the first set the intensity increases every 15 seconds, and in the second set the intensity increases every 30 seconds from level 6 to level 9. The rolling intervals are separated by a three-set cycle of 30-second intervals and a four-set cycle of 15-second intervals. Levels 8 and 9 are high-intensity interval training (HIIT). For safety's sake, encourage your participants to modify the intensity to a level that is challenging for them rather than try to keep up with other participants.

Level 6 (60 percent HR max)—Moderate
Level 7 (70 percent HR max)—Somewhat hard
Level 8 (80 percent HR max)—Hard
Level 9 (90 percent HR max)—Very hard

WARM-UP

Instructor's choice

A SET

Knee-high jog
Run tires
Jumping jacks
Cross-country ski
Kick forward
Heel jog

B SET

Knee-high jog with pumping arms
Run tires with shoulder blade squeeze
Jumping jacks, clap hands
Cross-country ski with windshield wiper arms
Kick forward with triceps extension
Heel jog with forearm press

C SET

Knee-high jog with reverse breaststroke, travel backward
Run tires with breaststroke, travel forward
Jumping jacks, clap hands, travel backward
Cross-country ski, travel forward
Kick forward with unison arm swing, travel backward
Heel jog with unison arm swing, travel forward

D SET INTERVALS

Rolling interval:

Work: Run 60 percent (15 seconds)
Sprint 70 percent (15 seconds)
Power run 80 percent (15 seconds)
Cross-country ski with power, travel forward 90 percent (15 seconds)
Recovery: Knee-high jog (1 minute)

3 sets:
Work: High kick 70 percent (30 seconds)
Recovery: Kick forward (30 seconds)

4 sets:
Work: Jumping jacks, faster 70 percent (15 seconds)

Recovery: Jumping jacks (15 seconds)
Rolling interval:
Work: Cross-country ski, full ROM 60 percent (30 seconds)
Cross-country ski, faster 70 percent (30 seconds)
Cross-country ski with rotation 80 percent (30 seconds)
Cross-country ski, arms sweep side to side 90 percent (30 seconds)
Recovery: Heel jog (1 minute)

E SET

Knee-high jog
Frog kick with elevation
Jumping jacks
Tuck ski together
Kick forward
Breaststroke kick with elevation

F SET

Run
Over the barrel, travel sideways R and L
Jumping jacks with diagonal turn
Cross-country ski, full ROM
High kick
Skate kick

G SET

Crossover knees
Inner-thigh lift
Jacks cross
Tuck ski with rotation
Crossover kick
Hopscotch

H SET

In, in, out, out
Cross-country ski 1×, jumping jacks 1×
R leg kicks forward and back
In, in, out, out
Cross-country ski 1×, jumping jacks 1×
L leg kicks forward and back

COOL-DOWN

(With dumbbells)
Cross-country ski, upright, diagonal and side lying, alternate R and L
Side-to-side extension

Side-to-side extension with legs in a diamond position

Cross-country ski, side lying, tuck and pike, alternate R and L

Cross-country ski, side lying, tuck, pike and crunch, alternate R and L

Stretch: quadriceps, hip flexors, hamstrings, outer thigh, inner thigh, pectorals

▶ Deep-Water Interval Lesson Plan 9

PF

RANDOM INTERVALS

EQUIPMENT
Deep-water belts, dumbbells

TEACHING TIP
In random intervals, the timing and duration varies so that it seems unpredictable to the participant. This example features two sets of rolling intervals back to back. In the first set the intensity increases every 30 seconds, and in the second set the intensity increases every 15 seconds from level 6 to level 9. Next is a four-set cycle of 30-second intervals. Finish with a Tabata cycle. Levels 8 and 9 are high-intensity interval training (HIIT). For safety's sake, encourage your participants to modify the intensity to a level that is challenging for them rather than try to keep up with other participants.

Level 6 (60 percent HR max)—Moderate
Level 7 (70 percent HR max)—Somewhat hard
Level 8 (80 percent HR max)—Hard
Level 9 (90 percent HR max)—Very hard

WARM-UP
Instructor's choice

A SET
Knee-high jog

Run tires

Jumping jacks

Cross-country ski

Kick forward

Heel jog

B SET
Knee-high jog with pumping arms

Run tires with shoulder blade squeeze

Jumping jacks, clap hands

Cross-country ski with windshield wiper arms

Kick forward with triceps extension

Heel jog with forearm press

C SET
Knee-high jog with reverse breaststroke, travel backward

Run tires with breaststroke, travel forward

Jumping jacks, clap hands, travel backward

Cross-country ski, travel forward

Kick forward with unison arm swing, travel backward

Heel jog with unison arm swing, travel forward

D SET INTERVALS
Rolling interval:

Work: Cross-country ski, full ROM 60 percent (30 seconds)

Cross-country ski, faster 70 percent (30 seconds)

Cross-country ski with rotation 80 percent (30 seconds)

Cross-country ski, arms sweep side to side 90 percent (30 seconds)

Recovery: Heel jog (1 minute)

Rolling interval:

Work: Run 60 percent (15 seconds)

Sprint 70 percent (15 seconds)

Power run 80 percent (15 seconds)

Cross-country ski with power, travel forward 90 percent (15 seconds)

Recovery: Bicycle (1 minute)

4 sets:

Work: High kick 7×, tuck, and turn 80 percent (30 seconds)

Recovery: Kick forward (30 seconds)

Tabata 8 sets (4 minutes):

Work: Frog kick with elevation and power 90 percent (20 seconds)

Recovery: Rest (10 seconds)

E SET
Knee-high jog

Frog kick with elevation

Jumping jacks

Tuck ski together

Kick forward

Breaststroke kick with elevation

F SET

Run

Over the barrel, travel sideways R and L

Jumping jacks with diagonal turn

Cross-country ski, full ROM

High kick

Skate kick

G SET

Crossover knees

Inner-thigh lift

Jacks cross

Tuck ski with rotation

Crossover kick

Hopscotch

H SET

In, in, out, out

Cross-country ski 1×, jumping jacks 1×

R leg kicks forward and back

In, in, out, out

Cross-country ski 1×, jumping jacks 1×

L leg kicks forward and back

COOL-DOWN

(With dumbbells)

Cross-country ski, upright, diagonal and side lying, alternate R and L

Side-to-side extension

Side-to-side extension with legs in a diamond position

Cross-country ski, side lying R, tuck and pike, alternate R and L

Cross-country ski, side lying R, tuck, pike and crunch, alternate R and L

Stretch: quadriceps, hip flexors, hamstrings, outer thigh, inner thigh, pectorals

▶ Deep-Water Cardio Lesson Plan 10

LAYER TECHNIQUE

EQUIPMENT

Deep-water belts, noodles

TEACHING TIP

The layer technique is a type of choreography in which you start with base moves and then repeat all the moves except one. That move is replaced with a different exercise. This lesson plan accelerates the layering process. The base moves are introduced in the warm-up. The first set repeats all of the base moves and then adds a variation. The second set repeats the variations, adds a new variation, and so on. Each succeeding variation is a little more complex than the previous one. Jacks tuck, hopscotch, and heel jog do not get new variations because they are transition moves that allow you to move smoothly from the previous exercise to the succeeding one. Three moves that may be new to participants are kayak row (see figure 7.29), tuck and down 2× and tuck and pike 2× (see figure 7.30), and holding one leg up as the other leg quad kicks and sweeps out (see figure 7.31).

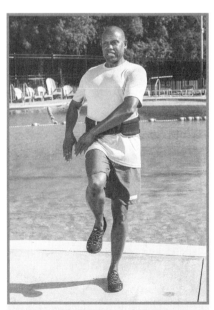

FIGURE 7.29 **Kayak row.**

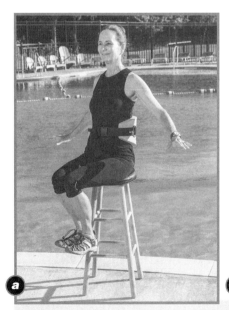

FIGURE 7.30 (*a*) **tuck and** (*b*) **pike.**

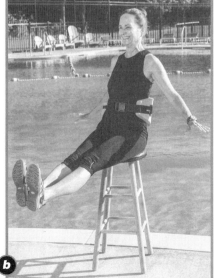

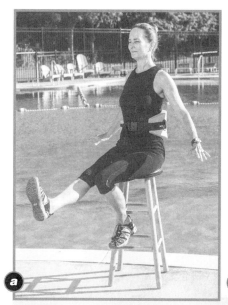 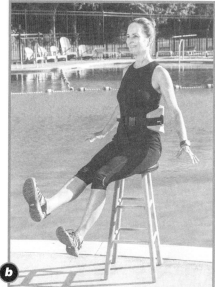 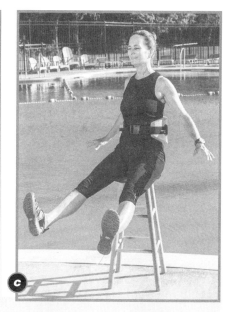

FIGURE 7.31 (*a*) hold R leg up, (*b*) L quad kick, and (*c*) sweep out.

WARM-UP

Jacks tuck

Jumping jacks

Inner-thigh lift

Hopscotch

Heel jog

Cross-country ski

Knee-high jog

Kick forward

A SET

Jacks tuck

Jumping jacks

Jumping jacks 1×, kick forward 1×

Inner-thigh lift

Inner-thigh lift R

Inner-thigh lift L

Hopscotch

Heel jog

Cross-country ski

Cross-country ski 3× and hold

Knee-high jog

Knee-high jog 3× and hold

Kick forward

Seated kick

B SET

Jacks tuck

Jumping jacks 1×, kick forward 1×

Jumping jacks 1×, skate kick 1×

Inner-thigh lift R

Inner-thigh lift L

Inner-thigh lift, doubles

Hopscotch

Heel jog

Cross-country ski 3× and hold

Cross-country ski 2× and cross-country ski with power 1×

Knee-high jog 3× and hold

Knee-high jog 3× and hold with kayak row

Seated kick

Hold R leg up, L quad kick

Hold L leg up, R quad kick

C SET

Jacks tuck

Jumping jacks 1×, skate kick 1×

Jumping jacks 2×, inner-thigh lift 1×

Inner-thigh lift, doubles

Inner-thigh lift R and hopscotch L, alternate

Inner-thigh lift L and hopscotch R, alternate

Hopscotch

Heel jog

Cross-country ski 2× and cross-country ski with power 1×

Cross-country ski with lat pull-down

Knee-high jog 3× and hold with kayak row

Tuck and hold

Hold R leg up, L quad kick

Hold L leg up, R quad kick

Hold R leg up, L quad kick 3× and down

Hold L leg up, R quad kick 3× and down

D SET

Jacks tuck

Jumping jacks 2×, inner-thigh lift 1×

Jumping jacks 2×, hopscotch 1×

Inner-thigh lift R and hopscotch L, alternate

Inner-thigh lift L and hopscotch R, alternate

Inner-thigh lift 1×, hopscotch 1×

Hopscotch

Heel jog

Cross-country ski with lat pull-down

Cross-country ski, tuck, diagonal turn, and center

Tuck and hold

Tuck and down 2×, tuck and pike 2×

Hold R leg up, L quad kick 3× and down

Hold L leg up, R quad kick 3× and down

Hold R leg up, L quad kick and sweep out

Hold L leg up, R quad kick and sweep out

COOL-DOWN

(With noodles)

Jumping jacks, plunge noodle in front

Knee-high jog, diagonal R, noodle under R arm

Side-to-side extension, noodle under R arm

Knee-high jog, diagonal L, noodle under L arm

Side-to-side extension, noodle under L arm

Swirl, noodle in both hands

Cross-country ski, noodle in L hand, travel sideways R

Cross-country ski, noodle in R hand, travel sideways L

Standing leg press R, foot on a noodle

Standing leg press to R side

Standing leg press L, foot on a noodle

Standing leg press to L side

Flutter kick, hold noodle overhead in a rainbow

Stretch: latissimus dorsi, upper back, hip flexors, gastrocnemius, hamstrings, inner thigh

▶ Deep-Water Interval Lesson Plan 10

PYRAMID

EQUIPMENT

Deep-water belts, noodles

TEACHING TIP

Deep-water cardio lesson plan 10 is modified to include interval training. In pyramid intervals in the preseason, the work time increases by 5 seconds in each set, but the recovery time stays at 45 seconds. The intensity level is 60 percent.

Level 6 (60 percent HR max)—Moderate

WARM-UP

Jacks tuck

Jumping jacks

Inner-thigh lift

Hopscotch

Heel jog

Cross-country ski

Knee-high jog

Kick forward

A SET

Jacks tuck

Jumping jacks

Jumping jacks 1×, kick forward 1×

Inner-thigh lift

Inner-thigh lift R

Inner-thigh lift L

Hopscotch

Heel jog

Cross-country ski

Cross-country ski 3× and hold

Knee-high jog

Knee-high jog 3× and hold

Kick forward

Seated kick

B SET INTERVALS

Work: Frog kick (15 seconds)

Recovery: Knee-high jog (45 seconds)

Work: Frog kick (20 seconds)

Recovery: Straddle jog (45 seconds)

Work: Frog kick (25 seconds)

Recovery: Run tires (45 seconds)

Work: Frog kick (30 seconds)

Recovery: Heel jog (45 seconds)

C SET

Jacks tuck

Jumping jacks 1×, kick forward 1×

Jumping jacks 1×, skate kick 1×

Inner-thigh lift R

Inner-thigh lift L

Inner-thigh lift, doubles

Hopscotch

Heel jog

Cross-country ski 3× and hold

Cross-country ski 2× and cross-country ski with power 1×

Knee-high jog 3× and hold

Knee-high jog 3× and hold with kayak row

Seated kick

Hold R leg up, L quad kick

Hold L leg up, R quad kick

D SET INTERVALS

Work: Jacks cross (15 seconds)

Recovery: Knee-high jog (45 seconds)

Work: Jacks cross (20 seconds)

Recovery: Straddle jog (45 seconds)

Work: Jacks cross (25 seconds)

Recovery: Run tires (45 seconds)

Work: Jacks cross (30 seconds)

Recovery: Heel jog (45 seconds)

E SET

Jacks tuck

Jumping jacks 1×, skate kick 1×

Jumping jacks 2×, inner-thigh lift 1×

Inner-thigh lift, doubles

Inner-thigh lift R and hopscotch L, alternate

Inner-thigh lift L and hopscotch R, alternate

Hopscotch

Heel jog

Cross-country ski 2× and cross-country ski with power 1×

Cross-country ski with lat pull-down

Knee-high jog 3× and hold with kayak row

Tuck and down

Hold R leg up, L quad kick

Hold L leg up, R quad kick

Hold R leg up, L quad kick 3× and down

Hold L leg up, R quad kick 3× and down

COOL-DOWN

(With noodles)

Jumping jacks, plunge noodle in front

Knee-high jog, diagonal R, noodle under R arm

Side-to-side extension, noodle under R arm

Knee-high jog, diagonal L, noodle under L arm

Side-to-side extension, noodle under L arm

Swirl, noodle in both hands

Cross-country ski, noodle in L hand, travel sideways R

Cross-country ski, noodle in R hand, travel sideways L

Standing leg press R, foot on a noodle

Standing leg press to R side

Standing leg press L, foot on a noodle

Standing leg press to L side

Flutter kick, hold noodle overhead in a rainbow

Stretch: latissimus dorsi, upper back, hip flexors, gastrocnemius, hamstrings, inner thigh

▶ Deep-Water Interval Lesson Plan 10

PYRAMID

EQUIPMENT

Deep-water belts, noodles

TEACHING TIP

In pyramid intervals in the transition season, the work time increases by 5 seconds in each set, but the recovery time stays at 30 seconds. The intensity level is 70 percent.

Level 7 (70 percent HR max)—Somewhat hard

WARM-UP

Jacks tuck

Jumping jacks

Inner-thigh lift

Hopscotch

Heel jog

Cross-country ski

Knee-high jog

Kick forward

A SET

Jacks tuck

Jumping jacks

Jumping jacks 1×, kick forward 1×

Inner-thigh lift

Inner-thigh lift R

Inner-thigh lift L

Hopscotch

Heel jog
Cross-country ski
Cross-country ski 3× and hold
Knee-high jog
Knee-high jog 3× and hold
Kick forward
Seated kick

B SET INTERVALS

Work: Jumping jacks, faster (15 seconds)
Recovery: Knee-high jog (30 seconds)
Work: Jumping jacks, faster (20 seconds)
Recovery: Straddle jog (30 seconds)
Work: Jumping jacks, faster (25 seconds)
Recovery: Run tires (30 seconds)
Work: Jumping jacks, faster (30 seconds)
Recovery: Heel jog (30 seconds)

C SET

Jacks tuck
Jumping jacks 1×, kick forward 1×
Jumping jacks 1×, skate kick 1×
Inner-thigh lift R
Inner-thigh lift L
Inner-thigh lift, doubles
Hopscotch
Heel jog
Cross-country ski 3× and hold
Cross-country ski 2× and cross-country ski with power 1×
Knee-high jog 3× and hold
Knee-high jog 3× and hold with kayak row
Seated kick
Hold R leg up, L quad kick
Hold L leg up, R quad kick

D SET INTERVALS

Work: Mini jacks, faster (15 seconds)
Recovery: Knee-high jog (30 seconds)
Work: Mini jacks, faster (20 seconds)
Recovery: Straddle jog (30 seconds)
Work: Mini jacks, faster (25 seconds)
Recovery: Run tires (30 seconds)
Work: Mini jacks, faster (30 seconds)
Recovery: Heel jog (30 seconds)

E SET

Jacks tuck
Jumping jacks 1×, skate kick 1×
Jumping jacks 2×, inner-thigh lift 1×
Inner-thigh lift, doubles
Inner-thigh lift R and hopscotch L alternate
Inner-thigh lift L and hopscotch R alternate
Hopscotch
Heel jog
Cross-country ski 2× and cross-country ski with power 1×
Cross-country ski with lat pull-down
Knee-high jog 3× and hold with kayak row
Tuck and down
Hold R leg up, L quad kick
Hold L leg up, R quad kick
Hold R leg up, L quad kick 3× and down
Hold L leg up, R quad kick 3× and down

F SET INTERVALS

Work: Star flutter kick, faster (15 seconds)
Recovery: Knee-high jog (30 seconds)
Work: Star flutter kick, faster (20 seconds)
Recovery: Straddle jog (30 seconds)
Work: Star flutter kick, faster (25 seconds)
Recovery: Run tires (30 seconds)
Work: Star flutter kick, faster (30 seconds)
Recovery: Heel jog (30 seconds)

COOL-DOWN

(With noodles)
Jumping jacks, plunge noodle in front
Knee-high jog, diagonal R, noodle under R arm
Side-to-side extension, noodle under R arm
Knee-high jog, diagonal L, noodle under L arm
Side-to-side extension, noodle under L arm
Swirl, noodle in both hands
Cross-country ski, noodle in L hand, travel sideways R
Cross-country ski, noodle in R hand, travel sideways L
Standing leg press R, foot on a noodle
Standing leg press to R side
Standing leg press L, foot on a noodle
Standing leg press to L side

Flutter kick, hold noodle overhead in a rainbow
Stretch: latissimus dorsi, upper back, hip flexors, gastrocnemius, hamstrings, inner thigh

▶ Deep-Water Interval Lesson Plan 10

PYRAMID

EQUIPMENT

Deep-water belts, noodles

TEACHING TIP

In pyramid intervals in the peak fitness season, the work time increases by 5 seconds in each set, but the recovery time stays at 15 seconds. The intensity level is 80 percent. Level 8 is high-intensity interval training (HIIT). For safety's sake, encourage your participants to modify the intensity to a level that is challenging for them rather than try to keep up with other participants.

Level 8 (80 percent HR max)—Hard

WARM-UP

Jacks tuck
Jumping jacks
Inner-thigh lift
Hopscotch
Heel jog
Cross-country ski
Knee-high jog
Kick forward

A SET

Jacks tuck
Jumping jacks
Jumping jacks 1×, kick forward 1×
Inner-thigh lift
Inner-thigh lift R
Inner-thigh lift L
Hopscotch
Heel jog
Cross-country ski
Cross-country ski 3× and hold
Knee-high jog
Knee-high jog 3× and hold
Kick forward
Seated kick

B SET INTERVALS

Work: Frog kick with elevation (15 seconds)
Recovery: Knee-high jog (15 seconds)
Work: Frog kick with elevation (20 seconds)
Recovery: Straddle jog (15 seconds)
Work: Frog kick with elevation (25 seconds)
Recovery: Run tires (15 seconds)
Work: Frog kick with elevation (30 seconds)
Recovery: Heel jog (15 seconds)
Work: Breaststroke kick with elevation (15 seconds)
Recovery: Knee-high jog (15 seconds)
Work: Breaststroke kick with elevation (20 seconds)
Recovery: Straddle jog (15 seconds)
Work: Breaststroke kick with elevation (25 seconds)
Recovery: Run tires (15 seconds)
Work: Breaststroke kick with elevation (30 seconds)
Recovery: Heel jog (15 seconds)

C SET

Jacks tuck
Jumping jacks 1×, kick forward 1×
Jumping jacks 1×, skate kick 1×
Inner-thigh lift R
Inner-thigh lift L
Inner-thigh lift, doubles
Hopscotch
Heel jog
Cross-country ski 3× and hold
Cross-country ski 2× and cross-country ski with power 1×
Knee-high jog 3× and hold
Knee-high jog 3× and hold with kayak row
Seated kick
Hold R leg up, L quad kick
Hold L leg up, R quad kick

D SET INTERVALS

Work: Bicycle, tandem, with power (15 seconds)
Recovery: Knee-high jog (15 seconds)
Work: Bicycle, tandem, with power (20 seconds)
Recovery: Straddle jog (15 seconds)
Work: Bicycle, tandem, with power (25 seconds)
Recovery: Run tires (15 seconds)
Work: Bicycle, tandem, with power (30 seconds)
Recovery: Heel jog (15 seconds)

Work: Tuck ski together (15 seconds)
Recovery: Knee-high jog (15 seconds)
Work: Tuck ski together (20 seconds)
Recovery: Straddle jog (15 seconds)
Work: Tuck ski together (25 seconds)
Recovery: Run tires (15 seconds)
Work: Tuck ski together (30 seconds)
Recovery: Heel jog (15 seconds)

E SET

Jacks tuck
Jumping jacks 1×, skate kick 1×
Jumping jacks 2×, inner-thigh lift 1×
Inner-thigh lift, doubles
Inner-thigh lift R and hopscotch L, alternate
Inner-thigh lift L and hopscotch R, alternate
Hopscotch
Heel jog
Cross-country ski 2× and cross-country ski with power 1×
Cross-country ski with lat pull-down
Knee-high jog 3× and hold with kayak row
Tuck and down
Hold R leg up, L quad kick
Hold L leg up, R quad kick
Hold R leg up, L quad kick 3× and down
Hold L leg up, R quad kick 3× and down

COOL-DOWN

(With noodles)

Jumping jacks, plunge noodle in front
Knee-high jog, diagonal R, noodle under R arm
Side-to-side extension, noodle under R arm
Knee-high jog, diagonal L, noodle under L arm
Side-to-side extension, noodle under L arm
Swirl, noodle in both hands
Cross-country ski, noodle in L hand, travel sideways R
Cross-country ski, noodle in R hand, travel sideways L
Standing leg press R, foot on a noodle
Standing leg press to R side
Standing leg press L, foot on a noodle
Standing leg press to L side

Flutter kick, hold noodle overhead in a rainbow
Stretch: latissimus dorsi, upper back, hip flexors, gastrocnemius, hamstrings, inner thigh

▶ Deep-Water Cardio Lesson Plan 11

TABATA TIMING 1

EQUIPMENT

Deep-water belts

TEACHING TIP

This lesson plan uses Tabata Timing for cardiorespiratory training. Each set begins with some basic exercises, knee-high jog (see figure 7.32), straddle jog (see figure 7.33), heel jog (see figure 7.34), and bicycle (see figure 7.35), using a variety of arm moves. Travel and stationary exercises alternate. At the end of each set is a Tabata Timing cycle in which two exercises are paired. One is more difficult because it is a longer-lever move or because it is performed faster. Have the participants do this exercise for 20 seconds and the easier exercise for 10 seconds, repeating the pair eight times. This lesson plan concludes with a game called You Be the Teacher just for fun.

WARM-UP

Instructor's choice

A SET

Knee-high jog, push forward, travel backward
Straddle jog, clap hands
Knee-high jog, hands cupped, travel forward
Straddle jog with shoulder blade squeeze

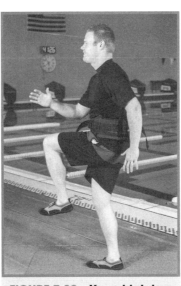

FIGURE 7.32 Knee-high jog.

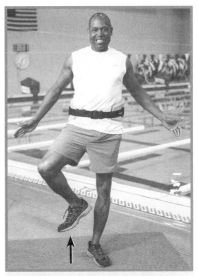

FIGURE 7.33 Straddle jog.

Knee-high jog, push forward, travel backward

Straddle jog, clap hands

Knee-high jog, hands cupped, travel forward

Straddle jog with shoulder blade squeeze

Tabata 8 sets (4 minutes):

Cross-country ski (20 seconds)

Tuck ski (10 seconds)

B SET

Straddle jog with reverse breaststroke, travel backward

Bicycle R leg

Straddle jog with breaststroke, travel forward

Bicycle L leg

Straddle jog with reverse breaststroke, travel backward

Bicycle R leg

Straddle jog with breaststroke, travel forward

Bicycle L leg

Tabata 8 sets (4 minutes):

Kick forward (20 seconds)

Flutter kick (10 seconds)

C SET

Heel jog with unison arm swing, travel backward

Jumping jacks with bowstring pull to R side

Heel jog with triceps kick back, travel forward

Jumping jacks with bowstring pull to L side

Heel jog with unison arm swing, travel backward

Jumping jacks with bowstring pull to R side

Heel jog with triceps kick back, travel forward

Jumping jacks with bowstring pull to L side

Tabata 8 sets (4 minutes):

Jumping jacks (20 seconds)

Run tires (10 seconds)

D SET

Bicycle with propeller scull, travel backward

Heel jog with arm curl

Bicycle with bicycle arms, travel forward

Heel jog with forearm press

Bicycle with propeller scull, travel backward

Heel jog with arm curl

Bicycle with bicycle arms, travel forward

Heel jog with forearm press

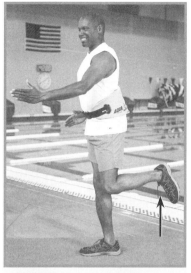
FIGURE 7.34 **Heel jog.**

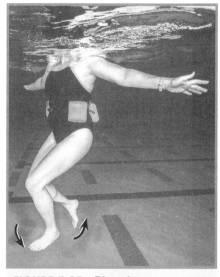
FIGURE 7.35 **Bicycle.**

Tabata 8 sets (4 minutes):

Cross-country ski (20 seconds)

Tuck ski (10 seconds)

COOL-DOWN: YOU BE THE TEACHER

(The class is in a big circle)

Ask one participant to lead the class in his or her favorite exercise. Then go around the circle until everyone has had a turn. Allow any participant who does not wish to lead an exercise to pass.

Stretch: hip flexors, quadriceps, gastrocnemius, outer thigh, hamstrings, lower back

▶ Deep-Water Interval Lesson Plan 11

TABATA TIMING 1

EQUIPMENT

Deep-water belts

TEACHING TIP

Deep-water cardio lesson plan 11 is modified to include interval training. In Tabata Timing during the preseason, the work phase is performed at level 7. During the recovery, the participant floats in place for 10 seconds to rest.

Level 7 (70 percent HR max)—Somewhat hard

WARM-UP

Instructor's choice

A SET

Knee-high jog, push forward, travel backward

Straddle jog, clap hands

Knee-high jog, hands cupped, travel forward

Straddle jog with shoulder blade squeeze

Knee-high jog, push forward, travel backward

Straddle jog, clap hands

Knee-high jog, hands cupped, travel forward

Straddle jog with shoulder blade squeeze

Tabata 8 sets (4 minutes):

    Work: Mini ski, faster 70 percent (20 seconds)

    Recovery: Rest (10 seconds)

B SET

Straddle jog with reverse breaststroke, travel
    backward

Bicycle R leg

Straddle jog with breaststroke, travel forward

Bicycle L leg

Straddle jog with reverse breaststroke, travel
    backward

Bicycle R leg

Straddle jog with breaststroke, travel forward

Bicycle L leg

Tabata 8 sets (4 minutes):

    Work: Knee-high jog, faster 70 percent (20 sec-
    onds)

    Recovery: Rest (10 seconds)

C SET

Heel jog with unison arm swing, travel backward

Jumping jacks with bowstring pull to R side

Heel jog with triceps kick back, travel forward

Jumping jacks with bowstring pull to L side

Heel jog with unison arm swing, travel backward

Jumping jacks with bowstring pull to R side

Heel jog with triceps kick back, travel forward

Jumping jacks with bowstring pull to R side

Tabata 8 sets (4 minutes):

    Work: Mini jacks, faster 70 percent (20 seconds)

    Recovery: Rest (10 seconds)

D SET

Bicycle with propeller scull, travel backward

Heel jog with arm curl

Bicycle with bicycle arms, travel forward

Heel jog with forearm press

Bicycle with propeller scull, travel backward

Heel jog with arm curl

Bicycle with bicycle arms, travel forward

Heel jog with forearm press

Tabata 8 sets (4 minutes):

    Work: Mini ski, faster 70 percent (20 seconds)

    Recovery: Rest (10 seconds)

COOL-DOWN: YOU BE THE TEACHER

(The class is in a big circle)

Ask one participant to lead the class in his or her favorite exercise. Then go around the circle until everyone has had a turn. Allow any participant who does not wish to lead an exercise to pass.

Stretch: hip flexors, quadriceps, gastrocnemius, outer thigh, hamstrings, lower back

▶ Deep-Water Interval Lesson Plan 11

TABATA TYPE 1

EQUIPMENT

Deep-water belts

TEACHING TIP

In Tabata intervals during the transition season, the work phase is performed at level 8. During the recovery, the participant floats in place for 10 seconds to rest. Level 8 is high-intensity interval training (HIIT), so you are doing Tabata Type rather than Tabata Timing. For safety's sake, encourage your participants to modify the intensity to a level that is challenging for them rather than try to keep up with other participants.

    Level 8 (80 percent HR max)—Hard

WARM-UP

Instructor's choice

A SET

Knee-high jog, push forward, travel backward

Straddle jog, clap hands

Knee-high jog, hands cupped, travel forward

Straddle jog with shoulder blade squeeze

Knee-high jog, push forward, travel backward

Straddle jog, clap hands

Knee-high jog, hands cupped, travel forward

Straddle jog with shoulder blade squeeze

Tabata 8 sets (4 minutes):

    Work: Cross-country ski with power 80 percent
    (20 seconds)

    Recovery: Rest (10 seconds)

B SET

Straddle jog with reverse breaststroke, travel backward

Bicycle R leg

Straddle jog with breaststroke, travel forward

Bicycle L leg

Straddle jog with reverse breaststroke, travel backward

Bicycle R leg

Straddle jog with breaststroke, travel forward

Bicycle L leg

Tabata 8 sets (4 minutes):

Work: Knee-high jog with elevation 80 percent (20 seconds)

Recovery: Rest (10 seconds)

C SET

Heel jog with unison arm swing, travel backward

Jumping jacks with bowstring pull to R side

Heel jog with triceps kick back, travel forward

Jumping jacks with bowstring pull to L side

Heel jog with unison arm swing, travel backward

Jumping jacks with bowstring pull to R side

Heel jog with triceps kick back, travel forward

Jumping jacks with bowstring pull to L side

Tabata 8 sets (4 minutes):

Work: Frog kick with elevation 80 percent (20 seconds)

Recovery: Rest (10 seconds)

D SET

Bicycle with propeller scull, travel backward

Heel jog with arm curl

Bicycle with bicycle arms, travel forward

Heel jog with forearm press

Bicycle with propeller scull, travel backward

Heel jog with arm curl

Bicycle with bicycle arms, travel forward

Heel jog with forearm press

Tabata 8 sets (4 minutes):

Work: Cross-country ski with rotation 80 percent (20 seconds)

Recovery: Rest (10 seconds)

COOL-DOWN: YOU BE THE TEACHER

(The class is in a big circle)

Ask one participant to lead the class in his or her favorite exercise. Then go around the circle until everyone has had a turn. Allow any participant who does not wish to lead an exercise to pass.

Stretch: hip flexors, quadriceps, gastrocnemius, outer thigh, hamstrings, lower back

▶ Deep-Water Interval Lesson Plan 11

TABATA TYPE 1

PF

EQUIPMENT

Deep-water belts

TEACHING TIP

In Tabata intervals during the peak fitness season, the work phase is performed at level 9. During the recovery, the participant floats in place for 10 seconds to rest. Level 9 is high-intensity interval training (HIIT), so you are doing Tabata Type rather than Tabata Timing. For safety's sake, encourage your participants to modify the intensity to a level that is challenging for them rather than try to keep up with other participants.

Level 9 (90 percent HR max)—Very hard

WARM-UP

Instructor's choice

A SET

Knee-high jog, push forward, travel backward

Straddle jog, clap hands

Knee-high jog, hands cupped, travel forward

Straddle jog with shoulder blade squeeze

Knee-high jog, push forward, travel backward

Straddle jog, clap hands

Knee-high jog, hands cupped, travel forward

Straddle jog with shoulder blade squeeze

Tabata 8 sets (4 minutes):

Work: Cross-country ski, arms sweep side to side 90 percent (20 seconds)

Recovery: Rest (10 seconds)

B SET

Straddle jog with reverse breaststroke, travel backward

Bicycle R leg

Straddle jog with breaststroke, travel forward

Bicycle L leg

Straddle jog with reverse breaststroke, travel backward

Bicycle R leg

Straddle jog with breaststroke, travel forward

Bicycle L leg

Tabata 8 sets (4 minutes):

Work: Bicycle with elevation and power 90 percent (20 seconds)

Recovery: Rest (10 seconds)

C SET

Heel jog with unison arm swing, travel backward

Jumping jacks with bowstring pull to R side

Heel jog with triceps kick back, travel forward

Jumping jacks with bowstring pull to L side

Heel jog with unison arm swing, travel backward

Jumping jacks with bowstring pull to R side

Heel jog with triceps kick back, travel forward

Jumping jacks with bowstring pull to L side

Tabata 8 sets (4 minutes):

Work: Frog kick with elevation and power 90 percent (20 seconds)

Recovery: Rest (10 seconds)

D SET

Bicycle with propeller scull, travel backward

Heel jog with arm curl

Bicycle with bicycle arms, travel forward

Heel jog with forearm press

Bicycle with propeller scull, travel backward

Heel jog with arm curl

Bicycle with bicycle arms, travel forward

Heel jog with forearm press

Tabata 8 sets (4 minutes):

Work: Helicopter ski with power 90 percent (20 seconds)

Recovery: Rest (10 seconds)

COOL-DOWN: YOU BE THE TEACHER

(The class is in a big circle)

Ask one participant to lead the class in his or her favorite exercise. Then go around the circle until everyone has had a turn. Allow any participant who does not wish to lead an exercise to pass.

Stretch: hip flexors, quadriceps, gastrocnemius, outer thigh, hamstrings, lower back

▶ Deep-Water Cardio Lesson Plan 12

TABATA TIMING 2

EQUIPMENT

Deep-water belts

TEACHING TIP

This lesson plan uses Tabata Timing all the way through except for the warm-up and the stretches. Sets A through F are cardiorespiratory training. Sets G and H are training for the upper body. Sets I and J are core strength training. Tabata cycles are four minutes long, and breaks after each cycle are one minute long, which means that the timing is specific. Instructors may wish to use a deck timer to help them manage the time. Two exercises in this lesson plan use the variation in tempo called syncopate, knee-high jog (see figure 7.36) and jumping jacks (see figure 7.37). Syncopate means slow, slow, quick, quick, quick.

WARM-UP

Instructor's choice

A SET

Tabata repeat 4× (4 minutes):

Knee lift, doubles (20 seconds)

Knee-high jog (10 seconds)

Knee-high jog, syncopate (20 seconds)

Knee-high jog (10 seconds)

One-minute break:

Knee-high jog with propeller scull, travel backward (30 seconds)

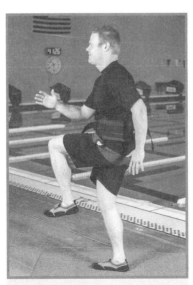

FIGURE 7.36 **Knee-high jog.**

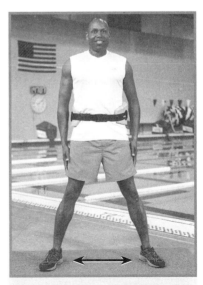

FIGURE 7.37 **Jumping jacks.**

Knee-high jog with propeller scull, travel forward (30 seconds)

B SET

Tabata repeat 4× (4 minutes):

R quad kick (20 seconds)

Kick forward (10 seconds)

L quad kick (20 seconds)

Kick forward (10 seconds)

One-minute break:

Flutter kick with reverse breaststroke, travel backward (30 seconds)

Flutter kick with breaststroke, travel forward (30 seconds)

C SET

Tabata repeat 4× (4 minutes):

Diamonds (20 seconds)

Straddle jog (10 seconds)

Cossack kick (20 seconds)

Straddle jog (10 seconds)

One-minute break:

Over the barrel, travel sideways R (30 seconds)

Over the barrel, travel sideways L (30 seconds)

D SET

Tabata repeat 4× (4 minutes):

Hopscotch (20 seconds)

Heel jog (10 seconds)

Skate kick (20 seconds)

Heel jog (10 seconds)

One-minute break:

Bicycle with propeller scull, travel backward (30 seconds)

Bicycle with propeller scull, travel forward (30 seconds)

E SET

Tabata repeat 4× (4 minutes):

Tuck ski, doubles (20 seconds)

Cross-country ski with knees bent 90 degrees (10 seconds)

Tuck ski (20 seconds)

Cross-country ski with knees bent 90 degrees (10 seconds)

One-minute break:

Knee-high jog with propeller scull, travel backward (30 seconds)

Crossover step, travel forward (30 seconds)

F SET

Tabata repeat 4× (4 minutes):

Jumping jacks (20 seconds)

Run tires (10 seconds)

Jumping jacks, syncopate (20 seconds)

Run tires (10 seconds)

One-minute break:

Knee-high jog with R shoulder sweep in, travel sideways R (30 seconds)

Knee-high jog with L shoulder sweep in, travel sideways L (30 seconds)

G SET

Tabata repeat 2× (4 minutes):

Knee-high jog, clap hands (20 seconds)

Bicycle (10 seconds)

Knee-high jog with standing row (20 seconds)

Bicycle R leg (10 seconds)

Knee-high jog with lat pull-down (20 seconds)

Bicycle (10 seconds)

Knee-high jog with arm lift to sides (20 seconds)

Bicycle L leg (10 seconds)

One-minute break:

Knee-high jog, push forward, travel backward (30 seconds)

Knee-high jog with crawl stroke, travel forward (30 seconds)

H SET

Tabata repeat 2× (4 minutes):

Straddle jog, push forward (20 seconds)

Inner-thigh lift (10 seconds)

Straddle jog, push across (20 seconds)

Inner-thigh lift R (10 seconds)

Straddle jog, open and close doors (20 seconds)

Inner-thigh lift (10 seconds)

Straddle jog with forearm press (20 seconds)

Inner-thigh lift L (10 seconds)

One-minute break:

Knee-high jog with R side arm curl, travel sideways R (30 seconds)

Knee-high jog with L side arm curl, travel sideways L (30 seconds)

I SET

Tabata repeat 2× (4 minutes):

Log jump, forward and back (20 seconds)

Seated kick (10 seconds)

Log jump, side to side (20 seconds)

Mermaid (10 seconds)

Figure-eight arms, legs hang (20 seconds)

Seated kick (10 seconds)

Brace core, arms down, turbulent hand movements (20 seconds)

Mermaid (10 seconds)

One-minute break:

Abdominal pike and spine extension (1 minute)

J SET

Tabata repeat 2× (4 minutes):

Crossover knees (20 seconds)

T-hang, contract abdominals (10 seconds)

Pelvic circles clockwise (20 seconds)

Tuck and hold (10 seconds)

Swirl (20 seconds)

T-hang, contract abdominals (10 seconds)

Pelvic circles counterclockwise (20 seconds)

Tuck and hold (10 seconds)

One-minute break:

Side-to-side extension (1 minute)

Stretch: quadriceps, gastrocnemius, hamstrings, outer thigh, pectorals, upper back

▶ **Deep-Water Interval Lesson Plan 12**

TABATA TIMING 2

EQUIPMENT

Deep-water belts

TEACHING TIP

Deep-water cardio lesson plan 12 is modified to include interval training. Set A is a cardiorespiratory transition into the Tabata intervals in sets B through F. Sets G and H are training for the upper body, and sets I and J are core strength training. In Tabata intervals during the preseason, the work phase is performed at level 7. During the recovery, the participant floats in place for 10 seconds to rest.

Level 7 (70 percent HR max)—Somewhat hard

Tabata cycles are four minutes long, and breaks after each cycle are one minute long, which means that the timing is specific. Instructors may wish to use a deck timer to help them manage the time.

WARM-UP

Instructor's choice

A SET

Tabata repeat 4× (4 minutes):

Knee lift, doubles (20 seconds)

Knee-high jog (10 seconds)

Knee-high jog, syncopate (20 seconds)

Knee-high jog (10 seconds)

One-minute break:

Knee-high jog with propeller scull, travel backward (30 seconds)

Knee-high jog with propeller scull, travel forward (30 seconds)

B SET

Tabata repeat 4× (4 minutes):

Work: Knee-high jog, faster 70 percent (20 seconds)

Recovery: Rest (10 seconds)

Work: Steep climb, faster 70 percent (20 seconds)

Recovery: Rest (10 seconds)

One-minute break:

Flutter kick with reverse breaststroke, travel backward (30 seconds)

Flutter kick with breaststroke, travel forward (30 seconds)

C SET

Tabata repeat 4× (4 minutes):

Work: Flutter kick, faster 70 percent (20 seconds)

Recovery: Rest (10 seconds)

Work: Star flutter kick, faster 70 percent (20 seconds)

Recovery: Rest (10 seconds)

One-minute break:

Over the barrel, travel sideways R (30 seconds)

Over the barrel, travel sideways L (30 seconds)

D SET

Tabata repeat 4× (4 minutes):

Work: Inner-thigh lift, faster 70 percent (20 seconds)

Recovery: Rest (10 seconds)

Work: Hopscotch, faster 70 percent (20 seconds)

Recovery: Rest (10 seconds)

One-minute break:

Bicycle with propeller scull, travel backward (30 seconds)

Bicycle with propeller scull, travel forward (30 seconds)

E SET

Tabata repeat 4× (4 minutes):

Work: Mini ski, faster 70 percent (20 seconds)

Recovery: Rest (10 seconds)

Work: Cross-country ski, faster 70 percent (20 seconds)

Recovery: Rest (10 seconds)

One-minute break:

Knee-high jog with propeller scull, travel backward (30 seconds)

Crossover step, travel forward (30 seconds)

F SET

Tabata repeat 4× (4 minutes):

Work: Mini jacks, faster 70 percent (20 seconds)

Recovery: Rest (10 seconds)

Work: Jumping jacks, faster 70 percent (20 seconds)

Recovery: Rest (10 seconds)

One-minute break:

Knee-high jog with R shoulder sweep in, travel sideways R (30 seconds)

Knee-high jog with L shoulder sweep in, travel sideways L (30 seconds)

G SET

Tabata repeat 2× (4 minutes):

Knee-high jog, clap hands (20 seconds)

Bicycle (10 seconds)

Knee-high jog with standing row (20 seconds)

Bicycle R leg (10 seconds)

Knee-high jog with lat pull-down (20 seconds)

Bicycle (10 seconds)

Knee-high jog with arm lift to sides (20 seconds)

Bicycle L leg (10 seconds)

One-minute break:

Knee-high jog, push forward, travel backward (30 seconds)

Knee-high jog with crawl stroke, travel forward (30 seconds)

H SET

Tabata repeat 2× (4 minutes):

Straddle jog, push forward (20 seconds)

Inner-thigh lift (10 seconds)

Straddle jog, push across (20 seconds)

Inner-thigh lift R (10 seconds)

Straddle jog, open and close doors (20 seconds)

Inner-thigh lift (10 seconds)

Straddle jog with forearm press (20 seconds)

Inner-thigh lift L (10 seconds)

One-minute break:

Knee-high jog with R side arm curl, travel sideways R (30 seconds)

Knee-high jog with L side arm curl, travel sideways L (30 seconds)

I SET

Tabata repeat 2× (4 minutes):

Log jump, forward and back (20 seconds)

Seated kick (10 seconds)

Log jump, side to side (20 seconds)

Mermaid (10 seconds)

Figure-eight arms, legs hang (20 seconds)

Seated kick (10 seconds)

Brace core, arms down, turbulent hand movements (20 seconds)

Mermaid (10 seconds)

One-minute break:

Abdominal pike and spine extension (1 minute)

J SET

Tabata repeat 2× (4 minutes):

Crossover knees (20 seconds)

T-hang, contract abdominals (10 seconds)

Pelvic circles clockwise (20 seconds)

Tuck and hold (10 seconds)

Swirl (20 seconds)

T-hang, contract abdominals (10 seconds)

Pelvic circles counterclockwise (20 seconds)

Tuck and hold (10 seconds)

One-minute break:

Side-to-side extension (1 minute)

Stretch: quadriceps, gastrocnemius, hamstrings, outer thigh, pectorals, upper back

▶ Deep-Water Interval Lesson Plan 12

TABATA TYPE 2

EQUIPMENT

Deep-water belts

TEACHING TIP

Set A is a cardiorespiratory transition into the Tabata intervals in sets B through F. Sets G and H are training for the upper body, and sets I and J are core strength training.

In Tabata intervals during the transition season, the work phase is performed at level 8. Level 8 is high-intensity interval training (HIIT), so you are doing Tabata Type rather than Tabata Timing. During the recovery, the participant floats in place for 10 seconds to rest. For safety's sake, encourage your participants to modify the intensity to a level that is challenging for them rather than try to keep up with other participants.

Level 8 (80 percent HR max)—Hard

Tabata cycles are four minutes long, and breaks after each cycle are one minute long, which means that the timing is specific. Instructors may wish to use a deck timer to help them manage the time.

WARM-UP

Instructor's choice

A SET

Tabata repeat 4× (4 minutes):
Knee lift, doubles (20 seconds)
Knee-high jog (10 seconds)
Knee-high jog, syncopate (20 seconds)
Knee-high jog (10 seconds)
One-minute break:
Knee-high jog with propeller scull, travel backward (30 seconds)
Knee-high jog with propeller scull, travel forward (30 seconds)

B SET

Tabata repeat 4× (4 minutes):
Work: High kick, power down 80 percent (20 seconds)
Recovery: Rest (10 seconds)
Work: High kick with power 80 percent (20 seconds)
Recovery: Rest (10 seconds)
One-minute break:
Flutter kick with reverse breaststroke, travel backward (30 seconds)
Flutter kick with breaststroke, travel forward (30 seconds)

C SET

Tabata repeat 4× (4 minutes):
Work: Frog kick with elevation 80 percent (20 seconds)

Recovery: Rest (10 seconds)
Work: Breaststroke kick with elevation 80 percent (20 seconds)
Recovery: Rest (10 seconds)
One-minute break:
Over the barrel, travel sideways R (30 seconds)
Over the barrel, travel sideways L (30 seconds)

D SET

Tabata repeat 4× (4 minutes):
Work: Inner-thigh lift with power 80 percent (20 seconds)
Recovery: Rest (10 seconds)
Work: Hopscotch with power 80 percent (20 seconds)
Recovery: Rest (10 seconds)
One-minute break:
Bicycle with propeller scull, travel backward (30 seconds)
Bicycle with propeller scull, travel forward (30 seconds)

E SET

Tabata repeat 4× (4 minutes):
Work: Cross-country ski with elevation 80 percent (20 seconds)
Recovery: Rest (10 seconds)
Work: Helicopter ski 80 percent (20 seconds)
Recovery: Rest (10 seconds)
One-minute break:
Knee-high jog with propeller scull, travel backward (30 seconds)
Crossover step, travel forward (30 seconds)

F SET

Tabata repeat 4× (4 minutes):
Work: Bicycle with power 80 percent (20 seconds)
Recovery: Rest (10 seconds)
Work: Bicycle, tandem with power 80 percent (20 seconds)
Recovery: Rest (10 seconds)
One-minute break:
Knee-high jog with R shoulder sweep in, travel sideways R (30 seconds)
Knee-high jog with L shoulder sweep in, travel sideways L (30 seconds)

G SET

Tabata repeat 2× (4 minutes):

Knee-high jog, clap hands (20 seconds)

Bicycle (10 seconds)

Knee-high jog with standing row (20 seconds)

Bicycle R leg (10 seconds)

Knee-high jog with lat pull-down (20 seconds)

Bicycle (10 seconds)

Knee-high jog with arm lift to sides (20 seconds)

Bicycle L leg (10 seconds)

One-minute break:

Knee-high jog, push forward, travel backward (30 seconds)

Knee-high jog with crawl stroke, travel forward (30 seconds)

H SET

Tabata repeat 2× (4 minutes):

Straddle jog, push forward (20 seconds)

Inner-thigh lift (10 seconds)

Straddle jog, push across (20 seconds)

Inner-thigh lift R (10 seconds)

Straddle jog, open and close doors (20 seconds)

Inner-thigh lift (10 seconds)

Straddle jog with forearm press (20 seconds)

Inner-thigh lift L (10 seconds)

One-minute break:

Knee-high jog with R side arm curl, travel sideways R (30 seconds)

Knee-high jog with L side arm curl, travel sideways L (30 seconds)

I SET

Tabata repeat 2× (4 minutes):

Log jump, forward and back (20 seconds)

Seated kick (10 seconds)

Log jump, side to side (20 seconds)

Mermaid (10 seconds)

Figure-eight arms, legs hang (20 seconds)

Seated kick (10 seconds)

Brace core, arms down, turbulent hand movements (20 seconds)

Mermaid (10 seconds)

One-minute break:

Abdominal pike and spine extension (1 minute)

J SET

Tabata repeat 2× (4 minutes):

Crossover knees (20 seconds)

T-hang, contract abdominals (10 seconds)

Pelvic circles clockwise (20 seconds)

Tuck and hold (10 seconds)

Swirl (20 seconds)

T-hang, contract abdominals (10 seconds)

Pelvic circles counterclockwise (20 seconds)

Tuck and hold (10 seconds)

One-minute break:

Side-to-side extension (1 minute)

Stretch: quadriceps, gastrocnemius, hamstrings, outer thigh, pectorals, upper back

▶ Deep-Water Interval Lesson Plan 12

TABATA TYPE 2

PF

EQUIPMENT

Deep-water belts

TEACHING TIP

Set A is a cardiorespiratory transition into the Tabata intervals in sets B through F. Sets G and H are training for the upper body, and sets I and J are core strength training.

In Tabata intervals during the peak fitness season, the work phase is performed at level 9. Level 9 is high-intensity interval training (HIIT), so you are doing Tabata Type rather than Tabata Timing. During the recovery, the participant floats in place for 10 seconds to rest. For safety's sake, encourage your participants to modify the intensity to a level that is challenging for them rather than try to keep up with other participants.

Level 9 (90 percent HR max)—Very hard

Tabata cycles are four minutes long, and breaks after each cycle are one minute long, which means that the timing is specific. Instructors may wish to use a deck timer to help them manage the time.

WARM-UP

Instructor's choice

A SET

Tabata repeat 4× (4 minutes):

Knee lift, doubles (20 seconds)

Knee-high jog (10 seconds)

Knee-high jog, syncopate (20 seconds)

Knee-high jog (10 seconds)

One-minute break:

Knee-high jog with propeller scull, travel backward (30 seconds)

Knee-high jog with propeller scull, travel forward (30 seconds)

B SET

Tabata repeat 4× (4 minutes):

Work: High kick with lat pull-down 90 percent (20 seconds)

Recovery: Rest (10 seconds)

Work: High kick, clap over and under 90 percent (20 seconds)

Recovery: Rest (10 seconds)

One-minute break:

Flutter kick with reverse breaststroke, travel backward (30 seconds)

Flutter kick with breaststroke, travel forward (30 seconds)

C SET

Tabata repeat 4× (4 minutes):

Work: Frog kick with double-arm press-down 90 percent (20 seconds)

Recovery: Rest (10 seconds)

Work: Frog kick 1×, tuck ski together 1× 90 percent (20 seconds)

Recovery: Rest (10 seconds)

One-minute break:

Over the barrel, travel sideways R (30 seconds)

Over the barrel, travel sideways L (30 seconds)

D SET

Tabata repeat 4× (4 minutes):

Work: Bicycle with elevation and power 90 percent (20 seconds)

Recovery: Rest (10 seconds)

Work: Breaststroke kick with elevation and power 90 percent (20 seconds)

Recovery: Rest (10 seconds)

One-minute break:

Bicycle with propeller scull, travel backward (30 seconds)

Bicycle with propeller scull, travel forward (30 seconds)

E SET

Tabata repeat 4× (4 minutes):

Work: Cross-country ski with rotation and power 90 percent (20 seconds)

Recovery: Rest (10 seconds)

Work: Helicopter ski with power 90 percent (20 seconds)

Recovery: Rest (10 seconds)

One-minute break:

Knee-high jog with propeller scull, travel backward (30 seconds)

Crossover step, travel forward (30 seconds)

F SET

Tabata repeat 4× (4 minutes):

Work: Hopscotch 1×, jumping jacks 1×, faster 90 percent (20 seconds)

Recovery: Rest (10 seconds)

Work: Jumping jacks, clap hands with power 90 percent (20 seconds)

Recovery: Rest (10 seconds)

One-minute break:

Knee-high jog with R shoulder sweep in, travel sideways R (30 seconds)

Knee-high jog with L shoulder sweep in, travel sideways L (30 seconds)

G SET

Tabata repeat 2× (4 minutes):

Knee-high jog, clap hands (20 seconds)

Bicycle (10 seconds)

Knee-high jog with standing row (20 seconds)

Bicycle R leg (10 seconds)

Knee-high jog with lat pull-down (20 seconds)

Bicycle (10 seconds)

Knee-high jog with arm lift to sides (20 seconds)

Bicycle L leg (10 seconds)

One-minute break:

Knee-high jog, push forward, travel backward (30 seconds)

Knee-high jog with crawl stroke, travel forward (30 seconds)

H SET

Tabata repeat 2× (4 minutes):

Straddle jog, push forward (20 seconds)

Inner-thigh lift (10 seconds)

Straddle jog, push across (20 seconds)

Inner-thigh lift R (10 seconds)

Straddle jog, open and close doors (20 seconds)

Inner-thigh lift (10 seconds)

Straddle jog with forearm press (20 seconds)

Inner-thigh lift L (10 seconds)

One-minute break:

Knee-high jog with R side arm curl, travel sideways R (30 seconds)

Knee-high jog with L side arm curl, travel sideways L (30 seconds)

I SET

Tabata repeat 2× (4 minutes):

Log jump, forward and back (20 seconds)

Seated kick (10 seconds)

Log jump, side to side (20 seconds)

Mermaid (10 seconds)

Figure-eight arms, legs hang (20 seconds)

Seated kick (10 seconds)

Brace core, arms down, turbulent hand movements (20 seconds)

Mermaid (10 seconds)

One-minute break:

Abdominal pike and spine extension (1 minute)

J SET

Tabata repeat 2× (4 minutes):

Crossover knees (20 seconds)

T-hang, contract abdominals (10 seconds)

Pelvic circles clockwise (20 seconds)

Tuck and hold (10 seconds)

Swirl (20 seconds)

T-hang, contract abdominals (10 seconds)

Pelvic circles counterclockwise (20 seconds)

Tuck and hold (10 seconds)

One-minute break:

Side-to-side extension (1 minute)

Stretch: quadriceps, gastrocnemius, hamstrings, outer thigh, pectorals, upper back

SECTION 2: STRENGTH TRAINING

▶ Deep-Water Strength Training 1

HAND POSITIONS AND LEVER LENGTH

P

EQUIPMENT

Deep-water belts

TEACHING TIP

In the preseason you want your participants to become aware that how they move their limbs through the water can increase or decrease the water's resistance. A hand sliced sideways through the water (see figure 7.38a) encounters minimal resistance. A closed fist (see figure 7.38b) encounters more resistance. But an open hand or a cupped hand position with the fingers relaxed and slightly apart (see figure 7.38c) will pull water more effectively and encounter the most resistance. In addition, a longer lever length will have more drag resistance and require more force than a shorter lever.

WARM-UP

Knee-high jog

Run tires

In, in, out, out

Jumping jacks

Jumping jacks 1×, kick forward 1×

Jacks tuck with reverse breaststroke, travel backward

Seated kick, travel forward

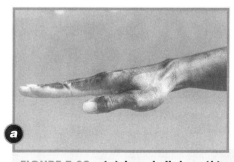
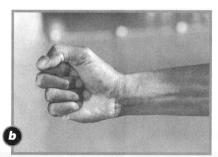
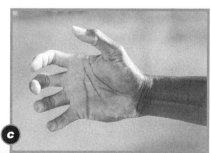

FIGURE 7.38 (*a*) hand slicing, (*b*) closed fist, (*c*) cupped hand.

Knee-high jog with propeller scull, travel backward

Skateboard R, travel forward

Knee-high jog with propeller scull, travel backward

Skateboard L, travel forward

A SET

Knee-high jog, R shoulder sweep in, hand slicing

Knee-high jog, L shoulder sweep in, hand slicing

Clamshells R

Clamshells L

Knee-high jog, R shoulder sweep in, hand cupped

Knee-high jog, L shoulder sweep in, hand cupped

R leg kicks side

L leg kicks side

Knee-high jog with hands fisted, one lap

B SET

Knee-high jog, R shoulder sweep out, hand slicing

Knee-high jog, L shoulder sweep out, hand slicing

Jacks tuck

Knee-high jog, R shoulder sweep out, hand open

Knee-high jog, L shoulder sweep out, hand open

Frog kick

Knee-high jog with hands cupped, one lap

C SET

Cross-country ski with R bowstring pull, hand
fisted

Cross-country ski with L bowstring pull, hand
fisted

R quad kick

L quad kick

Cross-country ski with R bowstring pull, hand
cupped

Cross-country-ski with L bowstring pull, hand
cupped

R leg kicks forward

L leg kicks forward

Knee-high jog with resistor arms, one lap

D SET

Knee-high jog with R arm curl, hand slicing

Knee-high jog with L arm curl, hand slicing

R hamstring curl

L hamstring curl

Knee-high jog with R arm curl, palm faces direction of motion

Knee-high jog with L arm curl, palm faces direction of motion

R leg kicks back

L leg kicks back

Knee-high jog, faster, with hands cupped, one lap

E SET

Knee-high jog with R forearm press, palm up,
hand slicing

Knee-high jog with L forearm press, palm up,
hand slicing

Flutter kick, point and flex feet

Knee-high jog with R forearm press, hand open

Knee-high jog with L forearm press, hand open

Mini ski, point and flex feet

Knee-high jog with hands cupped, one lap

F SET

Knee-high jog with figure-eight arms

Log jump, side to side

Crossover knees

Flutter kick

Knee-high jog with hand waves

Log jump, forward and back

Crossover step

Star flutter kick

Knee-high jog with wrist circles

Mermaid

Crossover step 3× and half turn

Swirl

Stretch: pectorals, upper back, latissimus dorsi,
hip flexors, hamstrings, outer thigh

▶ **Deep-Water Strength Training 2**

INERTIA
AND FRONTAL RESISTANCE

EQUIPMENT
Deep-water belts

TEACHING TIP
Changing movement or direction frequently is harder
than continuing with the same move. This lesson plan
pairs two upper-body exercises, such as breaststroke
and reverse breaststroke, alternating back and forth
between them to increase resistance. It does the same

with two lower-body exercises, such as kick forward (see figure 7.39) and skate kick (see figure 7.40). In a pyramid, you perform one exercise 8× and then its pair 8×, then 4×, then 2×, and you finally alternate one of each exercise.

WARM-UP
Instructor's choice

A SET
Knee-high jog with reverse breaststroke

Knee-high jog with breast-stroke

Kick forward

Skate kick

Knee-high jog with reverse breaststroke and breaststroke, pyramid 8×, 4×, 2×, 1×

Kick forward and skate kick, pyramid 8×, 4×, 2×, 1×

Knee-high jog with R shoulder sweep in, travel sideways R

Knee-high jog with L shoulder sweep in, travel sideways L

Kick forward, travel backward

Skate kick, travel forward

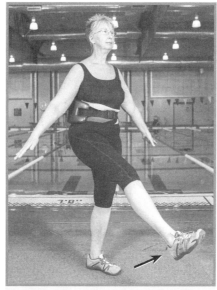

FIGURE 7.39 **Kick forward.**

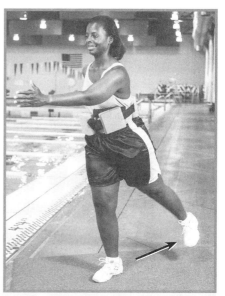

FIGURE 7.40 **Skate kick.**

B SET
Knee-high jog with double-arm press-down

Knee-high jog with lat pull-down

Cross-country ski

Jumping jacks

Knee-high jog with double-arm press-down and lat pull-down, pyramid 8×, 4×, 2×, 1×

Cross-country ski and jumping jacks, pyramid 8×, 4×, 2×, 1×

Knee-high jog with lat pull-down R, travel sideways R

Knee-high jog with lat pull-down L, travel sideways L

Cross-country ski, travel backward

Jumping jacks, clap hands, travel forward

C SET
Knee-high jog with unison push forward

Knee-high jog with standing row

Inner-thigh lift

Hopscotch

Knee-high jog with unison push forward and standing row, pyramid 8×, 4×, 2×, 1×

Inner-thigh lift and hopscotch, pyramid 8×, 4×, 2×, 1×

Knee-high jog with unison push forward, travel backward

Knee-high jog with standing row, travel forward

Inner-thigh lift, travel backward

Hopscotch, travel forward

D SET
Knee-high jog with arm curl

Knee-high jog with triceps extension

R quad kick

L quad kick

Skateboard R

Skateboard L

Knee-high jog with arm curl and triceps extension, pyramid 8×, 4×, 2×, 1×

R quad kick and skateboard R, pyramid 8×, 4×, 2×, 1×

L quad kick and skateboard L, pyramid 8×, 4×, 2×, 1×

Knee-high jog with propeller scull, travel backward

Knee-high jog with triceps kickback, travel forward

Cossack kick with sidestroke, travel sideways R and L

E SET

Bicycle R leg, travel forward

Bicycle L leg, travel forward

Bicycle 3× and hold

Log jump, side to side

Bicycle, side lying R, circle clockwise

Side-to-side extension

Bicycle, side lying L, circle counterclockwise

Tuck and hold sidesaddle R with reverse breast-stroke, travel backward

Tuck and hold sidesaddle L with breaststroke, travel forward

Seated swirl

Stretch: shoulders, pectorals, latissimus dorsi, quadriceps, gastrocnemius, hamstrings

▶ Deep-Water Strength Training 3

ACCELERATION 1

EQUIPMENT

Deep-water belts

TEACHING TIP

Acceleration, the primary means for overloading the muscles in the water, means pushing or pulling hard or applying force against the water's resistance. For example, reach forward and then pull hard in a standing row (see figure 7.41). Apply force when the leg kicks forward (see figure 7.42). Remind your participants to maintain their range of motion as they accelerate with their arms and legs and then to pause briefly before returning to the starting position.

WARM-UP

Instructor's choice

A SET

Knee-high jog with shoulder blade squeeze

Knee-high jog with standing row

Knee-high jog with arm lift to the sides, elbows bent

Cross-country ski with unison arm swing

Cross-country ski, clap hands (emphasize posterior deltoids)

Knee-high jog, one lap

B SET

Jumping jacks (emphasize latissimus dorsi)

Jumping jacks, palms touch in back

Knee-high jog, clap hands

Cross-country ski, clap hands (emphasize pectorals)

Knee-high jog with forearm press

Knee-high jog, one lap

C SET

Cross-country ski with forearm press, side to side

Knee-high jog with arm curl

Jumping jacks, open and close doors

Knee-high jog with jog press

Cross-country ski, push forward

Knee-high jog, one lap

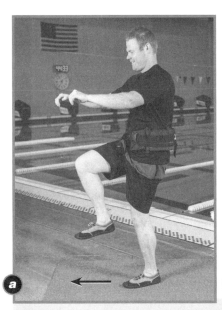
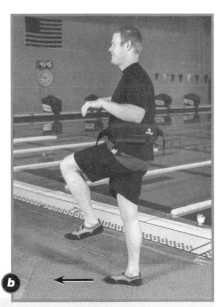

FIGURE 7.41 **Standing row: (a) start and (b) finish.**

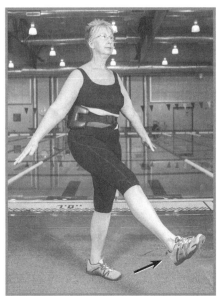

FIGURE 7.42 **Kick forward.**

D SET

Run to the ropes and run to the wall

Breaststroke with feet on the wall

Run to the ropes and run to the wall

Reverse breaststroke in a kneeling position with back to the wall

E SET

Knee-high jog with scull

Knee lift, straighten and power press-down

Cross-country ski with scull

R leg kicks side

L leg kicks side

Knee-high jog, one lap

F SET

Jumping jacks with scull

Jacks cross with scull

Mini cross with scull

Heel jog with scull

Knee-high jog, one lap

G SET

Bicycle with scull

R quad kick with scull

L quad kick with scull

Cossack kick with scull

Flutter kick, point and flex feet, with scull

Knee-high jog, one lap

H SET

Run to the ropes and run to the wall

Push off the wall with both feet and run back

Run to the ropes and run to the wall

Cross-country ski with back to the wall, heels tap the wall

I SET

Knee-high jog with resistor arms, travel forward

Knee-high jog with R arm press-down and L hand on hip, travel forward

Knee-high jog with L arm press-down and R hand on hip, travel forward

Bicycle R leg with breaststroke, travel forward

Bicycle L leg with breaststroke, travel forward

Crossover step

Crossover kick

Skate kick, crossover kick, sweep out and center

Swirl

Stretch: pectorals, upper back, triceps, lower back, hamstrings, outer thigh, hip flexors

▶ Deep-Water Strength Training 4

ACCELERATION 2

EQUIPMENT

Deep-water belts

TEACHING TIP

In deep water, participants' feet do not touch the floor, so they have to use acceleration to assist them in traveling. This lesson plan uses all the muscles of the upper and lower body to travel backward, forward, and sideways. An example is using the pectoralis major with a shoulder sweep in (see figure 7.43) to travel sideways. To knee-high jog in a bowtie pattern in I set, first jog with propeller scull to travel backward and then jog diagonally to the front R corner; jog with propeller scull to travel backward again and then jog diagonally to the front L corner.

WARM-UP

Instructor's choice

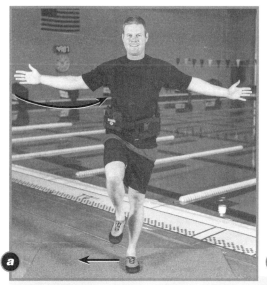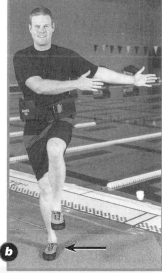

FIGURE 7.43 **Right shoulder sweep in: (*a*) start and (*b*) finish, travel sideways R.**

A SET

Knee-high jog with jog press

Straddle jog with shoulder blade squeeze

Run tires, reach side to side

Inner-thigh lift

Hopscotch

Jumping jacks

Jacks tuck

Tuck ski

Cross-country ski

B SET

Knee-high jog with propeller scull, travel backward

Knee-high jog with standing row, travel forward

Knee-high jog with propeller scull, travel backward

Knee-high jog with crawl stroke, travel forward

Knee-high jog with unison arm swing, travel backward and forward

C SET

Knee-high jog with L shoulder sweep out, travel sideways R

Knee-high jog with R shoulder sweep out, travel sideways L

Knee-high jog with propeller scull, travel backward

Knee-high jog with double-arm press-down, travel forward

Jumping jacks, travel sideways R and L

D SET

Knee-high jog, clap hands, travel backward

Power run

Knee-high jog with R shoulder sweep in, travel sideways R

Knee-high jog with L shoulder sweep in, travel sideways L

Knee-high jog with propeller scull, travel backward

Knee-high jog with forearm press out, travel forward

E SET

Knee-high jog with R side arm curl, travel sideways R

Knee-high jog with L side arm curl, travel sideways L

Knee-high jog with propeller scull, travel backward

Knee-high jog with triceps kickback, travel forward

Knee-high jog, push forward, travel backward

Power run

F SET

High kick, travel backward and forward

Jumping jacks, travel sideways R and L

Bent-knee jacks, travel backward and forward

G SET

Knee-high jog with propeller scull, travel backward

Skateboard R with breaststroke pull, travel forward

Knee-high jog with propeller scull, travel backward

Skateboard L with breaststroke pull, travel forward

Knee-high jog with propeller scull, travel backward

Bicycle with no arms, travel forward

Cossack kick with sidestroke, travel sideways R and L

H SET

Cross-country ski

Tuck ski

Jacks tuck

Jumping jacks

Hopscotch

Inner-thigh lift

Run tires, reach side to side

Straddle jog with shoulder blade squeeze

Knee-high jog with jog press

I SET

Crossover step

Knee-high jog

Knee-high jog, diagonal, travel sideways R and L

Knee-high jog, side lying, travel sideways R and L

Knee-high jog, travel in a bowtie pattern

Mermaid, circle clockwise and counterclockwise

Stretch: pectorals, upper back, triceps, lower back, hamstrings, outer thigh, hip flexors

► Deep-Water Strength Training 5
ͭ BUOYANT EQUIPMENT—NOODLES
PF

EQUIPMENT
Deep-water belts, noodles (figure 7.44)

TEACHING TIP
A noodle can be used as a piece of resistance equipment either held in the hands or placed under the foot. Perform 8 to 15 reps of each exercise, depending on the fitness level of your class. Use the noodle for support while performing the plank and side plank. In plank scissors, one leg is hyperextended and held for a few seconds. In side plank pliers, the top leg is abducted and held for a few seconds. If participants have shoulder issues, offer them the option to perform the exercises without equipment. These noodle exercises are a sampling and not a complete list of every possible noodle exercise.

WARM-UP
Knee-high jog with jog press

Jacks tuck

Seated kick

Tuck ski

Cross-country ski with knees bent 90 degrees

A SET
Knee-high jog with standing row, palms flat

Knee-high jog with breaststroke, palms flat

Cross-country ski

Jumping jacks

Knee-high jog with reverse breaststroke, palms flat

Knee-high jog with forearm press

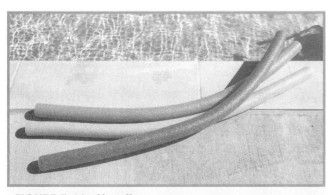

FIGURE 7.44   **Noodles.**

Knee-high jog with jog press

Skate kick with pumping arms

Jumping jacks

Bicycle with scull

Seated kick

B SET
Knee-high jog with propeller scull, travel backward

Tuck and hold with seated row, travel forward

Knee-high jog with propeller scull, travel backward

Tuck and hold with breaststroke, travel forward

Tuck and hold with unison arm swing, scoop forward, travel backward

Tuck and hold with unison arm swing, pressdown, travel forward

Tuck and hold with lat pull-down with elevation

Tuck and hold with reverse breaststroke, travel backward

Tuck and hold with forearm press, travel forward

Tuck and hold with triceps extension with elevation

Knee-high jog with propeller scull, travel backward

Skate kick, hands behind back, travel forward

Bent-knee jacks, emphasize in, travel backward

Bent-knee jacks, emphasize out, travel forward

Bicycle with propeller scull, travel backward

Bicycle, no hands, travel forward

Seated kick, toes pointed, travel backward

Seated kick, feet flexed, travel forward

C SET
(Noodle in hands)

Knee-high jog with standing row

Knee-high jog with double-arm press-down

Cross-country ski, noodle in L hand, travel sideways R

Cross-country ski, noodle in R hand, travel sideways L

Knee-high jog with lat pull-down, noodle in L hand, travel sideways R

Knee-high jog with lat pull-down, noodle in R hand, travel sideways L

Jumping jacks, touch ends in front

Jumping jacks with forearm press, noodle in back

Cross-country ski, push ends forward

Straddle jog with triceps extension

Knee-high jog, plunge L, travel sideways R

Knee-high jog, plunge R, travel sideways L

D SET

(Foot on a noodle)

Hip extension R

Hip extension L

Standing leg press R

Standing leg press L

Standing leg press to R side

Standing leg press to L side

E SET

(Sit on noodle like a swing)

Seated jacks

Seated kick

Seated kick with L shoulder sweep out, circle clockwise

Seated kick with R shoulder sweep out, circle counterclockwise

Point and flex feet

Hip hike

(Noodle in posterior sling)

Lower-body twist

(Noodle under knees)

Crunch, V position

(Noodle in hands under shoulder)

Plank

Plank scissors

Side plank R, noodle in R hand

Side plank pliers R

Side plank L, noodle in L hand

Side plank pliers L

Stretch: Swirl, pectorals, upper back, triceps, hamstrings, outer thigh, quadriceps

▶ Deep-Water Strength Training 6

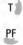

BUOYANT EQUIPMENT— DUMBBELLS

EQUIPMENT

Deep-water belts, dumbbells

TEACHING TIP

Buoyant dumbbells come in a variety of sizes (figure 7.45). The bigger the dumbbell is, the greater the resistance is. Start with the smaller size first. Make sure that participants are able to perform the exercises with the spine in neutral alignment before progressing to the next larger size. If participants have shoulder issues, offer them the option to perform the exercises without dumbbells. This lesson plan has three sets of strength-training exercises for the major muscle groups. Participants perform the first set slowly, the second set with power (acceleration), and the third set with buoyant dumbbells. Have them relax the shoulders and stretch the fingers after each dumbbell set. They should perform 8 to 15 reps of each exercise, depending on their fitness. Dumbbells work well for upper-body exercises, for stability during exercises for the abdominals and obliques, and in support of the plank position, but not for most leg exercises. Therefore, use acceleration to increase the intensity of the leg exercises. These dumbbell exercises are a sampling, not a complete list of every possible dumbbell exercise.

WARM-UP

Instructor's choice

A SET

Knee-high jog, clap hands, slow

Knee-high jog with scull

Knee-high jog, clap hands with power

Knee-high jog with scull

(With dumbbells) chest fly at 45-degree angle with flutter kick

Skateboard R with breaststroke pull, travel forward

Skateboard L with breaststroke pull, travel forward

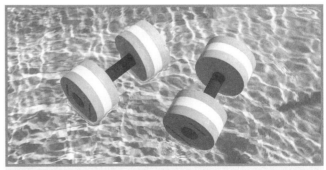

FIGURE 7.45 Dumbbells.

B SET

Cross-country ski with arm swing, slow

Knee-high jog with scull

Cross-country ski with unison arm swing with power

Knee-high jog with scull

(With dumbbells) cross-country ski with arm swing

Over the barrel, travel sideways R and L

C SET

Jumping jacks with lat pull-down, slow

Knee-high jog with scull

Jumping jacks with lat pull-down with power

Knee-high jog with scull

(With dumbbells) jumping jacks with lat pull-down

Knee-high jog, one lap

D SET

Straddle jog with triceps extension, slow

Knee-high jog with scull

Straddle jog with triceps extension with power

Knee-high jog with scull

(With dumbbells) straddle jog with triceps extension

Knee-high jog with sidestroke, travel sideways R and L

E SET

R knee swings forward and back

L knee swings forward and back

Knee-high jog with scull

R leg kicks forward and back

L leg kicks forward and back

Knee-high jog with scull

Cross-country ski with power

Power run, one lap

F SET

Clamshells R, slow

Clamshells L, slow

Knee-high jog with scull

Bent-knee jacks

Knee-high jog with scull

Frog kick with power

Knee-high jog with sidestroke, travel sideways R and L

G SET

Dog hike R

Dog hike L

Knee-high jog with scull

R leg kicks side

L leg kicks side

Knee-high jog with scull

Jacks cross with power

Knee-high jog, one lap

H SET

(With dumbbells) crunch, V position, slow

Knee-high jog with scull

(With dumbbells) abdominal pike

Knee-high jog with scull

(With dumbbells) abdominal pike and spine extension

Over the barrel, travel sideways R and L

I SET

(With dumbbells) side-to-side extension, slow

Knee-high jog with scull

(With dumbbells) side-to-side extension, faster

Knee-high jog with scull

(With dumbbells) side-to-side extension with legs in a diamond position

Skateboard R with breaststroke pull, travel forward

Skateboard L with breaststroke pull, travel forward

J SET

R leg lift with double-arm lift and hold

L leg lift with double-arm lift and hold

R leg lift side with arm lift to sides and hold

L leg lift side with arm lift to sides and hold

Clamshells R with shoulder sweep out and hold

Clamshells L with shoulder sweep out and hold

R hamstring curl with arm curl and hold

L hamstring curl with arm curl and hold

R knee lift, look L

L knee lift, look R

Stretch: pectorals, triceps, lower back, hamstrings, inner thigh, outer thigh

▶ **Deep-Water Strength Training 7**

PF

BUOYANT EQUIPMENT— DUMBBELLS (CONCENTRIC AND ECCENTRIC CONTRACTIONS)

EQUIPMENT
Deep-water belts, dumbbells

TEACHING TIP
Buoyant equipment can be used to target eccentric contractions by slowing down the dumbbells' return to the surface of the water. The muscles have to maintain their tension as they lengthen. In this lesson plan, three sets using dumbbells are performed for the targeted muscle groups. Participants perform the first set at a steady pace, the second set faster, and the third set fast during the concentric phase and slow during the eccentric phase. Have them relax the shoulders and stretch the fingers after each dumbbell set. They should perform 8 to 15 reps of each exercise, depending on their fitness. If participants have shoulder issues, offer them the option to perform the exercises without dumbbells. The upper-body sets are separated by leg exercises, using the dumbbells as stabilizers. Participants let them float on the surface of the water, keeping a loose grip on the bars and the shoulders relaxed. The last leg exercise of the set uses acceleration to increase the intensity. Cross the dumbbells and let them float on the water during this exercise. Dumbbells should not be used continuously for an entire class, so schedule a short break after the first two dumbbell sets and a long break after the fourth dumbbell set. Participants then pick up the dumbbells again for the abdominal exercises. These dumbbell exercises are a sampling, not a complete list of every possible dumbbell exercise.

WARM-UP
Instructor's choice

A SET
(With dumbbells)
Chest fly at 45-degree angle, with flutter kick
Cross-country ski with dumbbells as stabilizers
Chest fly, faster, at 45-degree angle, with flutter kick
Cross-country ski, faster, with dumbbells as stabilizers
Chest fly at 45-degree angle, fast concentric and slow eccentric, with flutter kick

Cross-country ski with elevation, no dumbbells

B SET
(With dumbbells)
Jumping jacks with lat pull-down
Bent-knee jacks with dumbbells as stabilizers
Jumping jacks with lat pull-down, faster
Bent-knee jacks, faster, with dumbbells as stabilizers
Jumping jacks with lat pull-down, fast concentric and slow eccentric
Frog kick with elevation, no dumbbells

C SET
Knee-high jog, one lap
Power run, one lap
Cross-country ski, one lap
Bicycle, one lap

D SET
(With dumbbells)
Cross-country ski with arm swing
Seated kick with dumbbells as stabilizers
Cross-country ski with arm swing, faster
Seated kick, faster, with dumbbells as stabilizers
Cross-country ski with arm swing, fast and slow, alternate
Mermaid with power, no dumbbells

E SET
(With dumbbells)
Straddle jog with triceps extension
Jumping jacks with dumbbells as stabilizers
Straddle jog with triceps extension, faster
Jumping jacks, faster, with dumbbells as stabilizers
Straddle jog with triceps extension, fast concentric and slow eccentric
Frog kick with elevation, no dumbbells

F SET
Knee-high jog, one lap
Power run, one lap
Cross-country ski, one lap
Bicycle, one lap

G SET
Cross-country ski with elevation
Tuck ski together
Tuck ski

Jacks cross
Jumping jacks
Jacks tuck
High kick
Kick forward
Flutter kick
Breaststroke kick
Frog kick
Cossack kick

H SET

Knee-high jog, one lap
Power run, one lap
Cross-country ski, one lap
Bicycle, one lap

I SET

(With dumbbells)
Abdominal pike and spine extension
Side-to-side extension
Plank
Side plank R
Side plank L
Stretch: pectorals, latissimus dorsi, triceps, hamstrings, outer thigh, quadriceps

▶ **Deep-Water Strength Training 8**

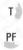

DRAG EQUIPMENT— WEBBED GLOVES

EQUIPMENT

Deep-water belts, webbed gloves

TEACHING TIP

Webbed gloves are one of the most popular pieces of resistance equipment (see figure 7.46). Participants are able to adjust the resistance by slicing through the water (see figure 7.47a), making a fist (see figure 7.47b), or opening out the hands (see figure 7.47c). They can focus on individual muscles by opening up the hand when the targeted muscle is contracting and then slicing to return to the starting position. Webbed gloves are so comfortable that experienced participants may wish to wear them during all of their classes except when they are using other handheld equipment. Participants with shoulder issues may choose to perform the exercises without webbed gloves. In this lesson plan, arm exercises alternate with leg exercises performed while sculling so that the upper-body muscles can rest between sets. The lesson plan concludes with some modified square dance moves just for fun. These exercises are a sampling, not a complete list of every possible exercise with webbed gloves.

WARM-UP

Instructor's choice

A SET

Knee-high jog, clap hands, sweep out and slice in
Flutter kick with scull
Knee-high jog, clap hands, sweep in and slice out
Flutter kick with scull
Knee-high jog, clap hands, faster
Flutter kick with scull

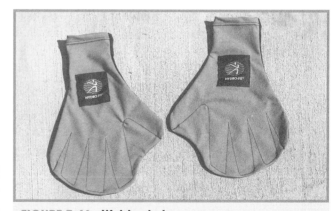

FIGURE 7.46 **Webbed gloves.**

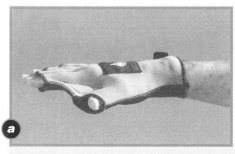 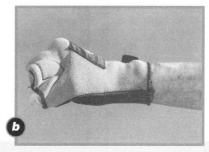 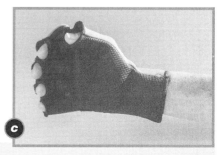

FIGURE 7.47 (*a*) slice, (*b*) fist, (*c*) open hand.

B SET

Cross-country ski with arm swing, scoop back and slice forward

Bicycle with scull

Cross-country ski with arm swing, scoop forward and slice back

Bicycle with scull

Cross-country ski with unison arm swing, palms face direction of motion, faster

Bicycle with scull

C SET

Jumping jacks with lat pull-down and slice up

Knee-high jog with scull

Jumping jacks with arm lift to sides and slice down

Knee-high jog with scull

Jumping jacks, faster

Knee-high jog with scull

D SET

Straddle jog with triceps extension and slice up

Jacks tuck

Straddle jog with arm curl and slice down

Jacks tuck

Straddle jog with arm curl, palms face direction of motion, faster

Jacks tuck

E SET

Clamshells R

Flutter kick with scull

Clamshells L

Flutter kick with scull

Bent-knee jacks, faster

Flutter kick with scull

F SET

R leg kicks forward and back

Bicycle with scull

L leg kicks forward and back

Bicycle with scull

Cross-country ski, faster

Bicycle with scull

G SET

Jumping jacks (emphasize abduction)

Knee-high jog with scull

Jumping jacks (emphasize adduction)

Knee-high jog with scull

Jacks cross, faster

Knee-high jog with scull

H SET

R quad kick

Jacks tuck

L quad kick

Jacks tuck

Seated kick, faster

Jacks tuck

I SET

Flutter kick, point and flex R foot

Abdominal pike

Flutter kick, point and flex L foot

Abdominal pike

Flutter kick point and flex feet, faster

Abdominal pike

J SET

(Square dance: Divide class into two lines facing each other. If you have an odd number of class participants, you will need to participate so that no one is left out.)

Partners run forward, shake R hands, and return

Partners run forward, shake L hands, and return

Partners run forward, do sa do, and return

Partners run forward, high-five, and return

Partners run forward, swing their partner R, and return

Partners run forward, swing their partner L, and return

Promenade (partners at the head of the two lines run forward and then run through the lines to the end; the other partners follow)

Stretch: pectorals, upper back, latissimus dorsi, outer thigh, hamstrings, hip flexors

▶ **Deep-Water Strength Training 9**

DRAG EQUIPMENT— MULTIPLANE DRAG EQUIPMENT

EQUIPMENT

Deep-water belts, multiplane drag equipment

TEACHING TIP

Not all multiplane drag equipment is appropriate for use in deep water. Choose a style that floats and will not sink to the bottom of the pool (see figure 7.48). The resistance should not be so great that the participant is unable to maintain proper alignment while using it. If there are participants with shoulder issues, offer them the option to perform the exercises without equipment. Usually, we think of strength training in terms of flexion and extension in the sagittal plane or abduction and adduction in the frontal plane. Including some exercises in diagonal patterns as well is beneficial (see figure 7.49). These multiplane drag equipment exercises are a sampling, not a complete list of every possible exercise with multiplane drag equipment.

WARM-UP

Instructor's choice

A SET

Knee-high jog with jog press

Run tires with scull

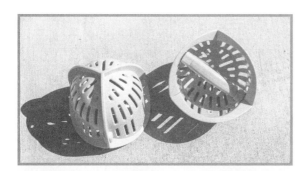

FIGURE 7.48 **Multiplane drag equipment**

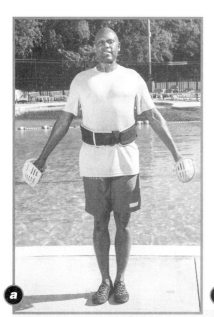
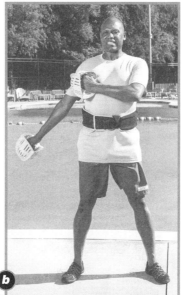

FIGURE 7.49 **(a) jumping jacks, (b) bring L arm across to R shoulder.**

Inner-thigh lift

Hopscotch

Jumping jacks

Jumping jacks with diagonal turn

Cross-country ski

Cross-country ski with rotation

B SET

(With multiplane drag equipment)

Straddle jog with chest fly

Cross-country ski

Straddle jog with chest fly, faster

Cross-country ski, faster

Jumping jacks with lat pull-down

Jumping jacks with lat pull-down, faster

Straddle jog, R shoulder sweep out

Straddle jog, L shoulder sweep out

C SET

Knee-high jog with jog press

Run tires with scull

Inner-thigh lift

Hopscotch

Jumping jacks

Jumping jacks with diagonal turn

Cross-country ski

Cross-country ski with rotation

D SET

(With multiplane drag equipment)

Knee-high jog, push forward R arm

Knee-high jog, push forward L arm

Knee-high jog, push forward R arm and L arm, alternate

Knee-high jog, unison push forward

Knee-high jog, pronate and supinate

E SET

(With multiplane drag equipment)

Jumping jacks, arms down at sides, bring R arm across to L shoulder

Jumping jacks, arms down at sides, bring L arm across to R shoulder

Jumping jacks, arms to sides 70 degrees, bring R arm down to L hip

Jumping jacks, arms to sides 70 degrees, bring L arm down to R hip

Inner-thigh lift R

Inner-thigh lift L
Jumping jacks with arm curl
Jumping jacks with triceps extension
Jumping jacks with forearm press
Inner-thigh lift

F SET

Knee-high jog with jog press
Run tires with scull
Inner-thigh lift
Hopscotch
Jumping jacks
Jumping jacks with diagonal turn
Cross-country ski
Cross-country ski with rotation

G SET

(With multiplane drag equipment)
Cross-country ski with R arm only
Cross-country ski with L arm only
Jumping jacks with R arm only
Jumping jacks with L arm only
Run one lap with resistor arms

H SET

Knee-high jog with jog press
Run tires with scull
Inner-thigh lift
Hopscotch
Jumping jacks
Jumping jacks with diagonal turn
Cross-country ski
Cross-country ski with rotation

I SET

(With multiplane drag equipment)
R knee lift with lat pull-down R
L knee lift with lat pull-down L
R knee lift with lat pull-down R and L knee lift
    with lat pull-down L, alternate
Tuck and hold, bring drag equipment together in
    front
Tuck and hold with lat pull-down
R leg lift, reach L arm forward
L leg lift, reach R arm forward
T-hang, pulse drag equipment down gently
Stretch: pectorals, upper back, latissimus dorsi,
    triceps, shoulders, gastrocnemius

▶ Deep-Water Strength Training 10

RUBBERIZED EQUIPMENT— BANDS (CONCENTRIC AND ECCENTRIC CONTRACTIONS)

EQUIPMENT

Deep-water belts, bands (see figure 7.50)

TEACHING TIP

Rubberized equipment is popular in land-based training and is now being used in the pool as well. The rubberized equipment used in the gym deteriorates quickly in chlorine, but manufacturers now make chlorine-resistant bands and loops specifically for use in the pool. The bands must be anchored to something, usually another body part, and the resistance is in the direction away from the anchor. Although putting a foot on a band or wrapping a loop around the ankles is possible, some participants may find it difficult or impossible to do that in deep water. The exercises in this lesson plan anchor the bands in ways that most participants are able to accomplish, such as bowstring pull (see figure 7.51), single arm press-down (see figure 7.52), arm lift to sides (see figure 7.53), and elbow sweep out (see figure 7.54). The lesson plan includes three sets of exercises for each muscle group. The first set is without equipment. The second set uses the bands. The third set adds a pause and a slow return to focus on eccentric muscle actions. If participants have shoulder issues, offer them the option to perform the exercises without bands. These band exercises are a sampling, not a complete list of every possible exercise with rubberized equipment.

WARM-UP

Knee-high jog
Tuck ski
Jacks tuck

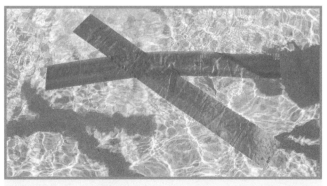

FIGURE 7.50 Bands.

Seated kick

Bent-knee jacks

A SET

Cross-country ski with R bowstring pull

Cross-country ski with L bowstring pull

Jumping jacks with double-arm press-down

Cross-country ski, push forward

Jumping jacks with power arms

Cross-country ski with alternating arm curl

Jumping jacks, open and close doors

Cross-country ski with forearm press side to side

B SET

Knee-high jog with propeller scull, travel backward and forward

Cross-country ski, travel backward and forward

Jumping jacks, clap hands, travel backward and forward

Seated kick, travel backward and forward

Clamshells R

Clamshells L

C SET

(With band)

Cross-country ski with R bowstring pull

Cross-country ski with L bowstring pull

Knee-high jog with R arm press-down

Knee-high jog with L arm press-down

Jumping jacks with chest press, band behind back

Seated kick with arm lift to sides, band under knees

Seated kick with arm curl, band under knees

Jumping jacks with R elbow sweep out

Jumping jacks with L elbow sweep out

Jumping jacks with forearm press out

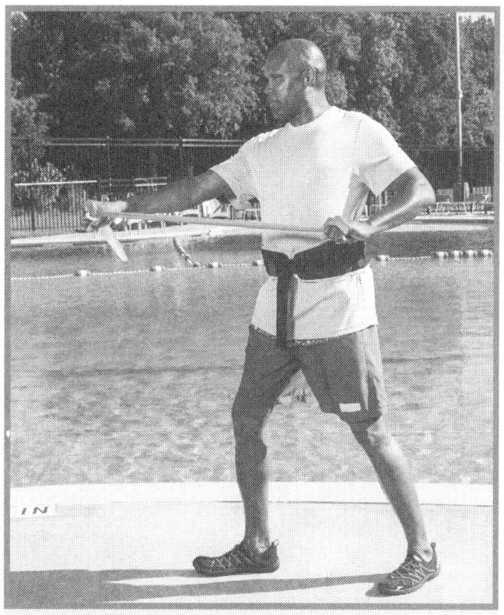

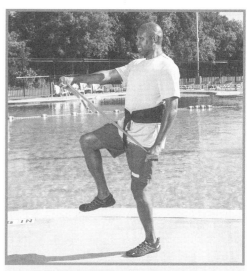

FIGURE 7.51   **Bowstring pull.**

FIGURE 7.52   **L arm press-down.**

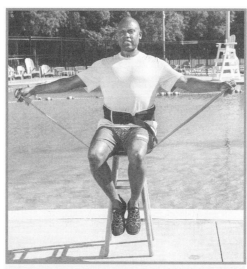

FIGURE 7.53   **Arm lift to sides.**

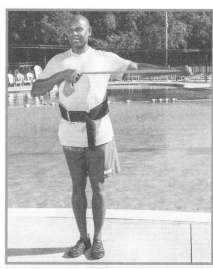

FIGURE 7.54   **L elbow sweep out.**

D SET

Knee-high jog with R shoulder sweep in, travel sideways R

Knee-high jog with L shoulder sweep in, travel sideways L

Cross-country ski with unison sidestroke, travel sideways R and L

Jumping jacks, travel sideways R and L

Cossack kick with sidestroke, travel sideways R and L

Clamshells R

Clamshells L

E SET

(With band, pause at the end range of motion, slow return)

Cross-country ski with R bowstring pull

Cross-country ski with L bowstring pull

Knee-high jog with R arm press-down

Knee-high jog with L arm press-down

Jumping jacks with chest press, band behind back

Seated kick with arm lift to sides, band under knees

Seated kick with arm curl, band under knees

Jumping jacks with R elbow sweep out

Jumping jacks with L elbow sweep out

Jumping jacks with forearm press out

F SET

Knee-high jog with quarter turn

Tuck ski with quarter turn

Jacks tuck with quarter turn

Mermaid, circle clockwise

Swirl in a yoga tree pose R

Swirl in a yoga tree pose L

G SET

Reverse bicycle, R leg with reverse breaststroke, travel backward

Skateboard R with breaststroke pull, travel forward

Reverse bicycle, L leg with reverse breaststroke, travel backward

Skateboard L with breaststroke pull, travel forward

Knee-high jog with propeller scull, travel backward

Bicycle, tandem, travel forward

Knee lift, straighten and power press-down R

Knee lift, straighten and power press-down L

Stretch: pectorals, upper back, latissimus dorsi, triceps, shoulders, hamstrings, hip flexors

▶ Deep-Water Strength Training 11

CIRCUIT CLASS 1

EQUIPMENT

Deep-water belts, bands (figure 7.55), noodles (figure 7.56)

TEACHING TIP

This circuit class gives participants the opportunity to use bands for the upper body and noodles for the

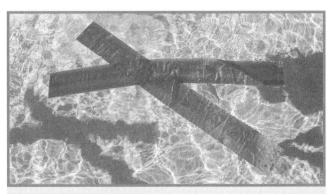

FIGURE 7.55 **Bands.**

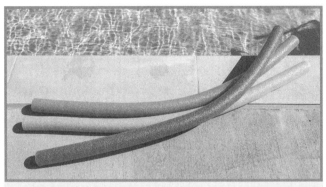

FIGURE 7.56 **Noodles.**

lower body and abdominal and obliques exercises. Have the participants do three sets of strength-training exercises for each targeted muscle group. Participants perform the first set slowly, the second set with power (acceleration), and the third set with equipment. If participants have shoulder issues, offer them the option to perform the exercises without equipment.

WARM-UP

Instructor's choice

A SET

Jumping jacks with shoulder blade squeeze, slow

Knee-high jog with scull

Jumping jacks with shoulder blade squeeze with power

Knee-high jog with scull

(With band) jumping jacks with bowstring pull to the R side

(With band) jumping jacks with bowstring pull to the L side

Skateboard R with breaststroke pull, travel forward

Skateboard L with breaststroke pull, travel forward

B SET

Jumping jacks with arm lift to sides, slow

Knee-high jog with scull

Jumping jacks with arm lift to sides with elbows bent, with power

Knee-high jog with scull

(With band) seated kick with arm lift to sides, band under knees

Over the barrel, travel sideways R and L

C SET

Jumping jacks with forearm press, slow

Knee-high jog with scull

Jumping jacks with forearm press with power

Knee-high jog with scull

(With band) jumping jacks with forearm press out

Knee-high jog, one lap

D SET

Seated leg press, slow

Knee-high jog with scull

Seated leg press with power

Knee-high jog with scull

(Foot on a noodle) standing leg press R

(Foot on a noodle) standing leg press L

Knee-high jog with sidestroke, travel sideways R and L

E SET

R quad kick, slow

L quad kick, slow

Knee-high jog with scull

R quad kick with power

L quad kick with power

Knee-high jog with scull

(Sit on noodle like a swing) seated kick

Power run, one lap

F SET

Clamshells R, slow

Clamshells L, slow

Knee-high jog with scull

Clamshells R with power

Clamshells L with power

Knee-high jog with scull

(Foot on a noodle) standing leg press to R side

(Foot on a noodle) standing leg press to L side

Knee-high jog with sidestroke, travel sideways R and L

G SET

Flutter kick, point and flex feet, slow

Knee-high jog with scull

Flutter kick, point and flex feet with power

Knee-high jog with scull

(Sit on a noodle like a swing) point and flex feet, alternate R and L

Knee-high jog, one lap

H SET

(Noodle under knees) crunch, slow

Knee-high jog with scull

(Noodle under knees) crunch, slower

Knee-high jog with scull

(Noodle in hands on surface of water) abdominal pike and spine extension

Over the barrel, travel sideways R and L

I SET

Swirl

Knee-high jog with scull

Seated swirl, pulse R 2× and L 2×

Knee-high jog with scull

(Straddle noodle and squeeze between thighs) seated swirl

Skateboard R with breaststroke pull, travel forward

Skateboard L with breaststroke pull, travel forward

J SET

Jacks tuck with reverse breaststroke, travel backward

Inner-thigh lift

Jacks tuck with breaststroke, travel forward

Cross-country ski and hold R with reverse breaststroke, travel backward

Helicopter ski

Cross-country ski and hold L with breaststroke, travel forward

Tuck and hold sidesaddle R with forearm press, travel backward

Seated swirl

Tuck and hold sidesaddle L with forearm press, travel forward

Stretch: upper back, latissimus dorsi, hamstrings, outer thigh, quadriceps, gastrocnemius

▶ Deep-Water Strength Training 12

CIRCUIT CLASS 2

T
PF

EQUIPMENT

Ankle cuffs (figure 7.57) or deep-water belts, webbed gloves (figure 7.58), multiplane drag equipment (figure 7.59)

TEACHING TIP

This circuit class uses ankle cuffs to add resistance for the lower body. When using ankle cuffs, be careful to choose two-legged, balanced exercises in an upright position. One-legged exercises and diagonal positions may be difficult for some participants to perform in good alignment while wearing cuffs. Ankle cuffs come in two sizes, regular cuffs and minicuffs. Experienced participants may choose to use cuffs instead of flotation belts. Newer participants should use the minicuffs and a flotation belt or use the flotation belt alone. They attach the cuffs or the flotation belt before entering the water and wear them for the entire class. In addition to the cuffs, two types of drag equipment are used to add resistance for the upper body, webbed gloves and multiplane drag equipment. Figure 7.59 shows two types of multiplane drag equipment that work well in deep water. If participants have shoulder issues, offer them the option to perform the exercises without equipment.

WARM-UP

(With ankle cuffs)
  Knee-high jog
  Bicycle
  Flutter kick
  Jacks tuck
  Tuck ski
  Bicycle
  Knee-high jog

A SET

  Seated kick
  Bicycle
  Cross-country ski
  Jumping jacks
  Frog kick
  Cossack kick

B SET

(With webbed gloves)
  Knee-high jog with standing row

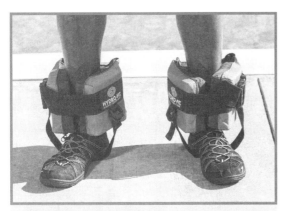

FIGURE 7.57 **Ankle cuffs.**

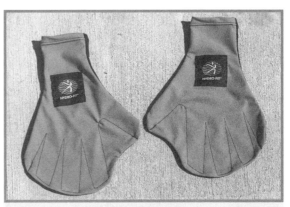

FIGURE 7.58 **Webbed gloves.**

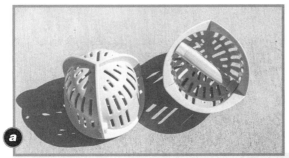

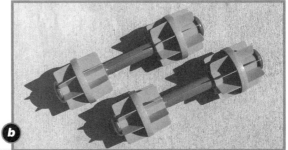

FIGURE 7.59 **(a) multiplane hand bells, (b) multiplane drag dumbbells.**

Straddle jog with double-arm press-down

Jumping jacks

Straddle jog, clap hands

Knee-high jog with R shoulder sweep in, travel sideways R

Knee-high jog with L shoulder sweep in, travel sideways L

Knee-high jog with L shoulder sweep out, travel sideways R

Knee-high jog with R shoulder sweep out, travel sideways L

Cross-country ski with forearm press side to side

Jumping jacks, open and close doors

Jumping jacks with arm curl, palms face direction of motion

C SET

Seated kick

Bicycle

Cross-country ski

Jumping jacks

Frog kick

Cossack kick

D SET

(With multiplane drag equipment)

Knee-high jog with standing row

Straddle jog with double-arm press-down

Jumping jacks

Straddle jog with chest fly

Knee-high jog with R shoulder sweep in, travel sideways R

Knee-high jog with L shoulder sweep in, travel sideways L

Knee-high jog with L shoulder sweep out, travel sideways R

Knee-high jog with R shoulder sweep out, travel sideways L

Cross-country ski with forearm press

Jumping jacks, open and close doors

Jumping jacks with triceps extension

E SET

Seated kick

Bicycle

Cross-country ski

Jumping jacks

Frog kick

Cossack kick

F SET

Seated kick

Tuck and hold R leg up with reverse breaststroke (see figure 7.60), travel backward

Tuck and hold with forearm press, travel forward

Seated kick

Tuck and hold L leg up with reverse breast-stroke, travel backward

Tuck and hold with forearm press, travel forward

Seated swirl

Cross-country ski

Cross-country ski and hold R with reverse breaststroke, travel backward

Cross-country ski and hold L with breaststroke, travel forward

Swirl

Bicycle

Reverse bicycle, travel backward

Bicycle, travel forward

Brace core, arms down, turbulent hand movements

Stretch: pectorals, shoulders, upper back, latissimus dorsi, triceps, hamstrings, hip flexors

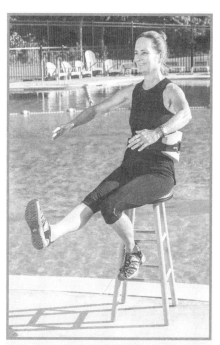

FIGURE 7.60 Hold R leg up with reverse breaststroke.

▶ **Deep-Water Strength Training 13**

FUNCTIONAL CORE STRENGTH

EQUIPMENT
Deep-water belts

TEACHING TIP
Functional core training involves practicing movements that allow people to perform the activities of daily life more easily. The exercises are designed to challenge the core in multiple planes to improve stability. This lesson plan challenges the core with one-arm moves and moves using no arms. When you use no arms, put the hands on the hips or abduct the arms 70 degrees and hold them there. You can also use one leg while keeping the other leg stable. Point and flex the feet to strengthen the ankles. Diagonal exercises, such as knee-high jog, diagonal (see figure 7.61) means leaning 45 degrees to the side while traveling sideways; be sure to maintain neutral alignment. Crossing the midline, such as with a crossover kick (see figure 7.62), also challenges the core. Traveling in a bowtie pattern involves traveling diagonally. Turning to a corner and jogging forward is not the same as traveling diagonally. Instead, continue to face forward while moving diagonally toward the corner. To make the bowtie, first travel backward, then travel diagonally to the R corner, travel backward again, and then travel diagonally to the L corner. The pattern can also be reversed: First, travel forward, then travel diagonally backward to the back R corner, travel forward again, and then travel diagonally backward to the back L corner.

WARM-UP
Instructor's choice

A SET
Knee-high jog with hands on hips

Flutter kick

Bicycle

Bicycle with R shoulder sweep in, travel sideways R

Bicycle with L shoulder sweep in, travel sideways L

Bicycle, diagonal, travel sideways R and L

Reverse bicycle, R leg with reverse breaststroke, travel backward

Bicycle R leg with breaststroke, travel forward

Flutter kick, point and flex feet

Reverse bicycle, L leg with reverse breaststroke, travel backward

Bicycle L leg with breaststroke, travel forward

Flutter kick with hands on hips

B SET
Knee-high jog with resistor arms, travel forward

Knee lift, straighten and power press-down

Crossover step

Straddle jog, clap hands, travel backward and forward

Over the barrel with arms to sides 70 degrees, travel sideways R and L

Knee-high jog, diagonal, travel sideways R and L

Knee-high jog with R arm press-down and L hand on hip, travel forward

Knee-high jog with L arm press-down and R hand on hip, travel forward

Knee-high jog, travel in a bowtie pattern

C SET
Skateboard R with breaststroke pull, travel forward

Skateboard L with breaststroke pull, travel forward

Cross-country ski

Cross-country ski with unison arm swing

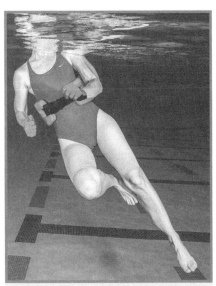

FIGURE 7.61 **Knee-high jog, diagonal.**

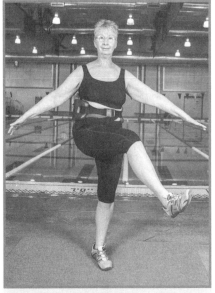

FIGURE 7.62 **Crossover kick.**

Cross-country ski with alternating sweep in, travel backward

Cross-country ski with alternating sweep out, travel forward

Tuck ski

Cross-country ski with rotation

Cross-country ski, arms sweep side to side

Tuck ski 3× and hold

Cross-country ski, diagonal, travel sideways R and L

Cross-country ski with forearm press

Crossover kick

Crossover kick and sweep out

Skate kick, crossover kick, sweep out and center

D SET

Jacks tuck

Jacks tuck with reverse breaststroke, travel backward

Inner-thigh lift

Jacks tuck with breaststroke, travel forward

Cross-country ski and hold R with reverse breaststroke, travel backward

Cross-country ski and hold L with breaststroke, travel forward

Seated kick with double-arm lift, travel backward

Seated kick with double-arm press-down, travel forward

Bent-knee jacks, travel backward

Tuck and hold sidesaddle R with forearm press, travel forward

Tuck and hold with reverse breaststroke, travel backward

Tuck and hold sidesaddle L with forearm press, travel forward

E SET

R leg kicks forward and back

L leg kicks forward and back

Clamshells R

Clamshells L

Tuck and hold with lat pull-down

Brace core, arms down, turbulent hand movements

Helicopter ski

Log jump, side to side

Bicycle, side lying R, circle clockwise

Bicycle, side lying L, circle counterclockwise

Side extension, tuck and pike, alternate R and L

Abdominal pike and spine extension

Log jump, forward and back

Seated swirl

Stretch: pectorals, upper back, lower back, hamstrings, hip flexors, neck

▶ Deep-Water Strength Training 14

BALANCE

EQUIPMENT

Deep-water belts, noodles

TEACHING TIP

One technique for improving balance is the unpredictable command. When your cues are unexpected, you help your participants learn to react. Quick reactions reduce the risk of falling. Unpredictable commands include performing an exercise with one arm and a different exercise with the other, using arm patterns that are not typical with a specific leg move such as performing jumping jacks with arm swing (see figure 7.63), changing direction at odd intervals, and traveling in one direction while looking in the opposite direction. You can increase the challenge by asking participants to do something mentally demanding while they exercise, such as counting or spelling backward or creating lists aloud. Noodle exercises are included at the end.

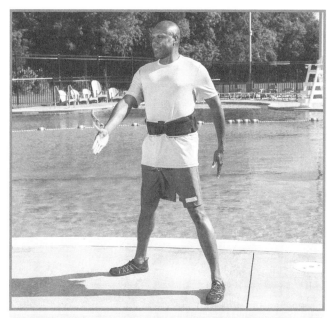

FIGURE 7.63 Jumping jacks with arm swing.

WARM-UP

Knee-high jog

Run tires

Inner-thigh lift

Jacks tuck

Tuck ski

Bicycle

Bicycle R leg

Bicycle L leg

A SET

Knee-high jog with propeller scull, travel backward and forward

Knee-high jog, diagonal, travel sideways R and L

Jumping jacks with R hand behind back

Jumping jacks with L hand behind back

Cross-country ski with R hand behind back

Cross-country ski with L hand behind back

Knee-high jog 3× and hold

Heel jog 3× and hold

R leg kicks forward and back

L leg kicks forward and back

B SET

Knee-high jog with R arm breaststroke and L arm crawl stroke

Knee-high jog with L arm breaststroke and R arm crawl stroke

Jumping jacks, R arm crosses in front and L arm crosses in back

Jumping jacks, L arm crosses in front and R arm crosses in back

Jumping jacks with arm swing

Cross-country ski with lat pull-down

Knee-high jog, travel backward, forward, and sideways with quick change of direction

R leg kicks side

L leg kicks side

C SET

(Travel in a bowtie pattern)

Knee-high jog with propeller scull, travel backward

Knee-high jog, travel diagonally to front R corner, look L

Knee-high jog with propeller scull, travel backward

Knee-high jog, travel diagonally to front L corner, look R

Over the barrel R, look L

Over the barrel L, look R

Jumping jacks, clap hands, travel backward

Cross-country ski, travel diagonally to front R corner

Jumping jacks, clap hands, travel backward

Cross-country ski, travel diagonally to front L corner

Knee-high jog with propeller scull, travel diagonally to back R corner

Knee-high jog, travel forward

Knee-high jog with propeller scull, travel diagonally to back L corner

Knee-high jog, travel forward

Clamshells R

Clamshells L

D SET

Knee-high jog, circle both thumbs clockwise

Knee-high jog, circle both thumbs counterclockwise

Jumping jacks 1×, inner-thigh lift 1×

Cross-country ski and tuck ski together, alternate

Helicopter ski

Knee-high jog, travel in a circle clockwise, look L

Knee-high jog, travel in a circle counterclockwise, look R

E SET

(With noodles)

Hip extension R, foot on a noodle

Hip extension L, foot on a noodle

Standing leg press R, foot on a noodle

Standing leg press L, foot on a noodle

Standing leg press to R side, foot on a noodle

Standing leg press to L side, foot on a noodle

Straddle noodle with front end between thighs

Raise and lower knees to find neutral spine

Reverse breaststroke, maintain neutral spine

Breaststroke, maintain neutral spine

Seated row, travel in a scatter pattern

Stretch: shoulders, upper back, lower back, outer thigh, quadriceps, gastrocnemius

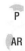

▶ Deep-Water Strength Training 15

PILATES FUSION

EQUIPMENT
Deep-water belts, dumbbells

TEACHING TIP
Joseph Pilates created the fitness regime named after him to develop deep torso strength and flexibility. Many of his exercises can be adapted for use in the water. When you combine these with other core strength exercises and alternate them with travel to keep participants from getting chilled, you have a Pilates fusion class. Perform the Pilates exercises slowly. An example of a slow Pilates exercise is pull one knee toward chest, lift and lower the other leg (see figure 7.64). Use dumbbells for support with other exercises, such as the plank and side plank (see figure 7.65). In plank scissors, one leg is hyperextended and held for a few seconds. In side plank pliers, the top leg is abducted and held for a few seconds.

WARM-UP
Knee-high jog

Jacks tuck

Straddle jog

Heel jog

Knee-high jog with propeller scull, travel backward and forward

Straddle jog with R shoulder sweep in, travel sideways R

Straddle jog with L shoulder sweep in, travel sideways L

Heel jog with propeller scull, travel backward and forward

A SET
Tilt pelvis forward and backward to find neutral

Rock pelvis side to side to find neutral

Brace core and sway legs side to side

Log jump, side to side

B SET
Reverse bicycle, R leg with reverse breaststroke, travel backward

Bicycle, R leg with breaststroke, travel forward

Reverse bicycle, L leg with reverse breaststroke, travel backward

Bicycle, L leg with breaststroke, travel forward

R leg kicks forward and back

L leg kicks forward and back

Cross-country ski with unison arm swing

Cross-country ski, arms sweep side to side

Knee-high jog with propeller scull, travel backward and forward

Straddle jog with R shoulder sweep in, travel sideways R

Straddle jog with L shoulder sweep in, travel sideways L

Heel jog with propeller scull, travel backward and forward

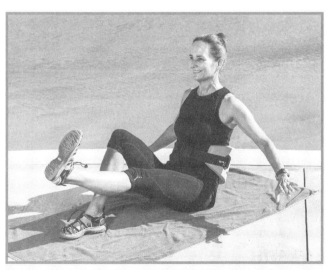

FIGURE 7.64 **Pull R knee toward chest, lift and lower L leg.**

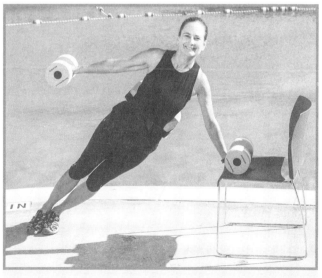

FIGURE 7.65 **Side plank.**

C SET

Seated kick, arms to sides 70 degrees

Bent-knee jacks, arms to sides 70 degrees

Seated kick, R shoulder sweep out, circle counterclockwise

Seated kick, L shoulder sweep out, circle clockwise

Hip hike

Seated swirl

Pike and hold

Pull R knee toward chest, lift and lower L leg

Pull L knee toward chest, lift and lower R leg

Pull R knee toward chest, hip roll

Pull L knee toward chest, hip roll

D SET

High kick and return

High kick and return with reverse breaststroke, travel backward

High kick and return with breaststroke, travel forward

Skate kick and return

Skate kick and return with reverse breaststroke, travel backward

Skate kick and return with breaststroke, travel forward

Jacks cross

Swirl with legs apart

Inner-thigh lift

Hopscotch

Inner-thigh lift R and hopscotch R, alternate

Inner-thigh lift L and hopscotch L, alternate

Knee-high jog with propeller scull, travel backward and forward

Straddle jog with R shoulder sweep in, travel sideways R

Straddle jog with L shoulder sweep in, travel sideways L

Heel jog with propeller scull, travel backward and forward

E SET

(With dumbbells)

R knee lift, lat pull-down R

L knee lift, lat pull-down L

R knee lift, lat pull-down R and L knee lift, lat pull-down L, alternate

Pull both knees up and bring dumbbells together in front

Pull both knees up with lat pull-down

R leg lift, dumbbells to sides

L leg lift, dumbbells to sides

Leg lift, R and L alternate, dumbbells to sides

Crossover kick toward opposite dumbbell

Leg circles in

Leg circles out

Ankle circles

Plank

Plank scissors

Side plank R

Side plank pliers R

Side plank L

Side plank pliers L

Abdominal pike and spine extension

T-hang and gently pulse dumbbells down

F SET

Knee-high jog with propeller scull, travel backward and forward

Straddle jog with R shoulder sweep in, travel sideways R

Straddle jog with L shoulder sweep in, travel sideways L

Heel jog with propeller scull, travel backward and forward

STRETCH

Knee-high jog with double-arm lift, sweep out, lat pull-down and reverse

Cross-country ski, slow and big

Helicopter ski

Bicycle

Swirl

Round out back and stretch chest with bicycle

Shoulder shrug

Look R and L

SECTION 3: FUN ACTIVITIES

Additional fun activities are described in the next section, Deep-Water Lesson Plans for Classes With Two Objectives.

▶ Deep-Water Fun Activities

AR CIRCUIT CLASS WITH PARTNERS

EQUIPMENT
Deep-water belts, noodles (figure 7.66), dumbbells (figure 7.67)

TEACHING TIP
The season for active recovery is a good time to try a circuit class with partners. These stations allow partners to cooperate on some activities and engage in a little friendly competition with others. Set up the equipment stations with three noodle exercises at one station and three dumbbell exercises at another station before class. The third station will be the wall with two exercises there. After your warm-up and a short cardio section, let the participants choose their partners. If you have an odd number of participants, you will need to get in the pool and be someone's partner so that no one is left out. Spend two minutes at each station doing the first exercise. Then go through the stations again doing the second exercise. Finish with the third exercises at the noodle and dumbbell stations. After the circuit has been completed, bring the class together for a second cardio set. Then ask everyone to choose a new partner and work through the stations again, spending one minute at each station instead of two. Before you know it, class time will be up and it will be time for stretching.

WARM-UP
Instructor's choice

A SET
Knee-high jog
Bicycle
Skate kick
Kick forward
Crossover kick
Crossover kick and sweep out
Seated kick
Jacks tuck
Frog kick
Frog kick with elevation
Run tires

B SET
Knee-high jog
Bicycle
Skate kick
Kick forward
Crossover kick
Crossover kick and sweep out, doubles
Seated kick
Jacks tuck
Breaststroke kick
Breaststroke kick with elevation
Heel jog

C SET
(Two minutes at each station; allow extra time to move to next station.)

Station 1 Noodles:
Bicycle race: Sit on noodle as if riding a bicycle and pedal with arms and legs; race until time is up.

Bicycle ride: Partner A is the handlebars with the noodle around his or her waist, and partner B is the bicycle rider, straddling the noodle. Halfway through they change positions.

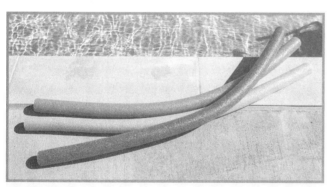
FIGURE 7.66   **Noodles.**

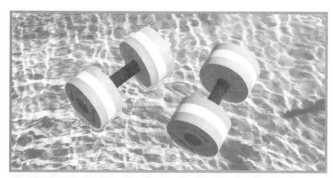
FIGURE 7.67   **Dumbbells.**

Canoe: Sit on noodle as if riding a bicycle. Partner A is in front of partner B as if in a canoe. Partner B holds the back end of partner A's noodle between his or her knees. Partners travel forward rowing with their arms. Halfway through they change positions.

Station 2 Dumbbells:

Push-ups: Partners face each other leaning forward 45 degrees with dumbbells in their hands under the shoulders and flutter kicking. Partners alternate pushing down.

Jumping jacks: When one partner does a lat pull-down, the other lifts the arms to sides.

Side-to-side extension: Partners face each other and coordinate so that both go to the same side at once.

Station 3 At the Wall:

Breaststroke and reverse: Partner A puts both feet on the wall and does a breaststroke. Partner B is in a kneeling position with back to the wall and does a reverse breaststroke. Halfway through they change positions.

Push off: Partners push off the wall with their feet, tuck, and run back.

D SET

Knee-high jog

Bicycle

Skate kick

Kick forward

Seated kick

Seated crossover kick

Seated crossover kick and sweep out

Jacks tuck

Tuck ski

Cross-country ski with elevation

Cross-country ski

E SET

(Repeat circuit with new partner, one minute at each station; allow extra time to move to next station.)

STRETCH

Knee-high jog

Flutter kick, point and flex feet

Swirl

Stretch R arm to the side and circle clockwise

Stretch L arm to the side and circle counterclockwise

R bowstring pull

L bowstring pull

Jacks cross, slow

Cross-country ski, slow and hold with quad stretch R

Cross-country ski, slow and hold with quad stretch L

Inhale and exhale

CHAPTER 8

Deep-Water Lesson Plans for Classes With Two Objectives

At times you may wish to combine two objectives in a single class, such as when your class meets only twice a week or during the recovery season. In that case, your class will start with a 5-minute warm-up and 30 minutes of cardiorespiratory fitness training. Then you can spend 20 minutes on your second objective. The second objective can be strength training, core strength training or fun activities. The class will end with 5 minutes of stretching. The following lesson plans are divided into two sections.

Section 1. 30-Minute Cardiorespiratory Fitness. The 12 lesson plans of continuous cardio in chapter 7, Deep-Water Lesson Plans for Classes With a Single Objective, have been shortened to 30 minutes.

Section 2. 20-Minute Aquatic Endings. The strength-training classes have been shortened to 20-minute sessions. Any of these 20 sessions can be used as an aquatic ending following one of the 30-minute cardio lesson plans.

Section 3. 20-Minute Fun Activities. This section includes four 20-minute sessions of fun activities and eight games. Use one of the fun activities or choose two or more games to play after your 30-minute cardio lesson plan during the recovery season or during any season to give your class a break when they have been working especially hard.

By mixing and matching the cardio in section 1 with the activities in section 2 and 3, you can create an almost endless variety of lesson plans for your two-objective classes.

SECTION 1: 30-MINUTE CARDIO-RESPIRATORY FITNESS

▶ Deep-Water 30-Minute Cardio Lesson Plan 1

MOVEMENT IN TWO PLANES

EQUIPMENT
Deep-water belts

WARM-UP
Knee-high jog

Run tires

Inner-thigh lift

Hopscotch

Jumping jacks

Jacks tuck

Tuck ski

Flutter kick

A SET
Flutter kick, diagonal, travel sideways R

Knee-high jog with paddlewheel

Flutter kick, diagonal, travel sideways L

Knee-high jog with paddlewheel

Knee-high jog with reverse breaststroke, travel backward

Kick forward with breaststroke, travel forward

Knee-high jog with reverse breaststroke, travel backward

Seated kick, travel forward

Flutter kick with reverse breaststroke, travel backward

Knee-high jog with pumping arms, travel forward

Knee lift, straighten and power press-down, travel forward

Knee-high jog with breaststroke, travel forward and knee-high jog, alternate

Knee-high jog, faster and knee-high jog, alternate

B SET
Inner-thigh lift

Jumping jacks

Frog kick

Jacks tuck

Hopscotch

C SET
Cross-country ski, diagonal, travel sideways R

Knee-high jog with hand waves

Cross-country ski, diagonal, travel sideways L

Knee-high jog with hand waves

Knee-high jog, push forward, travel backward

Cross-country ski, travel forward

Knee-high jog, push forward, travel backward

Tuck ski, travel forward

Cross-country ski, travel backward

Knee-high jog with crawl stroke, travel forward

Rock climb, travel forward

Knee-high jog with standing row, travel forward and knee-high jog, alternate

Knee-high jog, faster and knee-high jog, alternate

D SET
Inner-thigh lift

Jumping jacks

Frog kick

Jacks tuck

Hopscotch

20 minutes aquatic endings or fun activities

Stretch: hip flexors, quadriceps, gastrocnemius, hamstrings, inner thigh, outer thigh

▶ Deep-Water 30-Minute Cardio Lesson Plan 2

TURNS AND CIRCLES

EQUIPMENT
Deep-water belts

WARM-UP
Instructor's choice

A SET
Knee-high jog, R shoulder sweep out 2× and L shoulder sweep out 2×

Knee-high jog with unison arm swing

Jumping jacks, pulse out and jacks cross, alternate

Knee-high jog with reverse breaststroke, travel backward

Skateboard R with breaststroke pull, travel forward

Knee-high jog with reverse breaststroke, travel backward

Skateboard L with breaststroke pull, travel forward

Knee-high jog, push forward, travel backward

Crossover step, travel forward

Knee-high jog, push forward, travel backward

Crossover step, travel forward

Crossover kick

Crossover kick, doubles

Jacks cross 3-1/2× and half turn

Jacks cross, R leg in front, circle clockwise

Jacks cross, L leg in front, circle counterclockwise

Knee-high jog

B SET

Knee-high jog with double-arm press-down 2× and lat pull-down 2×

Jumping jacks with unison arm swing

Cross country ski and mini ski, alternate

Knee-high jog with reverse breaststroke, travel backward

Jacks tuck with breaststroke, travel forward

Knee-high jog with reverse breaststroke, travel backward

Jacks tuck with breaststroke, travel forward

Knee-high jog, push forward, travel backward

Jumping jacks with breaststroke, travel forward

Knee-high jog, push forward, travel backward

Jumping jacks with breaststroke, travel forward

Crossover kick, doubles

Crossover kick, doubles, one low and one high

Cross-country ski 3-1/2× and half turn

Helicopter ski

Knee-high jog

C SET

Knee-high jog, punch down R, L and punch across R, L

Cross-country ski with unison arm swing

Jumping jacks and mini cross, alternate

Knee-high jog with reverse breaststroke, travel backward

Cross-country ski, travel forward

Knee-high jog with reverse breaststroke, travel backward

Cross-country ski, travel forward

Knee-high jog, push forward, travel backward

Cross-country ski with alternating sweep out, travel forward

Knee-high jog, push forward, travel backward

Cross-country ski with alternating sweep out, travel forward

Crossover kick, doubles, one low and one high

Crossover kick and sweep out

Jacks cross 3-1/2× and half turn

Jacks cross, R leg in front, circle clockwise

Jacks cross, L leg in front, circle counterclockwise

Knee-high jog

20 minutes aquatic endings or fun activities

Stretch: shoulders, pectorals, hip flexors, gastrocnemius, hamstrings, outer thigh

▶ ### Deep-Water 30-Minute Cardio Lesson Plan 3

INCREASING COMPLEXITY
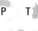

EQUIPMENT

Deep-water belts

WARM-UP

Instructor's choice

A SET

Jumping jacks

Jumping jacks with elbows bent

Inner-thigh lift

Straddle jog with shoulder blade squeeze

Skateboard R with breaststroke pull, travel forward

Skateboard L with breaststroke pull, travel forward

Bicycle with breaststroke, one lap

Cross-country ski with unison sidestroke, travel sideways R and L

Cross-country ski with unison arm swing

Cross-country ski with rotation

Knee-high jog

B SET

Jumping jacks

Jumping jacks, arms cross in front and in back

Hopscotch

Straddle jog with shoulder blade squeeze

Skateboard L with breaststroke pull, travel forward

Skateboard R with breaststroke pull, travel forward

Bicycle with bicycle arms, one lap
Cross-country ski, travel backward and forward
Cross-country ski, clap hands
Cross-country ski with rotation
Knee-high jog

C SET

Jumping jacks
Jumping jacks, palms touch in front and in back
Inner-thigh lift 1×, hopscotch 1×
Straddle jog with shoulder blade squeeze
Skateboard R with breaststroke pull, one lap
Skateboard L with breaststroke pull, one lap
Bicycle, tandem, one lap
Cross-country ski, diagonal, travel sideways R and L
Cross-country ski with forearm press
R leg kicks forward
L leg kicks forward
R leg kicks back
L leg kicks back
20 minutes aquatic endings or fun activities
Stretch: hamstrings, outer thigh, quadriceps, hip flexors, gastrocnemius, upper back

▶ **Deep-Water 30-Minute Cardio Lesson Plan 4**

BLOCK CHOREOGRAPHY WITH FIVE MOVES

EQUIPMENT

Deep-water belts

WARM-UP

Instructor's choice

A SET

Flutter kick
Kick forward
Jumping jacks
Heel jog
Cross-country ski

B SET

Flutter kick, punch forward and side
Chorus-line kick
Jumping jacks with diagonal turn

Skate kick with pumping arms
Cross-country ski, two easy and one with power

C SET

Flutter kick, push across and slice back
High kick
Jumping jacks, pulse out
R leg kicks forward and back
L leg kicks forward and back
Cross-country ski, four easy and four with power

D SET

Star flutter kick
Kick forward with lat pull-down
Jumping jacks, pulse in
Skate kick with pumping arms
Cross-country ski, two easy and one with power

E SET

Flutter kick, punch across
Crossover kick
Mini cross
R knee swings forward and back
L knee swings forward and back
Cross-country ski, four easy and four with power

F SET

Flutter kick
Seated kick
Bent-knee jacks
Heel jog
Cross-country ski with knees bent 90 degrees
20 minutes aquatic endings or fun activities
Stretch: quadriceps, hip flexors, inner thigh, hamstrings, pectorals, upper back

▶ **Deep-Water 30-minute Cardio Lesson Plan 5**

DOUBLE LADDER

EQUIPMENT

Deep-water belts

TEACHING TIP

In a double ladder, two exercises, such as jumping jacks and log jump, side to side, are paired. Perform each exercise for 10 seconds, then 20 seconds, and then 30 seconds, as if ascending a ladder. Next, descend the ladder, performing each exercise for 20 seconds and then 10 seconds. Each double ladder takes 3 minutes.

WARM-UP
Instructor's choice

A SET
Kick forward

Crossover kick

Cossack kick

Heel jog

Bicycle

Cross-country ski

Double ladder: 10, 20, 30, 20, and 10 seconds
    Jumping jacks
    Log jump, side to side

B SET
Kick forward, doubles

Crossover kick, doubles, one low and one high

Jumping jacks

Hopscotch, doubles

Bicycle, doubles

Tuck ski together

Double ladder: 10, 20, 30, 20, and 10 seconds
    Flutter kick
    Cross-country ski

C SET
High kick

Skate kick, crossover kick, sweep out and center

Jacks cross

Hopscotch

Bicycle, tandem

Double ladder: 10, 20, 30, 20, and 10 seconds
    Bicycle
    Frog kick

20 minutes aquatic endings or fun activities

Stretch: hamstrings, outer thigh, quadriceps, hip flexors, gastrocnemius, ankles

▶ Deep-Water 30-Minute Cardio Lesson Plan 6

 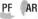

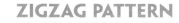
ZIGZAG PATTERN

EQUIPMENT
Deep-water belts

WARM-UP
Instructor's choice

A SET
In, in, out, out

Jumping jacks

Jumping jacks with diagonal turn

Crossover kick

Seated kick and high kick, alternate, travel backward

Knee-high jog, travel forward

Tuck and hold with reverse breaststroke, travel backward

Knee-high jog, travel in a zigzag

Skateboard R with breaststroke pull, travel forward

Skateboard L with breaststroke pull, travel forward

Kick forward

Seated kick

Tuck and hold, R shoulder sweep out and in

Tuck and hold, L shoulder sweep out and in

Knee-high jog

Knee-high jog, diagonal, travel sideways R and L

B SET
In, in, out, out

Jumping jacks

Jumping jacks with diagonal turn

Crossover kick, doubles, one low and one high

Seated kick and high kick, alternate, travel backward

Run 3× and hurdle 1×, travel forward

Tuck and hold with reverse breaststroke, travel backward

Cross-country ski, travel in a zigzag

Skate kick

Cross-country ski

Tuck ski together

Tuck and hold, R leg sweeps out and in

Tuck and hold, L leg sweeps out and in

Knee-high jog

Cross-country ski, diagonal, travel sideways R and L

C SET
In, in, out, out

Jumping jacks

Jumping jacks with diagonal turn

Crossover kick and sweep out

Seated kick and high kick, alternate, travel backward

Bicycle, tandem, travel forward

Tuck and hold with reverse breaststroke, travel backward

Bicycle, travel in a zigzag

Bicycle R leg

Bicycle L leg

Bicycle

Tuck ski

Seated kick 3× and hold, one leg sweeps out and in 1×

Knee-high jog

Bicycle, diagonal, travel sideways R and L

20 minutes aquatic endings or fun activities

Stretch: upper back, lower back, hamstrings, outer thighs, quadriceps, hip flexors

▶ Deep-Water 30-Minute Cardio Lesson Plan 7

CARDIO WITH WALL EXERCISES

EQUIPMENT
Deep-water belts

WARM-UP
Instructor's choice

A SET
Straddle jog, clap hands

Jumping jacks, clap hands

Inner-thigh lift

Jacks cross

Run to one side of the pool and back to the wall

Breaststroke with feet on the wall

Cross-country ski, travel backward

Knee-high jog, travel forward

Kick forward with propeller scull, travel backward

Knee-high jog, travel forward

Crossover kick

B SET
Straddle jog, palms touch in back

Jumping jacks, palms touch in back

Hopscotch

Jacks cross

Run to one side of the pool and back to the wall

Cross-country ski with both feet on the wall at twelve o'clock and six o'clock

Cross-country ski with reverse breaststroke, travel backward

Knee-high jog, travel forward

Kick forward with reverse breaststroke, travel backward

Knee-high jog, travel forward

Chorus-line kick

C SET
Straddle jog, open and close doors

Jumping jacks, open and close doors

Inner-thigh lift R and hopscotch L, alternate

Inner-thigh lift L and hopscotch R, alternate

Jacks cross

Run to one side of the pool and back to the wall

Reverse breaststroke in a kneeling position with back to the wall

Cross-country ski with unison arm swing, travel backward

Knee-high jog, travel forward

Kick forward with unison arm swing, travel backward

Knee-high jog, travel forward

Crossover kick, doubles, one low and one high

20 minutes aquatic endings or fun activities

Stretch: lower back, hamstrings, inner thigh, hip flexors, gastrocnemius, shoulders

▶ Deep-Water 30-Minute Cardio Lesson Plan 8

CHANGES

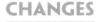

EQUIPMENT
Deep-water belts

WARM-UP
Instructor's choice

A SET
Knee-high jog with jog press

Run tires, reach side to side

Jumping jacks

Jacks tuck

Tuck and hold sidesaddle R with reverse breast-stroke, travel backward

Tuck and hold sidesaddle L with breaststroke, travel forward

Cross-country ski with R arm swing, L hand on hip

Knee-high jog with jog press

Run tires, reach side to side

Jumping jacks

Jacks tuck

Tuck and hold sidesaddle L with reverse breast-stroke, travel backward

Tuck and hold sidesaddle R with breaststroke, travel forward

Cross-country ski with L arm swing, R hand on hip

Cross-country ski 3× and hold

Cross-country ski 3× and tuck

Tuck ski

Jacks tuck

Knee-high jog

B SET

Knee-high jog, punch forward and side

Run tires with hand waves

Jumping jacks with diagonal turn

Jacks tuck 1×, seated kick 1×

Cross-country ski and hold R with reverse breaststroke, travel backward

Cross-country ski and hold L with breaststroke, travel forward

Helicopter ski

Knee-high jog, punch forward and side

Run tires with hand waves

Jumping jacks with diagonal turn

Jacks tuck 1×, seated kick 1×

Cross-country ski and hold L with reverse breast-stroke, travel backward

Cross-country ski and hold R with breaststroke, travel forward

Helicopter ski

Cross-country ski with rotation

Tuck ski with rotation

Cross-country ski, tuck, diagonal turn and center

Jacks tuck

Knee-high jog

20 minutes aquatic endings or fun activities

Stretch: hamstrings, hip flexors, quadriceps, gas-trocnemius, outer thigh, shoulders

▶ Deep-Water 30-Minute Cardio Lesson Plan 9

BLOCK CHOREOGRAPHY WITH SIX MOVES

EQUIPMENT
Deep-water belts

WARM-UP
Instructor's choice

A SET
Knee-high jog

Run tires

Jumping jacks

Cross-country ski

Kick forward

Heel jog

B SET
Knee-high jog with pumping arms

Run tires with shoulder blade squeeze

Jumping jacks, clap hands

Cross-country ski with windshield wiper arms

Kick forward with triceps extension

Heel jog with forearm press

C SET
Knee-high jog

Frog kick with elevation

Jumping jacks

Tuck ski together

Kick forward

Breaststroke kick with elevation

D SET
Run

Over the barrel, travel sideways R and L

Jumping jacks with diagonal turn

Cross-country ski, full ROM

High kick

Skate kick

E SET
Crossover knees

Inner-thigh lift

Jacks cross

Tuck ski with rotation

Crossover kick

Hopscotch

F SET

In, in, out, out

Cross-country ski 1×, jumping jacks 1×

R leg kicks forward and back

In, in, out, out

Cross-country ski 1×, jumping jacks 1×

L leg kicks forward and back

20 minutes aquatic endings or fun activities

Stretch: quadriceps, hip flexors, hamstrings, outer thigh, inner thigh, pectorals

▶ Deep-Water 30-Minute Cardio Lesson Plan 10

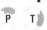

LAYER TECHNIQUE

EQUIPMENT

Deep-water belts

WARM-UP

Jacks tuck

Jumping jacks

Inner-thigh lift

Hopscotch

Heel jog

Cross-country ski

Knee-high jog

Kick forward

A SET

Jacks tuck

Jumping jacks

Jumping jacks 1×, kick forward 1×

Inner-thigh lift

Inner-thigh lift R

Inner-thigh lift L

Hopscotch

Heel jog

Cross-country ski

Cross-country ski 3× and hold

Knee-high jog

Knee-high jog 3× and hold

Kick forward

Seated kick

B SET

Jacks tuck

Jumping jacks 1×, kick forward 1×

Jumping jacks 1×, skate kick 1×

Inner-thigh lift R

Inner-thigh lift L

Inner-thigh lift, doubles

Hopscotch

Heel jog

Cross-country ski 3× and hold

Cross-country ski 2× and cross-country ski with power 1×

Knee-high jog 3× and hold

Knee-high jog 3× and hold with kayak row

Seated kick

Hold R leg up, L quad kick

Hold L leg up, R quad kick

C SET

Jacks tuck

Jumping jacks 1×, skate kick 1×

Jumping jacks 2×, inner-thigh lift 1×

Inner-thigh lift, doubles

Inner-thigh lift R and hopscotch L, alternate

Inner-thigh lift L and hopscotch R, alternate

Hopscotch

Heel jog

Cross-country ski 2× and cross-country ski with power 1×

Cross-country ski with lat pull-down

Knee-high jog 3× and hold with kayak row

Tuck and hold

Hold R leg up, L quad kick

Hold L leg up, R quad kick

Hold R leg up, L quad kick 3× and down

Hold L leg up, R quad kick 3× and down

20 minutes aquatic endings or fun activities

Stretch: latissimus dorsi, upper back, hip flexors, gastrocnemius, hamstrings, inner thigh

▶ Deep-Water 30-Minute Cardio Lesson Plan 11

TABATA TIMING 1

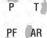

EQUIPMENT

Deep-water belts

WARM-UP

Instructor's choice

A SET

Knee-high jog, push forward, travel backward

Straddle jog, clap hands

Knee-high jog, hands cupped, travel forward

Straddle jog with shoulder blade squeeze

Knee-high jog, push forward, travel backward

Straddle jog, clap hands

Knee-high jog, hands cupped, travel forward

Straddle jog with shoulder blade squeeze

Tabata 8 sets (4 minutes):

Cross-country ski (20 seconds)

Tuck ski (10 seconds)

B SET

Straddle jog with reverse breaststroke, travel backward

Bicycle R leg

Straddle jog with breaststroke, travel forward

Bicycle L leg

Straddle jog with reverse breaststroke, travel backward

Bicycle R leg

Straddle jog with breaststroke, travel forward

Bicycle L leg

Tabata 8 sets (4 minutes):

Kick forward (20 seconds)

Flutter kick (10 seconds)

C SET

Heel jog with unison arm swing, travel backward

Jumping jacks with bowstring pull to R side

Heel jog with triceps kick back, travel forward

Jumping jacks with bowstring pull to L side

Heel jog with unison arm swing, travel backward

Jumping jacks with bowstring pull to R side

Heel jog with triceps kick back, travel forward

Jumping jacks with bowstring pull to L side

Tabata 8 sets (4 minutes):

Jumping jacks (20 seconds)

Run tires (10 seconds)

20 minutes aquatic endings or fun activities

Stretch: hip flexors, quadriceps, gastrocnemius, outer thigh, hamstrings, lower back

▶ Deep-Water 30-Minute Cardio Lesson Plan 12

TABATA TIMING 2

EQUIPMENT

Deep-water belts

WARM-UP

Instructor's choice

A SET

Tabata repeat 4× (4 minutes):

Knee lift, doubles (20 seconds)

Knee-high jog (10 seconds)

Knee-high jog, syncopate (20 seconds)

Knee-high jog (10 seconds)

One-minute break:

Knee-high jog with propeller scull, travel backward (30 seconds)

Knee-high jog with propeller scull, travel forward (30 seconds)

B SET

Tabata repeat 4× (4 minutes):

R quad kick (20 seconds)

Kick forward (10 seconds)

L quad kick (20 seconds)

Kick forward (10 seconds)

One-minute break:

Flutter kick with reverse breaststroke, travel backward (30 seconds)

Flutter kick with breaststroke, travel forward (30 seconds)

C SET

Tabata repeat 4× (4 minutes):

Diamonds (20 seconds)

Straddle jog (10 seconds)

Cossack kick (20 seconds)

Straddle jog (10 seconds)

One-minute break:

Over the barrel, travel sideways R (30 seconds)

Over the barrel, travel sideways L (30 seconds)

D SET

Tabata repeat 4× (4 minutes):

Hopscotch (20 seconds)

Heel jog (10 seconds)

Skate kick (20 seconds)

Heel jog (10 seconds)

One-minute break:

Bicycle with propeller scull, travel backward (30 seconds)

Bicycle with propeller scull, travel forward (30 seconds)

E SET

Tabata repeat 4× (4 minutes):

Tuck ski, doubles (20 seconds)

Cross-country ski with knees bent 90 degrees (10 seconds)

Tuck ski (20 seconds)

Cross-country ski with knees bent 90 degrees (10 seconds)

One-minute break:

Knee-high jog with propeller scull, travel backward (30 seconds)

Crossover step, travel forward (30 seconds)

F SET

Tabata repeat 4× (4 minutes):

Jumping jacks (20 seconds)

Run tires (10 seconds)

Jumping jacks, syncopate (20 seconds)

Run tires (10 seconds)

One-minute break:

Knee-high jog with R shoulder sweep in, travel sideways R (30 seconds)

Knee-high jog with L shoulder sweep in, travel sideways L (30 seconds)

20 minutes aquatic endings or fun activities

Stretch: quadriceps, gastrocnemius, hamstrings, outer thigh, pectorals, upper back

SECTION 2: 20-MINUTE AQUATIC ENDINGS

▶ Deep-Water 20-Minute Strength Training 1

HAND POSITIONS

EQUIPMENT

Deep-water belts

A SET

Knee-high jog, R shoulder sweep in, hand slicing

Knee-high jog, L shoulder sweep in, hand slicing

Knee-high jog, R shoulder sweep in, hand cupped

Knee-high jog, L shoulder sweep in, hand cupped

B SET

Knee-high jog, R shoulder sweep out, hand slicing

Knee-high jog, L shoulder sweep out, hand slicing

Knee-high jog, R shoulder sweep out, hand open

Knee-high jog, L shoulder sweep out, hand open

C SET

Cross-country ski with R bowstring pull, hand fisted

Cross-country ski with L bowstring pull, hand fisted

Cross-country ski with R bowstring pull, hand cupped

Cross-country-ski with L bowstring pull, hand cupped

D SET

Knee-high jog with R arm curl, hand slicing

Knee-high jog with L arm curl, hand slicing

Knee-high jog with R arm curl, palm faces direction of motion

Knee-high jog with L arm curl, palm faces direction of motion

E SET

Knee-high jog with R forearm press, palm up, hand slicing

Knee-high jog with L forearm press, palm up, hand slicing

Knee-high jog with R forearm press, hand open

Knee-high jog with L forearm press, hand open

▶ Deep-Water 20-Minute Strength Training 2

LEVER LENGTH

EQUIPMENT

Deep-water belts

A SET

Clamshells R

Clamshells L

R leg kicks side

L leg kicks side

B SET

Jacks tuck

Frog kick

Jacks tuck with reverse breaststroke, travel backward

Jacks tuck with breaststroke, travel forward

C SET

R quad kick

L quad kick

R leg kicks forward

L leg kicks forward

D SET

R hamstring curl

L hamstring curl

R leg kicks back

L leg kicks back

E SET

Flutter kick, point and flex feet

Mini ski, point and flex feet

Seated kick, toes pointed, travel backward

Seated kick, feet flexed, travel forward

▶ Deep-Water 20-Minute Strength Training 3

INERTIA AND FRONTAL RESISTANCE

EQUIPMENT

Deep-water belts

TEACHING TIP

In a pyramid, you perform one exercise 4× and then its pair 4×, then each exercise 2×, and finally you alternate one of each exercise.

A SET

Knee-high jog with reverse breaststroke

Knee-high jog with breaststroke

Kick forward

Skate kick

Knee-high jog with reverse breaststroke and breaststroke, pyramid 4×, 2×, 1×

Kick forward and skate kick, pyramid 4×, 2×, 1×

B SET

Knee-high jog with double-arm press-down

Knee-high jog with lat pull-down

Cross-country ski

Jumping jacks

Knee-high jog with double-arm press-down and lat pull-down, pyramid 4×, 2×, 1×

Cross-country ski and jumping jacks, pyramid 4×, 2×, 1×

C SET

Knee-high jog with unison push forward

Knee-high jog with standing row

Inner-thigh lift

Hopscotch

Knee-high jog with unison push forward and standing row, pyramid 4×, 2×, 1×

Inner-thigh lift and hopscotch, pyramid 4×, 2×, 1×

D SET

Knee-high jog with arm curl

Knee-high jog with triceps extension

R quad kick

L quad kick

Skateboard R

Skateboard L

Knee-high jog with arm curl and triceps extension, pyramid 4×, 2×, 1×

R quad kick and skateboard R, pyramid 4×, 2×, 1×

L quad kick and skateboard L, pyramid 4×, 2×, 1×

▶ Deep-Water 20-Minute Strength Training 4

ACCELERATION 1

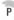

EQUIPMENT

Deep-water belts

A SET

Knee-high jog with shoulder blade squeeze

Knee-high jog with standing row

Knee-high jog with arm lift to the sides, elbows bent

Cross-country ski with unison arm swing

Cross-country ski, clap hands (emphasize posterior deltoids)

Knee-high jog, one lap

B SET

Jumping jacks (emphasize latissimus dorsi)

Jumping jacks, palms touch in back

Knee-high jog, clap hands

Cross-country, ski clap hands (emphasize pectorals)

Knee-high jog with forearm press

Knee-high jog, one lap

C SET

Cross-country ski with forearm press, side to side

Knee-high jog with arm curl

Jumping jacks, open and close doors

Knee-high jog with jog press

Cross-country ski, push forward

Run one lap

D SET

Run to the ropes and run to the wall

Breaststroke with feet on the wall

Run to the ropes and run to the wall

Reverse breaststroke in a kneeling position with back to the wall

▶ **Deep-Water 20-Minute Strength Training 5**

 ### ACCELERATION 2

EQUIPMENT

Deep-water belts

A SET

Knee-high jog with scull

Knee lift, straighten and power press-down

Cross-country ski with scull

R leg kicks side

L leg kicks side

Knee-high jog, one lap

B SET

Jumping jacks with scull

Jacks cross with scull

Mini cross with scull

Heel jog with scull

Knee-high jog, one lap

C SET

Bicycle with scull

R quad kick with scull

L quad kick with scull

Cossack kick with scull

Flutter kick, point and flex feet, with scull

Knee-high jog, one lap

D SET

Run to the ropes and run to the wall

Push off the wall with both feet and run back

Run to the ropes and run to the wall

Cross-country ski, back to the wall, heels tap the wall

▶ **Deep-Water 20-Minute Strength Training 6**

ACCELERATION 3

EQUIPMENT

Deep-water belts

A SET

Knee-high jog with propeller scull, travel backward

Knee-high jog with standing row, travel forward

Knee-high jog with propeller scull, travel backward

Knee-high jog with crawl stroke, travel forward

Knee-high jog with unison arm swing, travel backward and forward

B SET

Knee-high jog, clap hands, travel backward

Power run

Knee-high jog with propeller scull, travel backward

Knee-high jog with forearm press out, travel forward

Knee-high jog with propeller scull, travel backward

Knee-high jog with triceps kickback, travel forward

C SET

High kick, travel backward and forward

Jumping jacks, travel sideways R and L

Bent-knee jacks, travel backward and forward

D SET

Knee-high jog with propeller scull, travel backward

Skateboard R with breaststroke pull, travel forward

Knee-high jog with propeller scull, travel backward

Skateboard L with breaststroke pull, travel forward

Knee-high jog with propeller scull, travel backward

Bicycle with no arms, travel forward

Cossack kick with sidestroke, travel sideways R and L

▶ Deep-Water 20-Minute Strength Training 7

BUOYANT EQUIPMENT—NOODLES

T
PF

EQUIPMENT

Deep-water belts, noodles

A SET

(Noodle in hands)

Knee-high jog with standing row

Knee-high jog with double-arm press-down

Cross-country ski, noodle in L hand, travel sideways R

Cross-country ski, noodle in R hand, travel sideways L

Knee-high jog with lat pull-down, noodle in L hand, travel sideways R

Knee-high jog with lat pull-down, noodle in R hand, travel sideways L

Jumping jacks, touch ends in front

Jumping jacks with forearm press, noodle in back

Cross-country ski, push ends forward

Straddle jog with triceps extension

Knee-high jog, plunge L, travel sideways R

Knee-high jog, plunge R, travel sideways L

B SET

(Foot on a noodle)

Hip extension R

Hip extension L

Standing leg press R

Standing leg press L

Standing leg press to R side

Standing leg press to L side

C SET

(Sit on noodle like a swing)

Seated jacks

Seated kick

Seated kick with L shoulder sweep out, circle clockwise

Seated kick with R shoulder sweep out, circle counterclockwise

Point and flex feet

Hip hike

▶ Deep-Water 20-Minute Strength Training 8

BUOYANT EQUIPMENT— DUMBBELLS

T
PF

EQUIPMENT

Deep-water belts, dumbbells

A SET

Knee-high jog, clap hands

Knee-high jog with scull

(With dumbbells) chest fly at 45-degree angle with flutter kick

Knee-high jog with scull

B SET

Cross-country ski with arm swing

Knee-high jog with scull

(With dumbbells) cross-country ski with arm swing

Knee-high jog with scull

C SET

Jumping jacks with lat pull-down

Knee-high jog with scull

(With dumbbells) jumping jacks with lat pull-down

Knee-high jog with scull

D SET

Straddle jog with triceps extension

Knee-high jog with scull

(With dumbbells) straddle jog with triceps extension

Knee-high jog with scull

E SET

R leg kicks forward and back

L leg kicks forward and back

Knee-high jog with scull

Cross-country ski with power

Knee-high jog with scull

F SET

R leg kicks side

L leg kicks side

Knee-high jog

Jacks cross with power

Knee-high jog

H SET

(With dumbbells) abdominal pike and spine extension

(With dumbbells) side-to-side extension

▶ Deep-Water 20-Minute Strength Training 9

BUOYANT EQUIPMENT—DUMBBELLS (CONCENTRIC AND ECCENTRIC CONTRACTIONS)

PF

EQUIPMENT

Deep-water belts, dumbbells

A SET

(With dumbbells)

Chest fly at 45-degree angle, with flutter kick

Cross-country ski with dumbbells as stabilizers

Chest fly, faster, at 45-degree angle, with flutter kick

Cross-country ski, faster, with dumbbells as stabilizers

Chest fly at 45-degree angle, fast concentric and slow eccentric, with flutter kick

Cross-country ski with elevation, no dumbbells

B SET

(With dumbbells)

Jumping jacks with lat pull-down

Bent-knee jacks with dumbbells as stabilizers

Jumping jacks with lat pull-down, faster

Bent-knee jacks, faster, with dumbbells as stabilizers

Jumping jacks with lat pull-down, fast concentric and slow eccentric

Frog kick with elevation, no dumbbells

C SET

(With dumbbells)

Cross-country ski with arm swing

Seated kick with dumbbells as stabilizers

Cross-country ski with arm swing, faster

Seated kick, faster, with dumbbells as stabilizers

Cross-country ski with arm swing, fast and slow, alternate

Mermaid with power, no dumbbells

D SET

(With dumbbells)

Straddle jog with triceps extension

Jumping jacks with dumbbells as stabilizers

Straddle jog with triceps extension, faster

Jumping jacks, faster, with dumbbells as stabilizers

Straddle jog with triceps extension, fast concentric and slow eccentric

Frog kick with elevation, no dumbbells

▶ Deep-Water 20-Minute Strength Training 10

DRAG EQUIPMENT—WEBBED GLOVES

T
PF

EQUIPMENT

Deep-water belts, webbed gloves

A SET

Knee-high jog, clap hands, sweep out and slice in

Flutter kick with scull

Knee-high jog, clap hands, sweep in and slice out

Flutter kick with scull

Knee-high jog, clap hands, faster

Flutter kick with scull

B SET

Cross-country ski with arm swing, scoop back and slice forward

Bicycle with scull

Cross-country ski with arm swing, scoop forward and slice back

Bicycle with scull

Cross-country ski with unison arm swing, palms face direction of motion, faster

Bicycle with scull

C SET

Jumping jacks with lat pull-down and slice up

Knee-high jog with scull

Jumping jacks with arm lifts to sides and slice down

Knee-high jog with scull

Jumping jacks, faster

Knee-high jog with scull

D SET

Straddle jog with triceps extension and slice up

Jacks tuck

Straddle jog with arm curl and slice down

Jacks tuck

Straddle jog with arm curl, palms face direction of motion, faster

Jacks tuck

▶ Deep-Water 20-Minute Strength Training 11

T▶ DRAG EQUIPMENT—MULTIPLANE DRAG EQUIPMENT
PF

EQUIPMENT

Deep-water belts, multiplane drag equipment

A SET

Straddle jog with chest fly

Cross-country ski

Straddle jog with chest fly, faster

Cross-country ski, faster

Jumping jacks with lat pull-down

Jumping jacks with lat pull-down, faster

Straddle jog, R shoulder sweep out

Straddle jog, L shoulder sweep out

B SET

Knee-high jog, push forward R arm

Knee-high jog, push forward L arm

Knee-high jog, push forward R arm and L arm, alternate

Knee-high jog, unison push forward

Knee-high jog, pronate and supinate

C SET

Jumping jacks, arms down at sides, bring R arm across to L shoulder

Jumping jacks, arms down at sides, bring L arm across to R shoulder

Jumping jacks, arms to sides 70 degrees, bring R arm down to L hip

Jumping jacks, arms to sides 70 degrees, bring L arm down to R hip

Inner-thigh lift R

Inner-thigh lift L

Jumping jacks with arm curl

Jumping jacks with triceps extension

Jumping jacks with forearm press

Inner-thigh lift

D SET

Cross-country ski with R arm only

Cross-country ski with L arm only

Jumping jacks with R arm only

Jumping jacks with L arm only

Run one lap with resistor arms

▶ Deep-Water 20-Minute Strength Training 12

RUBBERIZED EQUIPMENT— BANDS (CONCENTRIC AND ECCENTRIC CONTRACTIONS)
PF

EQUIPMENT

Deep-water belts, bands

A SET

Cross-country ski with R bowstring pull

Cross-country ski with L bowstring pull

Knee-high jog with R arm press-down

Knee-high jog with L arm press-down

Jumping jacks with chest press, band behind back

Seated kick with arm lift to sides, band under knees

Seated kick with arm curl, band under knees

Jumping jacks with R elbow sweep out

Jumping jacks with L elbow sweep out

Jumping jacks with forearm press out

Knee-high jog

B SET

(Pause at the end range of motion, slow return)

Cross-country ski with R bowstring pull

Cross-country ski with L bowstring pull

Knee-high jog with R arm press-down

Knee-high jog with L arm press-down

Jumping jacks with chest press, band behind back

Seated kick with arm lift to sides, band under knees

Seated kick with arm curl, band under knees

Jumping jacks with R elbow sweep out

Jumping jacks with L elbow sweep out

Jumping jacks with forearm press out

▶ Deep-Water 20-Minute Strength Training 13

CIRCUIT CLASS 1

T

PF

EQUIPMENT

Deep-water belts, bands, noodles

A SET

(With band) jumping jacks with bowstring pull to the R side

(With band) jumping jacks with bowstring pull to the L side

Knee-high jog

(With band) seated kick with arm lift to sides, band under knees

Knee-high jog

(With band) jumping jacks with forearm press out

Knee-high jog

B SET

(Foot on a noodle) standing leg press R

(Foot on a noodle) standing leg press L

Knee-high jog

(Sit on noodle like a swing) seated kick

Knee-high jog

(Foot on a noodle) standing leg press to R side

(Foot on a noodle) standing leg press to L side

Knee-high jog

(Sit on a noodle like a swing) point and flex feet, alternate R and L

Knee-high jog

(Noodle in hands on surface of water) abdominal pike and spine extension,

Knee-high jog

(Straddle noodle and squeeze between thighs) seated swirl

Knee-high jog

▶ Deep-Water 20-Minute Strength Training 14

CIRCUIT CLASS 2

T

PF

EQUIPMENT

Ankle cuffs or deep-water belts, webbed gloves, multiplane drag equipment

A SET

(With ankle cuffs and webbed gloves)

Knee-high jog with standing row

Straddle jog with double-arm press-down

Jumping jacks

Straddle jog, clap hands

Knee-high jog with L shoulder sweep out, travel sideways R

Knee-high jog with R shoulder sweep out, travel sideways L

Cross-country ski with forearm press side to side

Jumping jacks with arm curl, palms face direction of motion

B SET

(With ankle cuffs)

Seated kick

Bicycle

Cross-country ski

Jumping jacks

Frog kick

Cossack kick

C SET

(With ankle cuffs and multiplane drag equipment)

Knee-high jog with standing row

Straddle jog with double-arm press-down

Jumping jacks

Straddle jog with chest fly

Knee-high jog with R shoulder sweep in, travel sideways R

Knee-high jog with L shoulder sweep in, travel sideways L

Cross-country ski with forearm press

Jumping jacks, open and close doors

▶ Deep-Water 20-Minute Strength Training 15

FUNCTIONAL CORE STRENGTH 1

EQUIPMENT
Deep-water belts

A SET
Knee-high jog with hands on hips
Flutter kick
Bicycle
Bicycle with R shoulder sweep in, travel sideways R
Bicycle with L shoulder sweep in, travel sideways L
Bicycle, diagonal, travel sideways R and L
Reverse bicycle, R leg with reverse breaststroke, travel backward
Bicycle R leg with breaststroke, travel forward
Flutter kick, point and flex feet
Reverse bicycle, L leg with reverse breaststroke, travel backward
Bicycle L leg with breaststroke, travel forward
Flutter kick with hands on hips

B SET
Knee-high jog with resistor arms, travel forward
Knee lift, straighten and power press-down
Crossover step
Straddle jog, clap hands, travel backward and forward
Over the barrel with arms to sides 70 degrees, travel sideways R and L
Knee-high jog, diagonal, travel sideways R and L
Knee-high jog with R arm press-down and L hand on hip, travel forward
Knee-high jog with L arm press-down and R hand on hip, travel forward
Knee-high jog, travel in a bowtie pattern

▶ Deep-Water 20-Minute Strength Training 16

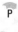

FUNCTIONAL CORE STRENGTH 2

EQUIPMENT
Deep-water belts

A SET
Jacks tuck
Jacks tuck with reverse breaststroke, travel backward
Inner-thigh lift
Jacks tuck with breaststroke, travel forward
Cross-country ski and hold R with reverse breaststroke, travel backward
Cross-country ski and hold L with breaststroke, travel forward
Seated kick with double-arm lift, travel backward
Seated kick with double-arm press-down, travel forward
Bent-knee jacks, travel backward
Tuck and hold sidesaddle R with forearm press, travel forward
Tuck and hold with reverse breaststroke, travel backward
Tuck and hold sidesaddle L with forearm press, travel forward

B SET
R leg kicks forward and back
L leg kicks forward and back
Clamshells R
Clamshells L
Tuck and hold with lat pull-down
Brace core, arms down, turbulent hand movements
Helicopter ski
Log jump, side to side
Bicycle, side-lying R, circle clockwise
Bicycle, side-lying L, circle counterclockwise
Side extension, tuck and pike, alternate R and L
Abdominal pike and spine extension
Log jump, forward and back
Seated swirl

▶ Deep-Water 20-Minute Strength Training 17

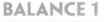

BALANCE 1

EQUIPMENT
Deep-water belts

A SET

Knee-high jog with R arm breaststroke and L arm crawl stroke

Knee-high jog with L arm breaststroke and R arm crawl stroke

Jumping jacks, R arm crosses in front, and L arm crosses in back

Jumping jacks, L arm crosses in front, and R arm crosses in back

Jumping jacks with arm swing

Cross-country ski with lat pull-down

Knee-high jog, travel backward, forward, and sideways with quick change of direction

R leg kicks side

L leg kicks side

B SET

(Travel in a bowtie pattern)

Knee-high jog with propeller scull, travel backward

Knee-high jog travel diagonally to front R corner, look L

Knee-high jog with propeller scull, travel backward

Knee-high jog travel diagonally to front L corner, look R

Over the barrel R, look L

Over the barrel L, look R

Jumping jacks, clap hands, travel backward

Cross-country ski, travel diagonally to front R corner

Jumping jacks, clap hands, travel backward

Cross-country ski, travel diagonally to front L corner

Knee-high jog with propeller scull, travel diagonally to back R corner

Knee-high jog, travel forward

Knee-high jog with propeller scull, travel diagonally to back L corner

Knee-high jog, travel forward

Clamshells R

Clamshells L

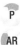

► **Deep-Water 20-Minute Strength Training 18**

BALANCE 2

EQUIPMENT

Deep-water belts, noodles

A SET

Knee-high jog 3× and hold

Heel jog 3× and hold

Knee-high jog, circle both thumbs clockwise

Knee-high jog, circle both thumbs counterclockwise

Jumping jacks 1×, inner-thigh lift 1×

Cross-country ski and tuck ski together, alternate

Helicopter ski

Knee-high jog, travel in a circle clockwise, look L

Knee-high jog, travel in a circle counterclockwise, look R

B SET

(With noodles)

Hip extension R, foot on a noodle

Hip extension L, foot on a noodle

Standing leg press R, foot on a noodle

Standing leg press L, foot on a noodle

Standing leg press to R side, foot on a noodle

Standing leg press to L side, foot on a noodle

Straddle noodle with front end between thighs

Raise and lower knees to find neutral spine

Reverse breaststroke, maintain neutral spine

Breaststroke, maintain neutral spine

Seated row, travel in a scatter pattern

► **Deep-Water 20-Minute Strength Training 19**

PILATES FUSION 1

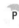

EQUIPMENT

Deep-water belts

A SET

Reverse bicycle, R leg with reverse breaststroke, travel backward

Bicycle, R leg with breaststroke, travel forward

Reverse bicycle, L leg with reverse breaststroke, travel backward

Bicycle, L leg with breaststroke, travel forward

R leg kicks forward and back

L leg kicks forward and back

Cross-country ski with unison arm swing

Cross-country ski, arms sweep side to side

Knee-high jog with propeller scull, travel backward and forward

Straddle jog with R shoulder sweep in, travel sideways R

Straddle jog with L shoulder sweep in, travel sideways L

Heel jog with propeller scull, travel backward and forward

B SET

Seated kick, arms to sides 70 degrees

Bent-knee jacks, arms to sides 70 degrees

Seated kick with R shoulder sweep out, circle counterclockwise

Seated kick with L shoulder sweep out, circle clockwise

Hip hike

Seated swirl

Pike and hold

Pull R knee toward chest, lift and lower L leg

Pull L knee toward chest, lift and lower R leg

Pull R knee toward chest, hip roll

Pull L knee toward chest, hip roll

Knee-high jog with propeller scull, travel backward and forward

Straddle jog with R shoulder sweep in, travel sideways R

Straddle jog with L shoulder sweep in, travel sideways L

Heel jog with propeller scull, travel backward and forward

▶ Deep-Water 20-Minute Strength Training 20

PILATES FUSION 2

EQUIPMENT

Deep-water belts, dumbbells

A SET

High kick and return

High kick and return with reverse breaststroke, travel backward

High kick and return with breaststroke, travel forward

Skate kick and return

Skate kick and return with reverse breaststroke, travel backward

Skate kick and return with breaststroke, travel forward

Jacks cross

Swirl with legs apart

Inner-thigh lift

Hopscotch

Inner-thigh lift R and hopscotch R, alternate

Inner-thigh lift L and hopscotch L, alternate

Knee-high jog with propeller scull, travel backward and forward

Straddle jog with R shoulder sweep in, travel sideways R

Straddle jog with L shoulder sweep in, travel sideways L

Heel jog with propeller scull, travel backward and forward

B SET

(With dumbbells)

R knee lift, lat pull-down R

L knee lift, lat pull-down L

R knee lift, lat pull-down R and L knee lift, lat pull-down L, alternate

Pull both knees up and bring dumbbells together in front

Pull both knees up with lat pull-down

Leg circles in

Leg circles out

Ankle circles

Plank

Plank scissors

Side plank R

Side plank pliers R

Side plank L

Side plank pliers L

Abdominal pike and spine extension

T-hang and gently pulse dumbbells down

SECTION 3: 20-MINUTE FUN ACTIVITIES

▶ Deep-Water 20-Minute Fun Activities 1

CIRCUIT CLASS WITH PARTNERS

EQUIPMENT

Deep-water belts, noodles, dumbbells

TEACHING TIP

Two minutes at each station; allow extra time to move to next station. If you have an odd number of class participants, you will need to participate so that no one is left out.

Station 1 Noodles:

Bicycle race: Sit on noodle as if riding a bicycle and pedal with arms and legs; race until time is up.

Bicycle ride: Partner A is the handlebars with the noodle around his or her waist, and partner B is the bicycle rider, straddling the noodle. Halfway through they change positions.

Canoe: Sit on noodle as if riding a bicycle. Partner A is in front of partner B as if in a canoe. Partner B holds the back end of partner A's noodle between his or her knees. Partners travel forward rowing with their arms. Halfway through they change positions.

Station 2 Dumbbells:

Push-ups: Partners face each other leaning forward 45 degrees with dumbbells in their hands under the shoulders and flutter kicking. Partners alternate pushing down.

Jumping jacks: When one partner does a lat pull-down, the other lifts the arms to sides.

Side-to-side extension: Partners face each other and coordinate so that both go to the same side at once.

Station 3 At the Wall:

Breaststroke and reverse: Partner A puts both feet on the wall and does a breaststroke. Partner B is in a kneeling position with back to the wall and does a reverse breaststroke. Halfway through they change positions.

Push-off: Partners push off the wall with their feet, tuck, and run back.

▶ Deep-Water 20-Minute Fun Activities 2

SQUARE DANCE

AR

EQUIPMENT

Deep-water belts

TEACHING TIP

Divide class into two lines facing each other. If you have an odd number of class participants, you will need to participate so that no one is left out.

A SET

Partners run forward, shake R hands, and return

Partners run forward, shake L hands, and return

Partners run forward, do sa do, and return
(Pass on R and move around partner while facing same direction.)

Partners run forward, high-five R, and return

Partners run forward, high-five L, and return

Partners run forward, high-ten, and return

Partners run forward, do sa do, and return

Partners run forward, hold R hands and kick, and return

Partners run forward, hold L hands and kick, and return

Partners run forward, hold both hands and Cossack kick, and return

Partners run forward, do sa do, and return

B SET

Partners run forward, swing their partner R, and return

Partners run forward, swing their partner L, and return

Partners run forward, swing their partner R and L, and return

Promenade
(Partners at the head of the two lines run forward and then run through the lines to the end; the other partners follow.)

Weave the ring
(Close the ends of the lines to form a circle and count off A, B, A, B, and so on. The A's circle clockwise, and the B's circle counterclockwise, weaving in and out of the ring.)

▶ Deep-Water 20-Minute Fun Activities 3

YOU BE THE TEACHER

AR

EQUIPMENT

Deep-water belts

TEACHING TIP

The class is in a big circle

Ask one participant to lead the class in his or her favorite cardio exercise. Then go around the circle until everyone has had a turn. Allow any participant who does not wish to lead an exercise to pass. The next time around the circle, ask for their favorite upper-body strength-training exercise, core strength exercise, lower-body strength-training exercise, stretch, and so on. Continue until 20 minutes are up.

▶ Deep-Water 20-Minute Fun Activities 4

MODIFIED SYNCHRONIZED SWIMMING

EQUIPMENT

Deep-water belts

TEACHING TIP

The class is in a big circle. Count off A, B, A, B, and so on. If you have an odd number of class participants, you will need to participate so that no one is left out.

A SET

Bicycle, travel clockwise around the circle

Flutter kick, A's do hand waves above the water

Bicycle, travel counterclockwise around the circle

Flutter kick, B's do hand waves above the water

Seated kick, travel toward the center of the circle

Seated leg press with propeller scull, travel backward

Tuck and hold with seated row, travel toward the center of the circle

Seated flutter kick with propeller scull, travel backward

B SET

Bicycle with L hand up, travel clockwise around the circle

Mermaid, circle clockwise

Bicycle with R hand up, travel counterclockwise around the circle

Mermaid, circle counterclockwise

Seated kick R, travel toward the center of the circle

Seated leg press with propeller scull, travel backward

Seated kick L, travel toward the center of the circle

Seated leg press with propeller scull, travel backward

C SET

A's bicycle toward the center of the circle; B's bicycle in place

A's bicycle and circle clockwise in the inner circle; B's bicycle and circle counterclockwise in the outer circle

A's seated flutter kick with propeller scull, travel backward; B's bicycle toward the center of the circle

B's bicycle and circle clockwise in the inner circle; A's bicycle and circle counterclockwise in the outer circle

B's seated flutter kick with propeller scull travel backward; A's bicycle in place

D SET

Bicycle with R hand in the center of the circle, travel clockwise around the circle

Mermaid, circle clockwise

Bicycle with L hand in the center of the circle, travel counterclockwise around the circle

Mermaid, circle counterclockwise

Tuck and hold with seated row, travel toward the center of the circle

Seated flutter kick with propeller scull, travel backward

A's link R arms with B to their R and circle clockwise

A's link L arms with B to their L and circle counterclockwise

Flutter kick, A's do hand waves above the water

Flutter kick, B's do hand waves above the water

Everyone flutter kicks with hand waves above the water

▶ Deep-Water Fun Activities

GAMES AND RELAY RACES

EQUIPMENT

Deep-water belts

TEACHING TIP

Choose one or more of these activities to play at the end of class.

1. Centipede (with noodles)

Everyone sits on a noodle as if riding a bicycle. They line up behind the instructor and hold the end of the noodle of the person in front of them with both hands. Everyone bicycles, and the instructor at the head of the line bicycles and does a breaststroke. Travel around the pool in straight lines, circles, spirals, or random patterns.

2. Bicycle race (with noodles)

Divide the group into two-person teams. One team member is the handlebars with the noodle around his or her waist, and the other team member is the bicycle rider, straddling the noodle. On signal, the person who is the handlebars in front runs and the bicycle rider bicycles to the end of the pool. Then they switch positions and return to the starting point. The first team to get to the starting point wins.

3. Rickshaw race (with noodles)

Divide the group into two-person teams. Each team has two noodles. The driver stands in front of the rider, holding the ends of the noodles under his or her arms. The rider holds the opposite ends of the two noodles under his or her arms. On signal, the drivers run to the end of the pool while the riders sit in a dining-room chair position enjoying the ride. Then they switch positions and return to the starting point. The first team to get to the starting point wins.

4. Choo-choo train relay (with noodles)

Divide the group into two teams. Each person has a noodle around his or her waist. The team members line up behind the first person in line, the engine, holding the ends of the noodle belonging to the person in front of them. They run to the back of the pool and return. The engine then goes to the end of the line, and the second person in line becomes the new engine. This continues until the original engine is again at the front. The first team to finish wins.

5. Kayak race (with noodles)

Everyone in the class sits on a noodle as if riding a bicycle and crosses his or her ankles. Participants row with their arms to the end of the pool and back. The first one to get to the starting line wins.

6. Pass the ball (with two balls)

Form a circle with an even number of players. You must participate if necessary to have an even number. Count off A, B, A, B, and so on. Give one ball to a player on team A on one side of the circle and a second ball to a player on team B on the opposite side of the circle. On signal, one team member passes the ball to the next, both balls traveling clockwise around the circle. The team whose ball overtakes the other team's ball wins the game.

7. Eye–hand coordination (with balls)

Form a circle and have the group pass one ball around the circle. Add another ball so that now they are passing two balls around the circle. Keep adding balls.

8. Ball toss (with one ball for every set of partners)

Position the class in two lines of partners, facing each other. If you have an odd number of class participants, you have to participate so that everyone has a partner. Each set of partners has a ball, which they toss back and forth. After one minute, the partners each take a step backward so that the distance between them increases. They keep moving backward every minute until they run out of room.

9. Ball sweep relay (with two balls and two kickboards)

Divide the group into two teams. Give each team a ball and a kickboard. The first person on each team sweeps the ball with the kickboard to the back of the pool and returns to his or her team. The person hands off the ball and kickboard to the next team member. The team members repeat until each person has had a turn. The first team to get back with the ball and kickboard wins.

10. Obstacle course (with kickboards, noodles, balls, and so on)

Divide the class into two groups. Arrange one group in various locations in an obstacle course. They can jog in place pushing the water to create turbulence or create turbulence by holding the ends of kickboards and pushing them forward. Two participants can each hold one end of a noodle in a rainbow. One or more can have balls. The second group runs through the human obstacle course. They run through the turbulence, run under the noodle rainbow, and stop to catch a ball and throw it back. Use your imagination with whatever equipment you have. When the second group completes the obstacle course, they become the obstacles and the first group runs through the course.

ABOUT THE AUTHOR

Christine Alexander has been a water fitness instructor since 1993. She teaches water fitness classes for the City of Plano Parks and Recreation Department and teaches an introductory course for water fitness instructors for the Parks and Recreation Department.

She is a nationally certified water fitness instructor through both the Aquatic Exercise Association (AEA) and the United States Water Fitness Association (USWFA). Alexander is the author of *Water Fitness Lesson Plans and Choreography* (Human Kinetics, 2011), has a blog at www.waterfitnesslessons.wordpress.com, and regularly contributes articles to AEA's *AKWA* magazine. She is also an AEA CEC provider, and is a board member for the Metroplex Association of Aquatic Professionals in Dallas, Texas.

Alexander lives in Plano, Texas, with her husband, Jim. In her free time, she enjoys weight training, cooking healthy meals, and organic gardening.

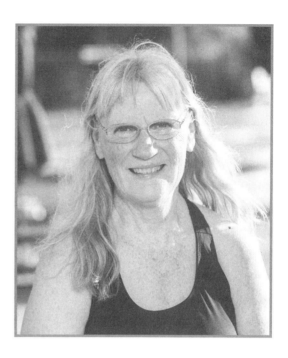

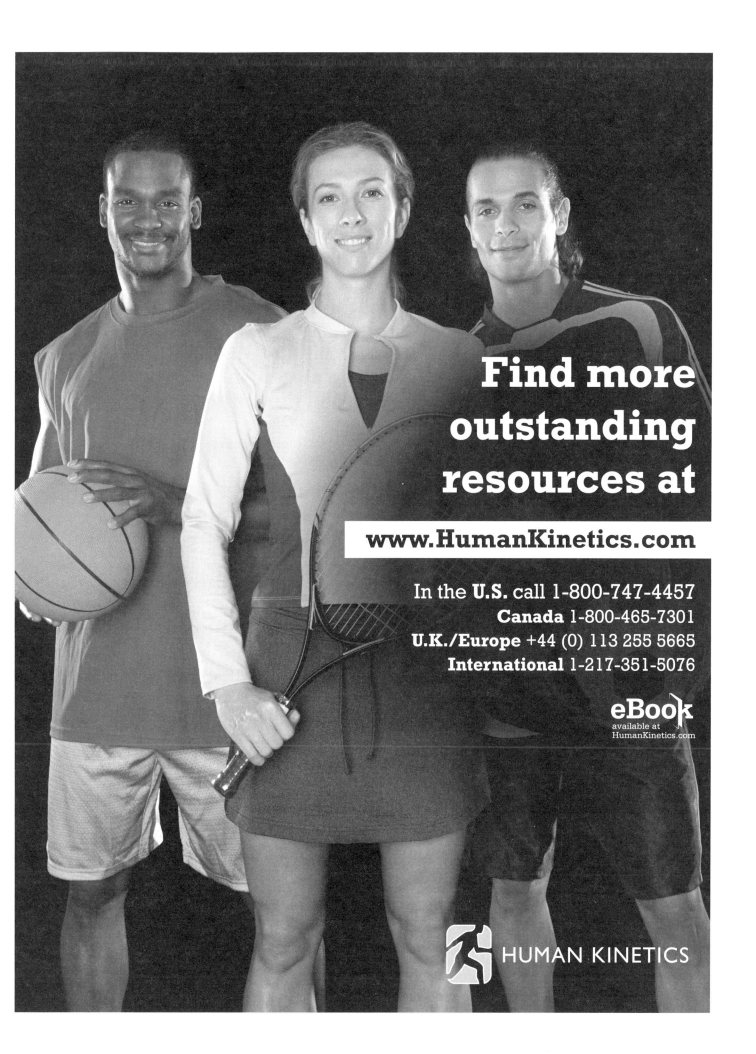